PRESCRIPTION FOR NUTRITIONAL HEALING

The A-to-Z Guide
to Supplements

PRESCRIPTION FOR NUTRITIONAL HEALING

The A-to-Z Guide to Supplements

Based on Part One of
Prescription for Nutritional Healing, Sixth Edition

PHYLLIS A. BALCH, CNC

AVERY

AN IMPRINT OF PENGUIN RANDOM HOUSE

NEW YORK

AVERY

an imprint of Penguin Random House LLC
penguinrandomhouse.com

Most Avery books are available at special quantity discounts for bulk purchase
for sales promotions, premiums, fund-raising, and educational needs. Special
books or book excerpts also can be created to fit specific needs. For details,
write SpecialMarkets@penguinrandomhouse.com.

Library of Congress Control Number: 2022939074

ISBN: 9780593541043

Printed in the United States of America
1st Printing

Book design by Shannon Nicole Plunkett

CONTENTS

AUTHOR'S ACKNOWLEDGMENTS

FROM THE FOURTH EDITION

There are many people who have come and gone in my life and have contributed to my books in many different ways, but I want to dedicate this to three loyal and true friends who are no longer with me: Judge Wendell W. Mayer, Charles R. Cripe, and Skeeners Balch. I also wish to acknowledge the following people, who both advised and supported me as I prepared and wrote the fourth edition of this book: my daughters, Ruby Hines and Cheryl Keene; my grandchildren, Lisa, Ryan, and Rachel; my brother, Al Henning; and my research and editing staff, Jeffrey W. Hallinger and Gary L. Loderhose and editor Amy Tecklenburg.

My gratitude also extends to Laurence Royse, DSc.; Aftab J. Ahmad, PhD, consulting molecular biologist; Philip Domenico, PhD, microbiologist and nutrition editor; Deborah A. Edson, RPh; James J. Gormley, editor in chief, *Remedies Magazine*; and also to members of the faculty of Southwest College of Naturopathic Medicine, Paul Mittman, ND, president, and Mona Morstein, ND, associate professor, all of whom graciously assisted in preparing and reviewing this book.

Finally, I would like to thank all the readers who have remained loyal throughout the years.

Phyllis A. Balch

PREFACE

A wise man should consider that health is the greatest of human blessings.

—Hippocrates

Socrates once said, "There is only one good, knowledge, and one evil, ignorance." This statement should guide us in all of our actions, especially where our health is concerned. Too many of us do not have the slightest idea of how to maintain good health. When illness strikes, we rely on our doctors to cure us. What we fail to realize is that "the cure" comes from within. Nature has provided us with a wondrous immune system, and all we have to do is take proper care of this inner healing force.

Does this sound too simple? Basically, it is simple; our modern lifestyles have gotten us off the right track, with fast foods, alcohol abuse, drug dependencies, a polluted environment, and high-tech stress. Nature intended to fuel our inner healing force with the right natural substances to enable the body to function up to its fullest potential. Nature's resources—whole foods, vitamins, minerals, enzymes, amino acids, phytochemicals, and other natural bounties—are designed for use in our immune systems. However, because most of us have a profound lack of knowledge as to what our bodies need to function properly, we find ourselves out of balance and susceptible to all sorts of illnesses.

All individuals should take an active role in the maintenance of their health, the prevention of disease, and the treatment of their disorders with the guidance of a health care professional. The more we take it upon ourselves to learn about nutrition, the better prepared we will be to take that active role. A good diet coupled with medical advice offers the best chance of living a healthy life. Attitude is also an important factor in the processes of health maintenance and healing. We must have a positive state of mind in order to bring harmony to the body. The realization that body (lifestyle), spirit (desire), and mind (belief) must come together is the first step to better health.

This book is the culmination of half a lifetime of study, work, and research. It is intended to provide you and your health care professional with a more natural approach to healing, which may be used in conjunction with your current medical treatment. A number of the suggestions offered, such as intravenous therapy, can be administered only by or under the supervision of a licensed physician. Also, because our body chemistries differ, some of us may have allergic reactions to certain supplements.

Before taking any nutritional supplement, check with your health care professional regarding its appropriateness. For your children, always check with their pediatrician first.

Should you experience an allergic reaction, especially abnormal bowel function (such as diarrhea), to any supplement, immediately discontinue use of the supplement. You should never attempt to treat yourself without professional advice.

No statement in this publication should be construed as a claim for cure, treatment, or prevention of any disease. It is also important to point out that you should not reject mainstream medical methods. Learn about your condition, and don't be afraid to ask questions. Feel free to get second and even third opinions from qualified health professionals. It is a sign of wisdom, not cowardice, to seek more knowledge through your active participation as a patient.

Every effort has been made to include the latest research available on nutritional healing. All the information in this book has been carefully researched, and the data have been reviewed and updated throughout the production process. Because this body of knowledge promises to continue growing and changing, we suggest that when questions arise about up-to-date information on treatment and prevention of disorders, you ask your health care provider. We will strive to keep abreast of new scientific information, treatments, and supplements.

Nearly nine hundred years ago, Moses Maimonides said, "The physician should not treat the ailment, but the patient who is suffering from it." This book was designed to meet the differing needs of individuals and to help each person create his or her own nutritional program.

About This Book

We have learned a great deal from traveling the country and speaking to so many of the people who have used our book *Prescription for Nutritional Healing*. That book was designed to be a comprehensive in-home guide that would help you to achieve and maintain the highest possible level of health and fitness through careful dietary planning and nutritional supplementation. However, we found we were frequently asked whether we could design a book that would provide basic information on a wide variety of today's dietary supplements, yet easily fit into a pocket or handbag to be taken to the store, on trips, or wherever needed—an edition that would incorporate up-to-date findings in the fields of nutrition and supplementation, from old standbys like vitamin C for the common cold to novel products with unique uses such as cordyceps, SAMe, and olive leaf extract. The answer to this question is *Prescription for Nutritional Healing: The A-to-Z Guide to Supplements*. This book was specifically created to provide on-the-go readers with authoritative information drawn from Part One of *Prescription for Nutritional Healing*, packaged in a handy reference guide that you can take along with you wherever you go. This volume provides all the information needed to design your own personal nutritional program as well as to use and understand today's supplements. What you will find here is a clear discussion of the basic principles of nutrition and health, as well as lists and explanations of the various types of nutrients, food supplements, and herbs found in health food shops and drugstores. Topics covered include vitamins, minerals, water, amino acids, antioxidants, enzymes, a wide variety of natural food supplements, and herbs.

Before you start any supplement regimen on a regular basis, test the supplements one at a time to find out if you have a reaction to any of them. Always listen to your body. If you experience unpleasant effects you suspect may be linked to a particular supplement, discontinue the supplement, or decrease the dosage or the frequency of use, or both.

Always take supplements with a full glass of water. Nutritional supplements are concentrated and can overburden the liver if you do not consume sufficient liquid with them. In addition, water enhances absorption and is needed to aid in carrying the nutrients to the cells.

If you follow a nutritional supplementation program for longer than a year, change brands periodically so that you do not develop an intolerance or build up a resistance to one or more of the ingredients in any given supplement. Remember, you can develop an intolerance to the ingredients in vitamins and other supplements just as you can to foods.

It is important for us to stress that the information offered in this book is not intended to replace appropriate medical advice and prescribed treatment. The use of any of the supplements recommended here should be approved and monitored by your medical doctor or other trained health care professional.

PRESCRIPTION FOR NUTRITIONAL HEALING

The A-to-Z Guide to Supplements

Introduction

The body is a complex organism that has the ability to heal itself—if only you listen to it and respond with proper nourishment and care. In spite of all the abuse our bodies endure—whether through exposure to environmental toxins, poor nutrition, cigarette smoking, alcohol consumption, or inactivity—they still usually serve us well for many years before signs of illness may start to appear. Even then, with a little help, they respond and continue to function. It is key to keep our immune systems up and running properly both to facilitate healing and to deal with new threats that develop, like the coronavirus.

The human body is the greatest machine on earth. Nerve signals travel through muscles at speeds as fast as 200 miles per hour. The brain puts out enough electric power to light a 60-watt lightbulb. If your leg muscles moved as fast as your eye muscles, you could walk over fifty miles in one day. According to scientists, bone is among the strongest building materials known to humankind.

Think of your body as being composed of millions of tiny little engines. Some of these engines work in unison; some work independently. All are on call twenty-four hours a day. In order for the engines to work properly, they require specific fuels. If the type of fuel given is the wrong blend, the engine will not perform to its maximum capacity. If the fuel is of a poor grade, the engine may sputter, hesitate, and lose power. If the engine is given no fuel at all, it will stop.

The fuel we give our bodies' engines comes directly from the things we consume. The foods we eat contain nutrients. These nutrients come in the form of vitamins, minerals, enzymes, water, amino acids, carbohydrates, and lipids. It is these nutrients that sustain life by providing us with the basic materials our bodies need to carry on their daily functions.

Individual nutrients differ in form and function, and in the amount needed by the body; however, they are all vital to our health. The actions that involve nutrients take place on microscopic levels, and the specific processes differ greatly. Nutrients are involved in all body processes, from combating infection to repairing tissue to thinking. Although nutrients have different specific functions, their common function is to keep us going.

Research has shown that each part of the body contains high concentrations of certain nutrients. A deficiency of those nutrients will cause the body part to malfunction and eventually break down—and, like dominoes, other body parts will follow. To keep this from happening, we need a proper diet and appropriate nutritional supplements. Brain function, memory, skin elasticity, eyesight, energy, the ratio of lean to fat tissue in the body, and overall health are all indications of how well the body is functioning. With the help of the proper nutrients, exercise, and a balanced diet, we can slow the aging process and greatly improve our chances for a healthier, pain-free—and possibly longer—life.

If we do not give ourselves the proper nutrients, we can impair the body's normal functions and cause ourselves great harm. Even if we show no signs of illness, we may not necessarily be healthy. It simply may be that we are not yet exhibiting any overt symptoms of illness. One problem most of us have is that we do not get the nutrients we need from our diets because most of the foods we consume are cooked and/or processed. Cooking food at high temperatures and conventional food processing destroy vital nutrients the body needs to function properly. The organic raw foods that supply these elements are largely missing from today's diet.

The past decade has brought to light much new knowledge about nutrition, its effects on the body, and the role it plays in disease. Phytochemicals, also known as phytonutrients, are one example of the results of this research.

Phytochemicals are compounds present in plants that make the plants biologically active. All fruits and vegetables contain phytochemicals. However, since few people eat enough fruits and vegetables to get the optimum amount of phytochemicals from diet alone, supplementation is recommended. Phytochemicals are not nutrients in the classic sense, but they determine a plant's color, flavor, and ability to resist disease. Researchers have identified literally thousands of phytochemicals and also have developed the technology to extract these chemical compounds and concentrate them into pills, powders, and capsules. These products are included under the term "nutraceuticals." The FDA uses the term "dietary supplement" to define natural compounds like phytochemicals.

Your body's nutritional needs are as unique to you as your appearance is. The first essential step toward wellness is to be sure you are getting the correct amounts of the proper nutrients. By understanding the principles of holistic nutrition and knowing what nutrients you need, you can improve the state of your health, ward off disease, and maintain a harmonious balance in the way nature intended. This book should provide you with a clear understanding of the vitamins, minerals, amino acids, enzymes, phytochemicals, and other nutrients you need, as well as important information on natural food supplements, herbs, and products that enhance nutrient activity. Eating a healthful diet and supplementing your diet with appropriate nutrients will help to assure that your organs, cells, and tissues get the fuel they need to operate properly. The nutrients suggested in this book promote healing and wellness by allowing the body to heal and reinvigorate itself.

Nutrition, Diet, and Wellness

UNDERSTANDING THE BASICS OF NUTRITION

Good nutrition is the foundation of good health. Everyone needs the four basic nutrients—water, carbohydrates, proteins, and fats—as well as vitamins, minerals, and other micronutrients.

To be able to choose the proper foods, and to better understand why those foods should be supported with supplements, you need to have a clear idea of the components of a healthy diet.

It is now a requirement in the United States that all packaged foods have a nutrition label that tells the consumer what is actually inside the package. This system may not be perfect, but it is a big improvement over no labeling at all, the situation that existed only a generation ago. Keep in mind that all fresh, minimally processed foods, such as grains purchased in bulk, meats, fruits, and vegetables, do not carry labels. However, they are inherently healthier than packaged foods because they have more beneficial nutrients and fewer harmful ones. For example, unlike processed items, these foods are naturally high in potassium and low in sodium.

Let's look at one of these generic labels and see what it tells us. Since January 2020, most food labels on packaged foods look like Figure 1.1 below:

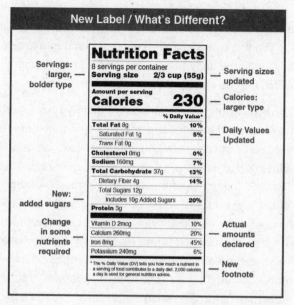

Figure 1.1

- The serving size is listed at the top of the label. All of the daily value percentages are based on this amount. It's good to keep in mind that the serving size listed on the label may not correspond with what many people consider a serving or portion of the product. However, the new food labels include serving sizes closer to what someone would eat as a meal or snack.

- There are 230 calories in this product. Fat provides 10 percent of the daily need. A rule of thumb is that fat should contribute no more than 30 percent of the total calories per serving, so this is acceptable.

- Note that the amounts of cholesterol, saturated fats, and trans fats are listed separately. Each is not an essential dietary nutrient and may increase the risk of heart disease. This food is low in cholesterol and saturated fat and has no trans fats.

- It's also important to pay attention to how much sodium the product contains and to maintain total intake below the suggested daily value. This food is low in sodium, which is good to help control high blood pressure.

- The label also gives the amount of dietary fiber (good), total sugars and added sugars (bad), and protein (you need some at each meal), and four selected vitamins and minerals that are most likely to be underconsumed (good). The food industry fought hard to have the FDA keep added sugars off the label but lost that battle. Consuming high amounts of added sugars leads to an increased risk of many common conditions like obesity, type 2 diabetes, and heart disease. Now it is easier to compute the daily intake of added sugars. The remaining sugars (total minus added) are naturally occurring, healthy, and often found in foods rich in other essential nutrients.

- The footnote gives target information for various nutrients based on a diet containing a total of 2,000 calories per day. This may or may not be useful to you, depending on your particular situation and calorie goal. It is also important to be aware that the percentages given are based on the need related to a 2,000-calorie diet and are not a percentage of the amount we actually recommend for good health or to maintain a healthy weight.

There is still some question as to the benefits of the revised food labeling system. Some are calling for a thorough assessment of whether the new labeling has actually enabled consumers to make healthier food choices. Some of the major food companies such as Kraft Foods and major grocery store chains such as Stop & Shop had created new labeling systems to help consumers make better choices, but these did not catch on. This section of the book will discuss the items shown on the nutrition label—and more—and also how they affect your health.

The Four Basic Nutrients

Water, carbohydrates, proteins, and fats are the basic building blocks of a good diet. By choosing the healthiest forms of each of these nutrients and eating them in the proper balance, you enable your body to function at its optimal level.

Water

The human body is two-thirds water. Water is an essential nutrient involved in every function of the body. It helps transport nutrients and waste products in and out of cells. It is necessary for all digestive, absorptive, circulatory, and excretory functions, as well as for the utilization of the water-soluble vitamins. It is also needed for the maintenance of proper body temperature. Each day the body loses up to 1 quart of water each from the kidneys and skin, about 1 cup from the lungs, and ½ cup from feces—a total of about 6 to 10 cups. To replace the water lost, males need to consume about 15 cups of fluid and females about 11 cups.

Ingesting an adequate amount of water each day—whether by food or water—is essential to maintain good health. Usually urine will be pale yellow in color if the body is sufficiently hydrated. It is possible to get a good portion of your daily intake of water—at least ten 8-ounce glasses—not from the tap, but from fruits and vegetables, which are loaded with water, some up to 90 percent water. Although studies have shown that beverages such as juices and sodas can be counted toward the daily fluid requirement, obtaining proper levels of fluids from fruits and vegetables and noncaloric beverages such as water and herbal tea is preferable, especially for weight control. For details on choosing the best water, see WATER later in this book. All liquids are not considered to be the same as water. Take, for example, sugar-sweetened beverages. Ironically, they dehydrate you rather than providing hydration.

Carbohydrates

Carbohydrates supply the body with the energy it needs to function. They are found almost exclusively in plant foods, such as fruits, vegetables, peas, grains, and beans. Milk and milk products are the only foods derived from animals that contain significant amounts of carbohydrates.

Carbohydrates are divided into two groups—simple carbohydrates and complex carbohydrates. *Simple carbohydrates,* sometimes called simple sugars, include fructose (fruit sugar), sucrose (table sugar), and lactose (milk sugar), as well as several other sugars. Fruits are one of the richest natural sources of simple carbohydrates. *Complex carbohydrates* are also made up of sugars, but the sugar molecules are strung together to form longer, more complex chains. Complex carbohydrates include fiber and starches. Foods rich in complex carbohydrates include vegetables, whole grains, peas, and beans.

Newer classifications for carbohydrates are based on their glycemic indexes (GI). The index is a scoring system to show how much glucose appears in the blood after eating a carbohydrate-containing food—the higher the number, the greater the blood sugar response. So a low GI food will cause a small rise, while a high GI food will trigger a dramatic spike. A GI of 70 or more is high, a GI of 56 to 69 is medium, and a GI of 55 or less is low. Most simple carbohydrates raise blood sugar levels more than complex ones, but not always. For example, white bread raises blood sugar more than table sugar because sugar has a lower GI. Eating foods with high glycemic indexes can lead to obesity, heart disease, and diabetes. (One source for the glycemic index of foods is www.health.harvard.edu/diseases-and-conditions/glycemic-index-and-glycemic-load-for-100-foods.) Simply put, adopting a low-glycemic-index diet is healthier. Low GI foods include fruits, vegetables, meat, oils, and dairy products. Most grain-based foods, especially those that are highly processed, have high glycemic indexes.

High GI foods are addictive and usually produce hunger within a couple of hours of eating them—yes, these foods make you hungry. A diet rich in high GI foods leads to overeating, obesity, and the risk of chronic conditions like type 2 diabetes and heart disease. If you are worried about the impact of a high GI diet, testing for hemoglobin A1c will provide a picture of how well your body is handling it. A doctor can interpret the results, but a low value (<5.7%) shows that your body can deal with the diet that you have been consuming for the past three months.

Carbohydrates are the main source of blood glucose, which is a major fuel for all of the body's cells and the only source of energy for the brain and red blood cells. Both simple and complex carbohydrates are converted into glucose. The glucose is then either used directly to provide energy for the body or stored in the liver for future use. If a person consumes more calories than his or her body is using, a portion of the carbohydrates consumed may be stored in the body as fat.

Due to complex chemical reactions in the brain, eating carbohydrates has a mild tranquilizing effect, and can be beneficial for people who suffer from seasonal affective disorder and/or depression.

When choosing carbohydrate-rich foods for your diet, choose unrefined foods such as fruits, vegetables, peas, beans, and whole-grain products, instead of refined, processed foods such as soft drinks, desserts, candy, and sugar. Refined foods offer few, if any, of the vitamins and minerals important to your health. Foods that are rich in nutrients are called nutrient-dense foods. A healthy diet should consist mainly of these foods and avoid those that are nutrient-poor. In addition, eating large amounts of simple carbohydrates found in refined foods, especially over a period of many years, can lead to a number of disorders, including diabetes and hypoglycemia (low blood sugar). Yet another problem is that foods high in refined simple sugars are often also high in fats, which should be limited in a healthy diet. This is why such foods—which include most cookies and cakes, as well as many snack foods—are usually loaded with calories.

A word is in order here regarding fiber, a very important form of carbohydrate. Referred to in the past as "roughage," dietary fiber is the part of a plant that is resistant to the body's digestive enzymes. As a result, only a relatively small amount of fiber is digested and absorbed in the intestines. There are two major types of dietary fiber: soluble and insoluble. The insoluble moves through the gastrointestinal tract and ends up in the stool. The soluble fiber is digested by intestinal bacteria, known as the microbiome. The bacteria consume the soluble fiber and produce healthy by-products like short-chain fatty acids, which are food for the intestinal cells.

Thus, both types of fiber deliver several important health benefits. First, insoluble fiber retains water, resulting in softer and bulkier stools that prevent constipation and hemorrhoids. A high-fiber diet, one rich in insoluble fiber, also reduces the risk of colon cancer, perhaps by speeding the rate at which stool passes through the intestine and by keeping the digestive tract clean. In addition, soluble fiber binds with certain substances that would normally result in the production of cholesterol and eliminates these substances from the body. In this way, a high-fiber diet helps lower blood cholesterol levels, reducing the risk of heart disease.

It is recommended that about 50 to 60 percent of your total daily calories come from carbohydrates. If much of your diet consists of healthy complex carbohydrates, you should easily fulfill the recommended daily minimum of 25 grams of fiber. Fiber should come primarily from a wide variety of fruits and vegetables. Whole grains are better than highly processed ones because they contain more fiber, either soluble or insoluble.

Protein

Protein is essential for growth and development. It provides the body with energy and is needed for the manufacture of hormones, antibodies, enzymes, and tissues. It also helps maintain the proper acid-alkali balance in the body.

When protein is consumed, the body breaks it down into amino acids, the building blocks of all proteins. Since protein is essential for life, other foods such as fruits and vegetables, which are alkaline-producing, need to be consumed to balance the body. Some of the amino acids from proteins are designated *nonessential.* This does not mean that they are unnecessary, but rather that they do not have to come from the diet because they can be synthesized by the body from other amino acids. Other amino acids are considered *essential,* meaning that the body cannot synthesize them and therefore must obtain them from the diet.

Whenever the body *makes* a protein—when it builds muscle, for instance—it needs a variety of amino acids for the protein-making process. These amino acids may come from dietary protein or from the body's own pool of amino acids. If a shortage of amino acids becomes chronic, which can occur if the diet is deficient in essential amino acids, the building of protein in the body stops, and the body suffers. The brain will trigger the muscle cells to release vital proteins to support the body. However, in extreme cases, some patients develop cachexia, which presents as weight loss, muscle atrophy, and severe fatigue and can result from a poor dietary protein intake. (For more information about amino acids, *see* AMINO ACIDS later in this book.)

Because of the importance of consuming proteins that provide all of the necessary amino acids, dietary proteins are considered to belong to two different groups, depending on the amino acids they provide. *Complete proteins,* which constitute the first group, contain ample amounts of all the essential amino acids. These proteins are found in meat, fish, poultry, cheese, eggs, and milk. Some plants provide complete proteins—for example, soy, quinoa, and legumes like chickpeas. *Incomplete proteins,* which constitute the second group, contain only some of the essential amino acids. These proteins are found in a variety of foods, including grains, legumes, and leafy green vegetables.

Although it is important to consume the full range of amino acids, both essential and nonessential, these do not have to come from meat, fish, poultry, and other complete-protein foods. In fact, because of their high fat content—as well as the use of anti-biotics and other chemicals in the raising of poultry and cattle—most of those foods should be eaten only in moderation. A group at the Harvard T. H. Chan School of Public Health avers that eating red meat shortens life. Many animal proteins are now available without hormones, or the animals are organically fed and hormone-free, so this risk can be mitigated by choosing these meats. It is best to trim all visible fat—including skin—from animal proteins and use low-fat or nonfat dairy products. Doing this will help reduce the risk of heart disease while still allowing for adequate intake of protein.

Fortunately, the dietary strategy called *mutual supplementation* enables you to combine partial-protein foods to make *complementary protein*—proteins that supply adequate amounts of all the essential amino acids. For instance, although beans and brown rice are both quite rich in protein, each lacks one or more of the necessary amino acids. However, when you combine beans and brown rice with each other, or when you combine either one with any of a number of protein-rich foods, you form a complete protein that is a high-quality substitute for meat. To make a complete protein, combine *beans* with any one of the following:

- Brown rice
- Corn
- Nuts
- Seeds
- Wheat

Or combine *brown rice* with any one of the following:

- Beans
- Nuts
- Seeds

Recent research indicates that it is possible to adequately meet your essential amino acid needs by eating an assortment of protein-containing foods over the course of the day and that there may be no need to combine proteins in one meal.

The problem is that many Americans eat too much protein, especially at one sitting, largely as the result of a diet high in meat and dairy products. Protein synthesis (manufacturing of new proteins for the body) works best when the protein is consumed on a regular basis throughout the day. Another problem is that Americans consume too few essential amino acids, which leads to increased hunger. If you have reduced the amount of meat and dairy foods in your diet, you should make sure to get 50 to 60 grams of high-quality protein each day. To make sure that you are getting enough variety of amino acids in your diet, add protein-rich foods to meals and snacks as often as possible. Eat bread with nut butters, for instance, or add nuts and seeds to salads and vegetable casseroles. Be aware that a combination of any grains, any nuts and seeds, any legumes (such as beans, peanuts, and peas), and a variety of mixed vegetables will make a complete protein.

All soybean products, such as tofu and soymilk, are complete proteins. These foods have high levels of fiber, and soy has been found to be the healthiest source of protein, more so than any other food. Soybean protein makes up 35 to 38 percent of its total calories, offers all eight essential amino acids, and is high in vitamin B_6. The average American consumes only about 10 milligrams of soy protein per day, although the American Heart Association suggests that consuming at least 25 grams per day may reduce the risk of heart disease. Available in most food stores, tofu, soy oil, soy flour, soy-based meat substitutes, soy cheese, and many other soy products are healthful ways to complement the meatless diet. Fermented soy products, such as miso, tempeh, fermented tofu, and soymilk, are now widely available and are loaded with isoflavones, which are immediately bioavailable, and they have more genistein (soy isoflavones) and nutrients than regular soy. They also fit in with Asian dietary practices. Fermentation yields more nutrients such as beta-glucan, glutathione, and the B vitamins than standard products.

Low-fat yogurt is the only animal-derived complete-protein source recommended for frequent use in the diet. Full-fat yogurt is loaded with saturated fats and should be avoided or used as a treat. Yogurt is made from milk that is curdled by bacteria; it contains *Lactobacillus acidophilus* and other "friendly" bacteria needed for the digestion of foods and the prevention of many disorders, including candidiasis. Yogurt is also a good source of calcium and other essential nutrients. Some yogurts have other healthy bacterial strains added to them.

Do not buy the sweetened, flavored yogurts that are sold in supermarkets. These products contain added sugar and, often, preservatives. Instead, either purchase fresh unsweetened yogurt from a health food store or make the yogurt yourself and sweeten it with fruit juices and other wholesome ingredients. Yogurt makers are relatively inexpensive and easy to use, and are available at most health food stores.

Fats

Although much attention has been focused on the need to reduce dietary fat, the body does need fat. During infancy and childhood, fat is necessary for normal brain development. Throughout life, it is essential to provide energy and support growth. Fat is in fact the most concentrated source of energy available to the body. However, after about two years of age, the body requires only small amounts of fat—much less than is provided by the average American diet. If you are an adult, about one-third of your calories should come from fat. Of that total, one-third should be saturated, one-third polyunsaturated (corn oil and fish oil), and one-third monounsaturated (olive oil).

Excessive fat intake is a major causative factor in obesity, high blood pressure, coronary heart disease, and colon cancer, and has been linked to a number of other disorders as well. To understand how fat intake is related to these health problems, it is necessary to understand the different types of fats available and the ways in which these fats act within the body. The types of fat included in your diet make all the difference as far as health. Fat itself is no longer considered to be a dietary enemy. In fact low-fat diets force increases in carbohydrate intake, which if drawn from refined sources, lead to worse health problems than including healthy fats.

Fats are composed of building blocks called *fatty acids.* There are three major categories of fatty acids—saturated, polyunsaturated, and monounsaturated. These classifications are based on the number of hydrogen atoms in the chemical structure of a given molecule of fatty acid.

Saturated fatty acids are found primarily in animal products, including dairy items such as whole milk, cream, butter, and cheese, and fatty meats like beef, veal, lamb, pork, and ham. The fat marbling you can see in beef and pork is composed of saturated fat. Some vegetable products—including coconut oil and palm kernel oil—are also high in saturates. The liver uses saturated fats to manufacture cholesterol. The excessive dietary intake of saturated fats can significantly raise the blood cholesterol level, especially the level of low-density lipoproteins (LDLs), or "bad cholesterol." Guidelines issued by the National Cholesterol Education Program (NCEP), and widely supported by most experts, recommend that the daily intake of saturated fats be kept below 7 percent of total caloric intake. However, for people who have severe problems with high blood cholesterol, even that level may be too high.

Polyunsaturated fatty acids are found in greatest abundance in corn, soybean, safflower, and sunflower oils. Certain fish oils are also high in polyunsaturates. Unlike the saturated fats, polyunsaturates may actually lower the total blood cholesterol level. In doing so, however, large amounts of polyunsaturates also have a tendency to reduce levels of high-density lipoproteins (HDLs), or "good cholesterol." For this reason—and because polyunsaturates, like all fats, are high in calories for their weight and volume—the NCEP guidelines state that an individual's intake of polyunsaturated fats should not exceed 10 percent of total caloric intake. Total fat intake should contribute 25 to 35 percent of total calorie intake.

The concept of "good" and "bad" fats has surfaced. Good fats are polyunsaturated and include those listed above. Added to this list are the omega-3 fats, which don't affect cholesterol levels, but may reduce the risk of heart disease by keeping blood flowing freely. Omega-3 fats are essential for life, but since the 1900s, people have been eating fewer of the foods that contain them. The polyunsaturated fats commonly consumed in the United States come from vegetable-based oils like corn, sunflower, and cottonseed oil and contain omega-6s. Although they are also essential, you need to consume only a teaspoon a day of these oils to meet your total omega-6 needs.

Over time, the intake of omega-6s has dwarfed that of omega-3s; our ancestors used to eat these fats in a one-to-one ratio. Many scientists believe that this shift in dietary intake of fats has led to depression and many of the chronic diseases of aging seen today, like heart disease, diabetes, and arthritis. The best way to balance your omega-3 to omega-6 ratio is to eat fish at least twice a week, and use canola oil rather than omega-6-rich vegetable oils. Most people have a ten-year store of omega-6 fats in their bodies. Therefore, it doesn't make sense to worry about getting enough every day. Olive oil contains hardly any essential fatty acids. Flax oil is rich in omega-3 fats, but only about 5 to 10 percent of the omega-3s in flax is usable by the body. Nevertheless, it is low in omega-6s, so it can be used, but only in uncooked items, as heat destroys the omega-3s.

Another caveat concerning polyunsaturated fats: vegetable shortening and stick margarine are made of liquid polyunsaturated fats, which means they should be healthful, but they are so highly processed that they are not. It is preferable to substitute soft-tub margarine, which is less processed than stick margarine, on your toast. It does not perform well when heated, however, so use stick margarine and vegetable shortenings when cooking—they are still preferable to butter.

Monounsaturated fatty acids are found mostly in vegetable and nut oils such as olive, peanut, and canola. These fats appear to reduce blood levels of LDLs without affecting HDLs in any way. However, this positive impact upon LDL cholesterol is relatively modest. The NCEP guidelines recommend that intake of monounsaturated fats can be up to 20 percent of total caloric intake.

Although most foods—including some plant-derived foods—contain a combination of all three types of fatty acids, one of the types usually predominates. Thus, a fat or oil is considered "saturated" or "high in saturates" when it is composed primarily of saturated fatty acids. Such saturated fats are usually solid at room temperature. Similarly, a fat or oil composed mostly of polyunsaturated fatty acids is called "polyunsaturated," while a fat or oil composed mostly of monounsaturated fatty acids is called "monounsaturated."

One other element, *trans-fatty acids,* was used in many food products. It was later found to increase the risk of heart disease. Also called *trans fats*, these substances occur when polyunsaturated oils are altered through hydrogenation, a process used to harden liquid vegetable oils into solid foods like margarine and shortening. As of June 2018, the FDA has banned the use of trans fats. Today you won't find many products that contain trans fats.

It is clear that if your goal is to lower blood cholesterol, polyunsaturated and monounsaturated fats are more desirable than saturated fats. Just as important, your total calories from fat should range between 25 to 35 percent of daily calories.

The Micronutrients: Vitamins and Minerals

Like water, carbohydrates, protein, and fats, and the enzymes required to digest them, vitamins and minerals are essential to life.

They are therefore considered nutrients and are often referred to as *micronutrients* simply because they are needed in relatively small amounts compared with the four basic nutrients.

Recommended Dietary Allowances (RDAs) were instituted in 1941 by the National Academy of Sciences' U.S. Food and Nutrition Board as a standard for the daily amounts of vitamins and minerals needed by a healthy person. These RDAs were the basis for the U.S. Recommended Daily Allowances (U.S. RDAs) adopted by the Food and Drug Administration (FDA). The U.S. RDA used to be the term that was used on food labels. However, the provisions of the Nutrition Labeling and Education Act and the Dietary Supplement Act of 1992 required a change in food product labeling to use a new reference term, Daily Value (DV), which began to appear on FDA-regulated product labels in 1994. Today you can look at any food or dietary supplement label and see the percent DV of all essential nutrients contained in the product. DVs are made up of two sets of references: Daily Reference Values (DRVs) and Reference Daily Intakes (RDIs).

DRVs are a set of dietary references that apply to fat, saturated fat, cholesterol, carbohydrate, protein, fiber, sodium, and potassium. RDIs are a set of dietary references based on the Recommended Dietary Allowances for essential vitamins and minerals and, in selected groups, protein. The term *RDI* replaces *U.S. RDA*.

Starting in 1998 the Food and Nutrition Board of the Institute of Medicine began publishing new information about nutrient requirements. These were referred to as the Dietary Reference Intakes (DRIs), and later adopted by the Food and Drug Administration to serve as the basis of the DVs on the new food labels. The nutrient DVs on food labels are appropriate for anyone aged four years and older.

The amounts of these nutrients defined by the DRI give us about twice the amount needed to ward off vitamin deficiency diseases such as beriberi, rickets, scurvy, and night blindness. What they do not account for are the amounts needed to maintain maximum health, rather than borderline health. Moreover, they are not good at providing an individual's need, but rather population norms.

Scientific studies have shown that taking dosages of vitamins above the DRIs helps our body work better. The DRIs therefore are not very useful for determining what our intake of different vitamins should be. We prefer to speak in terms of *optimum daily intakes* (ODIs)—the amounts of nutrients needed for vibrant good health. This entails consuming larger amounts of vitamins than the DRIs. The nutrient doses recommended on pages 23–26 are ODIs. By providing our bodies with an optimum daily amount of necessary vitamins, we can enhance our health. The dosages outlined in this book will enable you to design a vitamin program that is custom-tailored for the individual. Many nutrients with a DRI also have a corresponding Tolerable Upper Level of Intake (UL), which is usually higher than the DRI and the DV but that has been found to be safe. (To learn the ULs for all vitamins and minerals, go to http://fnic.nal.usda.gov.) The one exception is magnesium; its UL is lower than the recommendation. Consult your health care provider about an appropriate amount to take. Otherwise, do not take more than the UL for any nutrient (unless your health care provider recommends that you do) because it is not safe to do so based on what we know today. Some nutrients do not have corresponding ULs. This means only that no upper toxic limit has been identified and does not mean that large amounts are safe.

FDA'S GOOD MANUFACTURING PRACTICES

Ideally, all of us would get all the nutrients we need for optimal health from fresh, healthful foods. In reality, however, this is often difficult, if not impossible. In our chemically polluted and stress-filled world, our nutritional requirements have been increasing, but the number of calories we require has been *decreasing,* as our general level of physical activity has declined. This means we are faced with needing somehow to get more nutrients from less food. At the same time, many of our foods are depleted of certain nutrients. Modern farming practices have resulted in soils that are lacking in selenium and other nutrients. The main problem is that people just aren't eating nutrient-rich foods according to the Dietary Guidelines for Americans 2015–2020.

Harvesting and shipping practices are dictated not by nutritional considerations but by marketing demands. Add to this extensive processing, improper storage, and other factors, and it is little wonder that many of the foods that reach our tables cannot meet our nutritional needs. Getting even the DRI of vitamins from today's diet has become quite hard to do. This means that for optimum health, it is necessary to take nutrients in supplement form. Dr. Bruce Ames, a well-known nutritional scientist, argues that low dietary intakes of vitamins and minerals are widespread in the United States and that this may accelerate chronic diseases of aging like cancer.

Given the nature of the food supply, everyone would benefit from taking dietary supplements. And supplements have become much safer. Since July 2008, all companies that manufacture dietary supplements must follow Good Manufacturing Practices (GMPs). The FDA has established guidelines for manufacturing procedures so that you actually get the nutrients that are advertised on the label. Also, the new requirements dictate that the products must be clean and free of harmful bacteria and other toxins. The FDA now requires manufacturers to store all the ingredients used in a product after the product has been sold. Each product must have a name and phone number to call if a user becomes ill. The batch number of the product then can be matched to the stored ingredients to help figure out why someone has had an adverse reaction. Some companies have gone beyond GMPs and enlisted the services of NSF, an independent third-party testing organization that tests dietary supplements. Dietary supplements that engage NSF undergo a higher level of scrutiny. Companies that pass the stricter assessment can put an NSF-certified sticker on their products.

Nutrients and Dosages for Maintaining Good Health

The table on pages 23–26—which includes not just vitamin and mineral supplements, but other supplements as well—should be used as a guideline. Although the amounts listed as ODIs are safe (they will not cause toxicity), they should be varied according to a person's size and body weight. People who are active and exercise; those who are under great stress, on restricted diets, or mentally or physically ill; women who take oral contraceptives; those on medication; those who are recovering from surgery; and smokers and those who consume alcoholic beverages—all may need larger-than-normal amounts of certain nutrients.

In addition to a proper diet, exercise and a positive attitude are two important elements that are needed to prevent sickness and disease. If your lifestyle includes each of these, you will feel good and have more energy—something we all deserve. Nature has the answers we need to maintain our health, but you need to know what nutrients you are taking to make sure all the pieces of the puzzle fit together.

If you are not used to taking supplements, especially in larger-than-normal doses, your body may need time to adjust. Always take a multivitamin/multimineral supplement with food—if possible, with the biggest meal of the day—to avoid stomach upset and foster better absorption of the nutrients. Otherwise, if the tablet can be split in two, take half in the morning and half at the evening meal.

Daily dosages are suggested; however, before using any supplements, you should consult with your health care provider. The dosages given here are for adults and children weighing 100 pounds and over. Appropriate dosages for children vary according to age and weight. A child weighing between 70 and 100 pounds should be given three-quarters the adult dose; a child weighing less than 70 pounds (and *over* the age of six years) should be given one-half the adult dose. A child under the age of six years should be given nutritional formulas designed specifically for young children. Follow the dosage directions on the product label. Many products have not been directly tested for use by children, so be sure to check with the child's health care provider before giving any supplement to a child. Besides vitamins and minerals, other nutrients that have been tested in children include *Andrographis paniculata*, cranberry, echinacea, evening primrose oil, garlic, ivy leaf, and valerian.

I recommend using only quality supplements from a reputable source. Lower-priced supplements can mean lower quality, with higher levels of fillers and other undesirable ingredients. Give your body the best—it deserves it. Of course, it is better to take the supplements than not, so if you can't afford the higher-quality vitamins, then use the lower-cost ones.

For your reference, both milligrams (mg) and micrograms (mcg) refer to specific weights. The old system of using an international unit (IU) was the amount of a vitamin, mineral, or other substance that elicited a certain biological activity. It is easy to convert IU to the newer system using these guidelines:

- Vitamin A: 1 IU = 0.3 mcg vitamin A

- Vitamin D: 1 IU = 0.025 mcg

- Vitamin E: 1 IU = 0.9 mg d-alpha-tocopherol (based on the synthetic form)

Nutrients with a corresponding DV do not have a constraint as to how the nutrient is delivered. For example, calcium that comes from milk or a supplement of carbonate or citrate are considered to be the same, despite each having different absorption rates. Studies have found that people who regularly take supplements typically have a better quality of life, a lower risk of heart attack and diabetes, and lower blood pressure compared to those who do not take supplements.

NUTRIENT	OPTIMUM DAILY INTAKE*	DAILY VALUE (DV)	TOLERABLE UPPER LEVEL OF INTAKE (UL) PER DAY FOR ADULTS
Vitamins with DVs			
Vitamin A (retinol and carotenoids)	1,500–3,000 mcg (formerly 5,000–10,000 IU)	900 mcg (formerly 3,000 IU)	3,000 mcg
Thiamine (B_1)	50–100 mg	1.2 mg	Not determined
Riboflavin (B_2)	15–50 mg	1.3 mg	Not determined
Niacin (B_3)	16–35 mg	16 mg	35 mg
Pantothenic acid	50–100 mg	5 mg	Not determined
Vitamin B_6	50–100 mg	1.7 mg	100 mg
Vitamin B_{12}	200–400 mcg	2.4 mcg	Not determined
Biotin		30 mcg	
Choline	At least 550 mg	550 mg	3,500 mg
Folic acid	400–800 mcg	400 mcg (as dietary folate equivalents)	1,000 mcg
Vitamin C	1,000–2,000 mg	90 mg	2,000 mg
Vitamin D	At least 20 mcg (formerly 400 IU)	20 mcg (formerly 800 IU)	100 mcg
Vitamin E	90 mg (formerly 200 IU)	15 mg (formerly 33 IU)	1,000 mg
Vitamin K		120 mcg	
Vitamins without DVs			No DVs established
Inositol	50–200 mg		
Para-aminobenzoic acid (PABA)	10–50 mg		
Bioflavonoids (mixed)	200–500 mg		
Hesperidin	50–100 mg		
Rutin	25 mg		

NUTRIENT	OPTIMUM DAILY INTAKE*	DAILY VALUE (DV)	TOLERABLE UPPER LEVEL OF INTAKE (UL) PER DAY FOR ADULTS
Minerals with DVs			
Calcium	1,800–2,000 mg	1,300 mg	2,000 mg
Chloride		2,300 mg	3,600 mg
Chromium	150–400 mcg	35 mcg	Not determined
Copper	2–3 mg	0.9 mg	10 mg (10,000 mcg)
Iodine	150–225 mcg	150 mcg	1,100 mcg
Iron**	18–30 mg	18 mg	45 mg
Magnesium	420 mg	420 mg	350 mg
Manganese	3–10 mg	2.3 mg	11 mg
Molybdenum	45–100 mcg	45 mcg	2,000 mcg
Phosphorus		1,250 mg	4,000 mg
Potassium	At least 1,250 mg	4,700 mg	Not determined
Selenium	100–200 mcg	55 mcg	400 mcg
Sodium		2,300 mg	2,300 mg
Zinc	30–50 mg	11 mg	40 mg
Minerals without DVs			
Boron (picolinate or citrate)	3–6 mg		20 mg
Vanadium (vanadyl sulfate)	200 mcg–1 mg		1.8 mg
Amino acids (essential)		mg per pound body weight per day (based on 154-pound person)	No upper limits established
Histidine		1,540 mg	
Isoleucine		3,080 mg	
Leucine		6,006 mg	

NUTRIENT	OPTIMUM DAILY INTAKE*	DAILY VALUE (DV)	TOLERABLE UPPER LEVEL OF INTAKE (UL) PER DAY FOR ADULTS
Lysine		4,620 mg	
Methionine + cysteine		2,310 mg	
Phenylalanine + tyrosine		3,850 mg	
Threonine		2,310 mg	
Tryptophan		616 mg	
Valine		4,004 mg	
Total essential amino acids		~28 grams	

Amino acids (nonessential)***

NUTRIENT	OPTIMUM DAILY INTAKE*	DAILY VALUE (DV)	TOLERABLE UPPER LEVEL OF INTAKE (UL) PER DAY FOR ADULTS
Acetyl-L-carnitine		100–500 mg	
Acetyl-L-cysteine		100–500 mg	
L-carnitine		500 mg	
Taurine		100–500 mg	

*Be careful not to confuse milligrams (mg) with micrograms (mcg). A microgram is 1/1,000 of a milligram, or 1/1,000,000 of a gram.

**You should take iron supplements only if you have been diagnosed with a deficiency of this mineral. Always take iron supplements separately, rather than in a multivitamin and mineral formula.

***See AMINO ACIDS for more information. You should not take individual amino acids on a regular basis unless you are using them for the treatment of a specific disorder. Requirements are for a minimum and obtained from the WHO Technical Report Series 935, 2002.

OPTIONAL SUPPLEMENTS****	OPTIMUM DAILY INTAKES
Chondroitin sulfate	As directed on label.
Coenzyme Q_{10}	30–100 mg
Cryptoxanthin	110 mcg
Essential fatty acids (EFAs) (primrose oil, flaxseed oil, salmon oil, and fish oil are good sources)	As directed on label.
Flavonoids (citrus fruits and berries)	As directed on label.
Garlic	As directed on label.
Ginkgo biloba (herb)	As directed on label.
Glucosamine sulfate	As directed on label.
Lecithin	200–500 mg
Lutein/lycopene	As directed on label.
Pectin	50–100 mg
Phosphatidylcholine	As directed on label.
Phosphatidylserine	As directed on label.
Pycnogenol or grape seed extract (OPCs)	As directed on label.
Quercetin	70–140 mg
RNA-DNA	100 mg
Silicon	As directed on label.
Soy isoflavones (genistein)	As directed on label.
Superoxide dismutase (SOD)	As directed on label.
Zeaxanthin	90 mcg

****See NATURAL FOOD SUPPLEMENTS for more information.

Other supplements that you may wish to take for increased energy include the following:

- Bee pollen.
- Coenzyme A.
- Coenzyme 1 (nicotinamide adenine dinucleotide with high-energy hydrogen, or NADH; sold under the brand name Enada).
- Free-form amino acid.
- Kyo-Green from Wakunaga of America.
- N, N-Dimethylglycine (DMG).
- Octacosanol.
- Siberian ginseng.
- Spirulina.
- Wheat germ.

In addition, there are many good formulas on the market specifically formulated to help meet the nutritional needs of infants and children.

Synergy and Deficiency

Data compiled by the U.S. Department of Agriculture indicate that at least 40 percent of the people in this country routinely consume a diet containing only 60 percent of the Recommended Daily Allowance (RDA) of each of ten selected nutrients. This means that close to half of the population (and very likely more) suffer from a deficiency of at least one important nutrient. Specially, 40 percent of men and 29 percent of women have vitamin deficiencies, and 54 percent of men and 44 percent of women have mineral deficiencies.

A poll of 37,000 Americans conducted by Food Technology found that half of them were deficient in vitamin B_6 (pyridoxine), 42 percent did not consume sufficient amounts of calcium, 39 percent had an insufficient iron intake, and 25 to 39 percent did not obtain enough vitamin C. The poll found that 90 percent of people don't get enough folate, vitamin D, and vitamin E. In children, more than 80 percent are deficient in vitamins A, D, and E. Based on the most recent information from 2015 to 2020, the nutrients that are most underconsumed are vitamins A, C, D, E, choline, calcium, magnesium, iron, potassium, and fiber. Of this group, not getting enough of some (vitamin D, calcium, potassium, and fiber) leads to adverse health outcomes. Additional research has shown that a vitamin deficiency may not affect the whole body, but only specific cells. For example, those who smoke may suffer from a vitamin C deficiency, but only in the lung area.

Whenever you seek to correct a vitamin or mineral deficiency, you must recognize that nutrients work synergistically. This means that there is a cooperative action between certain vitamins and minerals, which work as catalysts, promoting the absorption and assimilation of other vitamins and minerals. Correcting a deficiency in one vitamin or mineral requires the addition of others, not simply replacement of the one in which you are deficient. This is why taking a single vitamin or mineral may be ineffective or even dangerous, and why a balanced vitamin and mineral preparation should always be taken in addition to any single supplements. The following table indicates which vitamins and minerals are necessary to correct certain deficiencies. The best way to avoid interfering with the natural synergies among nutrients is to take supplements with meals, unless otherwise instructed. Food stimulates the natural digestive processes and contains natural nutrients to foster the digestion and absorption of nutrients from food and supplements.

VITAMINS	SUPPLEMENTS NEEDED FOR ASSIMILATION
Vitamin A	Choline, essential fatty acids, zinc, vitamins C, D, and E.
Vitamin B complex	Calcium, vitamins C and E.
Vitamin B_1 (thiamine)	Manganese, vitamin B complex, vitamins C and E.
Vitamin B_2 (riboflavin)	Vitamin B complex, vitamin C.
Vitamin B_3 (niacin)	Vitamin B complex, vitamin C.
Vitamin B_5 (pantothenic acid)	Vitamin B complex, vitamins A, C, and E.
Vitamin B_6 (pyridoxine)	Potassium, vitamin B complex, vitamin C.
Biotin	Folic acid, vitamin B complex, pantothenic acid (vitamin B_5), vitamin B_{12}, vitamin C.
Choline	Vitamin B complex, vitamin B_{12}, folic acid, inositol.
Inositol	Vitamin B complex, vitamin C.
Para-aminobenzoic acid (PABA)	Vitamin B complex, folic acid, vitamin C.
Vitamin C	Bioflavonoids, calcium, magnesium.
Vitamin D	Calcium, choline, essential fatty acids, phosphorus, vitamins A and C.
Vitamin E	Essential fatty acids, manganese, selenium, vitamin A, vitamin B_1 (thiamine), inositol, vitamin C.
Essential fatty acids	Vitamins A, C, D, and E.

MINERALS	SUPPLEMENTS NEEDED FOR ASSIMILATION
Calcium	Boron, essential fatty acids, lysine, magnesium, manganese, phosphorus, vitamins A, C, D, and E.
Copper	Cobalt, folic acid, iron, zinc.
Iodine	Iron, manganese, phosphorus.
Magnesium	Calcium, phosphorus, potassium, vitamin B_6 (pyridoxine), vitamins C and D.
Manganese	Calcium, iron, vitamin B complex, vitamin E.
Phosphorus	Calcium, iron, manganese, sodium, vitamin B_6 (pyridoxine).
Silicon	Iron, phosphorus.
Sodium	Calcium, potassium, sulfur, vitamin D.
Sulfur	Potassium, vitamin B_1 (thiamine), pantothenic acid (vitamin B_5), biotin.
Zinc	Calcium, copper, phosphorus, vitamin B_6 (pyridoxine).

There are certain cautions that you should take into account when taking supplements. Antibiotics interfere with the natural balance of normal intestinal flora needed to produce vitamin K, which is necessary for normal blood clotting and maintaining the integrity of the bones. Too much coffee and/or caffeine-containing soft drinks can interfere with calcium metabolism. On the plus side, coffee has been shown to prolong life, possibly by reducing the chances of developing heart disease or diabetes.

Aspirin can irritate the gastrointestinal tract and may cause gastrointestinal bleeding. Aspirin can also interfere with the absorption of B vitamins and vitamin C. If you are taking aspirin daily for cardiovascular health, it is better to take baby aspirin—studies have shown that it is less irritating to the gastrointestinal tract, and it works just as well as ordinary aspirin. Baby aspirin usually has 80 milligrams of aspirin, but check with your health care provider before using aspirin in this way.

BASIC GUIDELINES FOR SELECTING AND PREPARING FOODS

Clearly, a healthy diet must provide a proper balance of the four essential nutrients, as well as a rich supply of vitamins, minerals, and other micronutrients. The EAT-Lancet diet offers a sound way to get a nutrient-rich diet. This diet optimizes health while preserving the planet. However, it is not enough simply to purchase foods that are high in complex carbohydrates with low-glycemic indexes, fiber, and complementary proteins, and low in saturated fats. Food also must be free of harmful additives, and it must be prepared in a way that preserves its nutrients and avoids the production of harmful substances.

When nutritionists talk about diet, they are referring to live whole foods—unprocessed food with nothing added or taken away. Whole foods are more healthful because they usually contain no potentially harmful ingredients. In addition, plant foods are full of hundreds of phytochemicals that can help prevent disease and keep the body healthy. These are our frontline defenders against cancer and free radicals. (*See* PHYTOCHEMICALS on page 33.) Foods known to supply important phytochemicals include soybeans and soy products, broccoli, citrus peels, flax, garlic, green tea, grapes, and tomatoes. In order to optimize your phytochemical intake, you need to consume a biodiverse diet. To achieve biodiversity in your diet, simply eating a lot of fruits and vegetables is not enough. A biodiverse diet includes not only consuming at least 8 to 10 servings (½ cup per serving) per day, but also making sure there is as much diversity within food groups as possible.

Limit Intake or Avoid Foods That Contain Additives and Artificial Ingredients

Additives are placed in foods for a number of reasons: to lengthen shelf life; to make a food more appealing by enhancing color, texture, or taste; to facilitate food preparation; or to otherwise make the product more marketable.

Certain additives, like sugar, are derived from natural sources. Other additives, like aspartame (in NutraSweet and Equal), are made synthetically. Sweeteners derived from natural sources include sucralose, the compound used in Splenda. Sucralose is synthesized from sucrose (sugar) and appears to be inert metabolically, which would make it ideal for people with diabetes. However, sucralose might be stored in the body simply because this synthetic molecule is never found in nature and the body is not equipped to metabolize it. We would advise limiting the use of this additive/artificial sweetener. Although many additives are used in very small amounts, it has been estimated that the average American consumes about 5 pounds of additives per year. If you include sugar—the food processing industry's most used additive—the number jumps to 135 pounds a year. Anyone whose diet is high in processed products clearly consumes a significant amount of additives and artificial ingredients.

At their best, additives and artificial ingredients simply add little or no nutritional value to a food product. At their worst, some additives could pose a threat to your health. The history of additive use includes a number of products that were once deemed safe but later were banned or allowed only if accompanied by warnings. The artificial sweeteners cyclamate and saccharin are just two examples of such products. Other additives, like monosodium glutamate (MSG) and aspartame, are used without warnings per se, but packages of food that contain them are now marked in the United States with sometimes cryptic statements, such as PHENYLKETONURICS: CONTAINS PHENYL-ALANINE, which appears on packets of Equal, NutraSweet, and other products containing aspartame. These products may cause problems for some sensitive people. The warning is there to protect children born with PKU (phenylketonuria). This condition is identified at birth so those who have it know they have it. The long-term effects of most sugar-substitute additives, including sucralose, are unknown. A safer sugar substitute is an extract made from the herb *Stevia rebaudiana*, which is available in health food stores. Stevia is derived from the leaf of a plant and is commercially available. It is a natural sweetener that does not affect blood sugar levels and yields a pleasant sweet taste. In 2009, the FDA granted stevia GRAS (Generally Recognized as Safe) status.

Increase Your Consumption of Raw Produce

The most healthful fruits and vegetables are those that have been grown organically—without the use of insecticides, herbicides, artificial fertilizers, or growth-stimulating chemicals. Organic produce can be found in select health food stores, as well as in some supermarkets and greenmarkets and through food co-ops.

When choosing your produce, look for fruits and vegetables that are at the peak of ripeness. These contain more vitamins and enzymes than do foods that are underripe or overripe, or that have been stored for any length of time. The longer a food is kept in storage, the more nutrients it loses.

Once you get your organic produce home, running water and a vegetable brush are probably all that will be needed to get it ready for the table. If the produce is not organic, however, you will want to wash it more thoroughly to rid it of any chemical residues. Use a soft vegetable brush to scrub the foods, and then let them soak in water for ten minutes.

You can also clean produce with nontoxic rinsing preparations, which are available in reputable health food stores. If the products are waxed, peel them, because wax cannot be washed away. Remove as thin a layer of peel as possible.

Most fruits and vegetables should be eaten in their entirety, as all of the parts, including the skin, contain valuable nutrients. When eating citrus fruits, remove the rinds, but eat the white part inside the skin for its vitamin C and bioflavonoid content.

Although most people usually cook their vegetables before eating, both fruits and vegetables should be eaten raw if possible. All enzymes and most vitamins are extremely sensitive to heat and are usually destroyed in the cooking process.

PHYTOCHEMICALS

For many years, researchers have recognized that diets high in fruits, vegetables, grains, and legumes appear to reduce the risk of a number of diseases, including cancer, heart disease, diabetes, and high blood pressure, when compared with diets high in meat. It was discovered that the disease-preventing effects of these foods are partly due to antioxidants—specific vitamins, minerals, and enzymes that help prevent cancer and other disorders by protecting cells against damage from oxidation. Now researchers have discovered that fruits, vegetables, grains, and legumes contain yet another group of health-promoting nutrients. Called *phytochemicals,* these substances appear to be powerful ammunition in the war against cancer and other disorders.

Phytochemicals are the biologically active substances in plants that are responsible for giving them color, flavor, and natural disease resistance. To understand how phytochemicals protect the body against cancer, it is necessary to understand that cancer formation is a multistep process. Phytochemicals seem to fight cancer by blocking one or more of the steps that lead to cancer.

For instance, cancer can begin when a carcinogenic molecule—from the food you eat or the air you breathe—invades a cell. But if sulforaphane, a phytochemical found in broccoli, also reaches the cell, it activates a group of enzymes that whisk the carcinogen out of the cell before it can cause any harm.

Other phytochemicals are known to prevent cancer in other ways. Flavonoids, found in citrus fruits and berries, keep cancer-causing hormones from latching on to cells in the first place. Also, consuming a flavonoid-rich diet over a lifetime has been shown to reduce the chances of developing dementia, including Alzheimer's disease. Genistein, found in soybeans, kills tumors by preventing the formation of the capillaries needed to nourish them. Indoles, found in cruciferous vegetables such as Brussels sprouts, cauliflower, and cabbage, increase immune activity and make it easier for the body to excrete toxins. Saponins, found in kidney beans, chickpeas, soybeans, and lentils, may prevent cancer cells from multiplying. P-coumaric acid and chlorogenic acid, found in tomatoes, interfere with certain chemical unions that can create carcinogens. The list of these protective substances goes on and on. Tomatoes alone are believed to contain an estimated 10,000 different phytochemicals. Carotenoids like those found in tomatoes are shown to reduce age-related cognitive decline.

Although no long-term human studies have shown that specific phytochemicals stop cancer, research on phytochemicals supports the more than two hundred studies that link lowered cancer risk with a diet rich in grains, legumes, fruits, and vegetables. Moreover, animal and in vitro studies have demonstrated how some phytochemicals prevent carcinogens from promoting the growth of specific cancers. For instance, the phytochemical phenethyl isothiocyanate (PEITC), found in cabbage and turnips, has been shown to inhibit the growth of lung cancer in rats and mice. Among other things, PEITC protects the cells' DNA from a potent carcinogen found in tobacco smoke.

Researchers have been able to isolate some phytochemicals, and a number of companies are now selling concentrates that contain phytochemicals obtained from vegetables such as broccoli. These may be used as supplemental sources of some of these nutrients.

However, such pills should *not* be seen as replacements for fresh whole foods. Because *several thousand* phytochemicals are currently known to exist, and because new ones are being discovered all the time, no supplement can possibly contain all of the cancer-fighters found in a shopping basket full of fruits and vegetables.

Fortunately, it is easy to get a healthy dose of phytochemicals at every meal. Almost every grain, legume, fruit, and vegetable tested has been found to contain these substances. Moreover, unlike many vitamins, these substances do not appear to be destroyed by cooking or other processing. Genistein, the substance found in soybeans, for instance, is also found in soybean products such as tofu and miso soup. Similarly, the phytochemical PEITC, found in cabbage, remains intact even when the cabbage is made into coleslaw or sauerkraut. The flavonoid content of foods has recently become available. Of course, by eating much of your produce raw or only lightly cooked, you will be able to enjoy the benefits not just of phytochemicals, but of all the vitamins, minerals, and other nutrients that fresh whole foods have to offer.

If fresh produce is unavailable, use frozen fruits and vegetables instead. Avoid highly processed food items because they usually contain significant amounts of salt and sugar and other unhealthy additives. If raw produce does not agree with you, steam your vegetables lightly in a steamer, cooking pan, or wok just until slightly tender.

If fresh fruits and vegetables are not an option, it is still better to eat them than not—regardless of the form they come in. Many of the published studies on the health benefits of fruits and vegetables were based on consumption of any type (organic and nonorganic) and any state (fresh, frozen, canned, and juice).

Avoid Overcooking Your Foods

As just discussed, cooking foods for all but brief periods of time can destroy many valuable nutrients. More alarming is that when foods are cooked to the point of browning or charring, the organic compounds they contain undergo changes in structure, producing carcinogens.

Barbecued meats seem to pose the worst health threat in this regard. When burning fat drips onto an open flame, polycyclic aromatic hydrocarbons (PAHs)—dangerous carcinogens—are formed. When amino acids and other chemicals found in muscle are exposed to high temperatures, other carcinogens, called heterocyclic aromatic amines (HAAs), are created. In fact, many of the chemicals used to produce cancer in laboratory animals have been isolated from cooked proteins.

It is important to note, though, that cooked meats do not pose the only threat. Even browned or burned bread crusts contain a variety of carcinogenic substances.

The dangers posed by the practice of cooking foods at high temperatures or until browned or burned should not be dismissed. Although eating habits vary widely from person to person, it seems safe to assume that many people consume many grams of overcooked foods a day. By comparison, only half a gram of this same dangerous burned material is inhaled by someone who smokes two packs of cigarettes a day. Clearly, by eating produce raw or only lightly cooked, and by greatly limiting your consumption of meat, you will be doing much to decrease your risk of cancer and possibly other disorders.

SAFE SUGAR SUBSTITUTES— DO THEY EXIST?

Americans are obsessed with sugar and eat more than twice the recommended amount of 50 grams daily. On average, sugar consumption is six cups each week. It is consumed in ways that are obvious, such as in sugared cereals, carbonated beverages, cakes, or when added to coffee or tea. Sugar is also hidden in foods that you wouldn't expect, like catsup. Excess sugar intake leads to chronic conditions like obesity, diabetes, and heart disease. To help consumers still get the sweet flavor, the food industry has developed artificial sweeteners. Most notable is aspartame (found in Equal and NutraSweet), which may have its own health risks.

Two natural high-intensity sweeteners are available that will satisfy a sweet tooth without carrying any health risks. These are stevia and monk fruit. These are deemed safe by the FDA, provide no calories, and have no impact on blood sugar levels.

STEVIA
Stevia is from the leaf of a South American plant and is 200 to 400 times sweeter than table sugar. The only parts of the plant that are safe to consume are the steviol glycosides, which are natural constituents of stevia leaves (from *Stevia rebaudiana* Bertoni). Stevia leaf and crude stevia extracts are not permitted for sale, because animal studies indicate that they may cause cancer.

The sweetest part of the steviol glycosides is rebaudioside A (also known as Reb A). Reb A tastes similar to sugar, has the same duration of sweetness, and is free of aftertaste. A popular version is a stevia that is 75 percent Reb A. Reb A does not cause cancer and helps with blood sugar control.

MONK FRUIT
Monk fruit is commonly known as *luo han guo* and is a plant native to Southern China.

Monk fruit extract (from *Siraitia grosvenorii* Swingle) has a sweet flavor similar to sugar with no aftertaste. The fruit contains varying levels of mogrosides, which are compounds in the fruit that taste sweet. Monk fruit varies in sweetness based on the mogroside content, with higher concentrations producing more sweetness. Look for products containing the highest-grade monk fruit (grade V out of V), which is 100 to 250 times sweeter than sugar. It has no known side effects.

Besides tasting sweet, monk fruit has only a few calories and no effect on blood sugar levels. In addition, monk fruit contains antioxidants, which rid the body of harmful oxygen particles. No other natural sweetener has this property. The high-grade monk fruit offers the most antioxidant protection of any monk fruit or any other natural sweetener.

To get a sweet flavor, choose products that contain both stevia and monk fruit. Sometimes a little sugar is added to enhance the flavor, but at much smaller amounts than would ordinarily be used.

Use the Proper Cooking Utensils

Although raw foods have many advantages over cooked ones, nourishing soups and a variety of other dishes can be made healthfully. One of the ways to ensure wholesome cooked food is the careful selection of cookware.

When preparing foods, use only glass, stainless steel, or iron pots and pans. Do not use aluminum cookware or utensils. Foods cooked or stored in aluminum produce a substance that neutralizes the digestive juices, leading to acidosis and ulcers. Worse, the aluminum in the cookware can leach from the pot into the food. When the food is consumed, the aluminum is absorbed by the body, where it accumulates in the brain and nervous system tissues. Excessive amounts of these aluminum deposits have been implicated in Alzheimer's disease.

Other cookware to be avoided includes all pots and pans with nonstick coatings. Too often, the metals and other substances in the pots' finish flakes or leaches into the food. Ultimately, these chemicals end up in your body.

BASIC NUTRITIONAL GUIDE

A diet high in nutrients is the key to good health. Use the following table as a guide when deciding which types of food to include in your diet and which ones to avoid in order to maintain good health.

TYPE OF FOOD	FOODS TO AVOID OR LIMIT INTAKE OF	ACCEPTABLE FOODS
Beans	Canned pork and beans, canned beans with salt or preservatives.	All beans (especially soy) cooked without animal fat or salt.
Beverages	Alcoholic drinks, coffee, cocoa, pasteurized and/or sweetened juices and fruit drinks, sodas, tea (except herbal and green tea).	Herbal teas, fresh vegetable and fruit juices, grain beverages (often sold as coffee substitutes), mineral or distilled water.
Dairy products	All soft cheeses, all pasteurized or artificially colored cheese products, ice cream.	Raw goat cheese, nonfat cottage cheese, kefir, unsweetened yogurt, goat's milk, raw or skim milk, buttermilk.
Eggs	Fried or pickled.	Boiled or poached (limit of four weekly).
Fish	All fried fish, all shellfish, salted fish, anchovies, herring, fish canned in oil.	All freshwater whitefish, salmon, broiled or baked fish, water-packed tuna. (Limit tuna to two servings a week to avoid excessive mercury intake.)
Fruits	Canned, bottled, or frozen fruits with sweeteners added; oranges.	All fresh, frozen, stewed, or dried fruits without sweeteners (except oranges, which are acidic and highly allergenic), unsulfured fruits, home-canned fruits.
Grains	All white flour products, white rice, pasta, crackers, cold cereals, instant types of oatmeal and other hot cereals.	All whole grains and products containing whole grains: cereals, breads, muffins, whole-grain crackers, cream of wheat or rye cereal, buckwheat, millet, oats, brown rice, wild rice. (Limit yeast breads to 3 servings per week.)

TYPE OF FOOD	FOODS TO AVOID OR LIMIT INTAKE OF	ACCEPTABLE FOODS
Meats	Beef; all forms of pork; hot dogs; luncheon meats; smoked, pickled, and processed meats; corned beef; duck; goose; spareribs; gravies; organ meats.	Skinless turkey and chicken, lamb. (Limit meat to three 3-ounce servings per week.)
Nuts	All salted or roasted nuts; peanuts (if suffering from a related disorder).	All fresh raw nuts (peanuts in moderation only).
Oils (fats)	All saturated fats, hydrogenated margarine, refined processed oils, shortenings, hardened oils.	All cold-pressed oils: corn, safflower, sesame, olive, flaxseed, soybean, sunflower, and canola oils; margarine made from these oils; eggless mayonnaise.
Seasonings	Black or white pepper, salt, hot red peppers, all types of vinegar except pure natural apple cider vinegar.	Garlic, onions, cayenne, Spike, all herbs, dried vegetables, apple cider vinegar, tamari, miso, seaweed, dulse.
Soups	Canned soups made with salt, preservatives, MSG, or fat stock; all creamed soups.	Homemade bean (salt- and fat-free), lentil, pea, vegetable, barley, brown rice, onion.
Sprouts and seeds	All seeds cooked in oil or salt.	All slightly cooked sprouts (except alfalfa, which should be raw and washed thoroughly), wheatgrass, all raw seeds.
Sweets	White, brown, or raw cane sugar, corn syrups, chocolate, sugar candy, fructose (except that in fresh whole fruit), all syrups (except pure maple syrup), all sugar substitutes, jams and jellies made with sugar.	Barley malt or rice syrup, small amounts of raw honey, pure maple syrup, stevia, unsulfured blackstrap molasses.
Vegetables	All canned or frozen with salt or additives.	All raw, fresh, frozen (no additives), or home-canned without salt (undercook vegetables slightly).

Limit Your Use of Salt

Although some sodium is essential for survival, inadequate sodium intake is a rare problem. (Symptoms of salt deficiency include light-headedness and muscle fatigue.) We need 2,300 mg daily, but those with high blood pressure may need less. The American Heart Association recommends 1,500 milligrams of sodium a day for most adults to stay healthy. This is enough to accomplish all the vital functions that sodium performs in the body—helping maintain normal fluid levels, healthy muscle function, and proper acidity (pH) of the blood. Excessive sodium intake can cause fluid to be retained in the tissues, which can lead to hypertension (high blood pressure) and can aggravate many medical disorders, including congestive heart failure, certain forms of kidney disease, and premenstrual syndrome (PMS).

One of the best ways to limit the sodium in your diet is to limit your consumption of processed and fast foods, which often contain excessively high amounts of sodium. Cooking at home is a perfect opportunity to control your salt intake. Last, if you can see it, avoid it—for example, in salty snacks such as pretzels and potato chips.

Vitamins

INTRODUCTION

Vitamins are essential to life. They contribute to good health by
regulating the metabolism and assisting the biochemical processes that release energy from digested food. They are considered
micronutrients because the body needs them in relatively small
amounts compared with nutrients such as carbohydrates, proteins, fats, and water.

Enzymes are essential chemicals that are the foundation of
human bodily functions. (*See* ENZYMES later in this book.) They
are catalysts (activators) in the chemical reactions that are continually taking place within the body. As coenzymes, vitamins
work with enzymes, thereby allowing all the activities that occur within the body to be carried out as they should be. Whole,
fresh raw foods are a good source of enzymes.

Of the major vitamins, some are soluble in water and others
in oil. Water-soluble vitamins must be taken into the body daily,
as they cannot be stored and are excreted within four hours to
one day. These include vitamin C and the B-complex vitamins.
Oil-soluble vitamins can be stored for longer periods of time in
the body's fatty tissue and the liver. These include vitamins A,
D, E, and K. Both types of vitamins are needed by the body for
proper functioning.

SYNTHETIC VERSUS NATURAL

Make sure you are getting at least 100 percent of all essential vitamins from the foods you eat with a diet rich in fruits and vegetables. Once this has been accomplished, most people will need more from supplements to achieve optimal health. Vitamin supplements can be divided into two groups—synthetic and natural. Synthetic vitamins are produced in laboratories from isolated chemicals that mirror their counterparts found in nature. Natural vitamins are derived from food sources. Although there are no major chemical differences between a vitamin found in food and one created in a laboratory, synthetic supplements contain the isolated vitamins only, while natural supplements may contain other nutrients not yet discovered. This is because these vitamins are in their natural state. If you are deficient in a particular nutrient, the chemical source will work, but you will not get the benefits of the vitamin as found in whole foods. Supplements that are not labeled natural also may include coal tars, artificial coloring, preservatives, sugars, and starch, as well as other additives. You should beware of such harmful elements.

However, you should also note that a bottle of "natural" vitamins might contain vitamins that have not been extracted from a natural food source. It is necessary to read labels carefully to make sure the products you buy contain nutrients from food sources, with none of the artificial additives mentioned above.

Studies have shown that protein-bonded vitamins, as found in natural whole-food supplements, are absorbed, utilized, and retained in the tissues better than supplements that are not protein-bonded. Chemical-derived vitamins are not protein-bonded. Vitamins and minerals in food are bonded to proteins, lipids, carbohydrates, and bioflavonoids. Few studies are available to show the superiority of synthetic forms over what is found naturally in foods. Lycopene from tomato soup or tomato paste was absorbed the same as lycopene from a tablet.

Dr. Abram Hoffer, one of the "founding fathers" of orthomo-
lecular medicine (a school of medicine that emphasizes the role
of nutrition in health), has explained:

> Components [of food] do not exist free in nature; nature does
> not lay down pure protein, pure fat, or pure carbohydrates.
> Their molecules are interlaced in very complex three-
> dimensional structures, which even now have not been fully
> described. Intermingled are the essential nutrients such as
> vitamins and minerals, again not free, but combined in complex
> molecules.
>
> Using a natural form of vitamins and minerals in nutritional
> supplements is the objective of the protein-bonding process.
> Taking supplements with meals helps to assure a supply of other
> nutrients needed for better assimilation as well.

WHAT'S ON THE SHELVES

Over-the-counter vitamin supplements come in various forms, combinations, and amounts. They are available in tablet, capsule, gel
capsule, powder, sublingual (under the tongue), lozenge, nano particles, and liquid forms. They can also be administered by injection.

In most cases, it is a matter of personal preference as to how
you take them; however, due to slight variations in how rapidly
the supplements are absorbed and assimilated into the body, we
will sometimes recommend one form over another. These recommendations are given throughout the book.

Vitamin supplements are usually available as isolated vitamins or in combination with other nutrients. It is important to
select your vitamins based upon what you really need. A program designed for health maintenance would be different from
one designed to overcome a specific disorder. Some 50 percent of
Americans are now taking supplements on a regular basis.

If you find one supplement that meets your needs, remember to
take it daily. If it does not contain a large enough quantity of what

you want, you may consider taking more than one. Just make sure that you are aware of the increased dosage of the other nutrients it may contain. If there is no single supplement that provides you with what you are looking for, consider taking a combination of different supplements. This book lists each supplement separately, so you will know what each does and the amount needed. But you may find a supplement that contains several needed nutrients in one tablet or capsule. In fact, a good multivitamin (and multimineral) should be a part of everyone's diet after he or she reaches a certain age, with additional supplements as necessary.

Because the potency of most vitamins may be decreased by sunlight, make sure that the container holding your vitamins is dark enough to shield its contents properly. Some people may be sensitive to plastic and may need to purchase vitamins in glass containers. Vitamin supplements should be kept in a cool, dark place.

All vitamin supplements work best when taken in combination with food. Unless specified otherwise, oil-soluble vitamins should be taken before meals, and water-soluble ones should be taken after meals. (This applies when you are taking individual supplements only. Multivitamins have both water-soluble and fat-soluble elements.) If you are concerned about getting the full potency from your supplements, you may want to try using raw-food-created vitamins made from a single-cell yeast, *Saccharomyces cerevisiae*. This yeast creates vitamins and minerals that are not isolated or synthesized, but that come from nutrient-dense whole foods. One of the best sources of raw-food-created vitamins is Garden of Life.

VITAMINS FROM A TO Z

Vitamin A and the Carotenoids

Vitamin A prevents night blindness and other eye problems, as well as some skin disorders, such as acne. It enhances immunity, may help to heal gastrointestinal ulcers, and is needed for the maintenance and repair of epithelial tissue, of which the skin and mucous membranes are composed.

It is important in the formation of bones and teeth, aids in fat storage, and protects against colds, flu, and infections of the kidneys, bladder, lungs, and mucous membranes. Vitamin A acts as an antioxidant, helping to protect the cells against cancer and other diseases (*see* ANTIOXIDANTS later in this book) and is necessary for new cell growth. It guards against heart disease and stroke and lowers cholesterol levels. People receiving radiation treatment for cervical cancer, prostate cancer, or colorectal cancer have benefited from taking oral vitamin A. Radiation-induced anal ulcers can be a problem with such treatment programs, and a vitamin A megadose (30,000 mcg; 100,000 international units daily) significantly reduced symptoms in 88 percent of people undergoing such regimens. Girls with frequent urinary tract infections benefited from vitamin A by having fewer days with a fever, less frequent urination, and a faster return to appetite compared to a group who did not get vitamin A. This important vitamin also slows the aging process. The body cannot utilize protein without vitamin A. Vitamin A is a well-known wrinkle eliminator. Applied topically in the form of tretinoin (the active ingredient in Retin-A and Renova), vitamin A reduces fine lines in the skin and helps to fade age spots.

A deficiency of vitamin A can cause dry hair and/or skin, dryness of the conjunctiva and cornea, poor growth, and/or night blindness. Other possible results of vitamin A deficiency include abscesses in the ears; insomnia; fatigue; reproductive difficulties; sinusitis, pneumonia, and frequent colds and other respiratory infections; skin disorders, including acne; and weight loss.

The *carotenoids* are a class of compounds related to vitamin A. In some cases, they can act as precursors of vitamin A; some act as antioxidants or have other important functions.

The best-known subclass of the carotenoids is the carotenes, of which beta-carotene is the most widely known. Also included in this group are alpha-carotene, gamma-carotene, and lycopene. When food or supplements containing beta-carotene are consumed, the beta-carotene is converted into vitamin A in the liver. According to some reports, beta-carotene appears to aid in cancer prevention by scavenging, or neutralizing, free radicals. One study reported in the *Journal of the National Cancer Institute*, published in May 2003, found that people who took beta-carotene supplements and who smoked and drank alcohol doubled their risk of precancerous colorectal tumors, while for those who also took the supplements but who didn't smoke or drink, there was a 44 percent *decrease* in their risk. Other types of carotenoids that have been identified are the xanthophylls (including beta-cryptoxanthin, canthaxanthin, lutein, and zeaxanthin); the limonoids (including limonene); and the phytosterols (including perillyl alcohol). Evidence suggests that greater consumption of lutein reduces the risk of cataracts and age-related macular degeneration (AMD), and that taking lutein supplements can slow the progress of these disorders, although it does not appear to reverse them if they are already established. High lutein consumption has also been reported to decrease the incidence of prostate cancer.

Science has not yet discovered all of the carotenoids, although one source documents six hundred different carotenoids identified so far. Combinations of carotenoids have been shown to be more beneficial than individual carotenoids taken alone.

Taking large amounts of vitamin A, more than 30,000 mcg (100,000 international units) daily, over long periods can be toxic to the body, mainly to the liver. Toxic levels of vitamin A are associated with abdominal pain, amenorrhea (cessation of menstruation), enlargement of the liver and/or spleen, gastrointestinal disturbances, hair loss, itching, joint pain, nausea and vomiting, water on the brain, elevated liver enzymes, and small cracks and scales on the lips and at the corners of the mouth. Excessive intake of vitamin A during pregnancy has been linked to birth defects, including cleft palate and heart defects. It is better to take beta-carotene during pregnancy. If you have a particular disorder that calls for taking high doses of vitamin A, use an emulsified form, which puts less stress on the liver.

No overdose can occur with beta-carotene, although if you take too much, your skin may turn slightly yellow-orange in color. Beta-carotene does not have the same effect as vitamin A in the body and is not harmful in larger amounts unless your liver cannot convert beta-carotene into vitamin A. There is mixed evidence (mostly from studies done in Europe) as to whether too much vitamin A may increase the risk of osteoporosis. In the United States, women usually don't have a problem with getting too much vitamin A because manufacturers mix beta-carotene with vitamin A. However, women who are worried about osteoporosis should consult a health care provider before taking vitamin A. It is important to take only *natural* beta-carotene or a natural carotenoid complex. Betatene is the trade name for a type of carotenoid complex extracted from sea algae. Different manufacturers use it as an ingredient in various products.

Sources

Vitamin A can be obtained from animal livers, fish liver oils, and green and yellow fruits and vegetables. Foods that contain significant amounts include apricots, asparagus, beet greens, broccoli, cantaloupe, carrots, collards, dandelion greens, dulse (a red seaweed), fish liver and fish liver oil, garlic, kale, mustard greens, papayas, peaches, pumpkin, red peppers, spinach, spirulina, sweet potatoes, Swiss chard, turnip greens, watercress, and yellow squash. It is also present in the following herbs: alfalfa, borage leaves, burdock root, cayenne (capsicum), chickweed, eyebright, fennel seed, hops, kelp, lemongrass, mullein, nettle, oat straw, paprika, parsley, peppermint, plantain, raspberry leaf, red clover, rose hips, sage, uva ursi, violet leaves, watercress, and yellow dock. Animal sources of vitamin A are up to six times as strong as vegetable sources, but you should exercise caution if you choose to eat organ meats. A plant-based diet better promotes overall health.

Comments

Antibiotics, laxatives, and some cholesterol-lowering drugs interfere with the absorption of vitamin A.

Cautions

If you have liver disease, do not take a daily dose of over 3,000 mcg (10,000 international units) of vitamin A in pill form, or any amount of cod-liver oil. If you are pregnant, do not take more than 3,000 mcg (10,000 international units) of vitamin A daily because of reported problems in fetal development. Children should not take excess vitamin A unless prescribed by a physician. For most people, beta-carotene is the best source of vitamin A because it is converted by the liver into only the amount of vitamin A that the body actually needs. However, if you have diabetes or hypothyroidism, there is a good possibility your body cannot convert beta-carotene into vitamin A. Consuming large amounts of beta-carotene may therefore place unnecessary stress on your liver.

Vitamin B Complex

The B vitamins help to maintain the health of the nerves, skin, eyes, hair, liver, and mouth, as well as healthy muscle tone in the gastrointestinal tract and proper brain function.

B-complex vitamins act as coenzymes, helping enzymes to react chemically with other substances, and are involved in energy production. They may be useful for alleviating depression or anxiety as well. Adequate intake of the B vitamins is very important for elderly people because these nutrients are not as well absorbed as we age. There have even been cases of people diagnosed with Alzheimer's disease whose problems were later found to be due to a deficiency of vitamin B_{12} plus the B-complex vitamins. The B vitamins should always be taken together, but up to two to three times more of one B vitamin than another can be taken for a period of time if needed for a particular disorder. There are spray and sublingual forms that are absorbed more easily, which are good choices for older adults and those with absorption problems.

Because the B vitamins work together, a deficiency in one often indicates a deficiency in another. Although the B vitamins are a team, they will be discussed individually.

Vitamin B$_1$ (Thiamine)

Thiamine (thiamine hydrochloride) enhances circulation and assists in blood formation and carbohydrate metabolism, and in the production of hydrochloric acid, which is important for proper digestion. Thiamine also optimizes cognitive activity and brain function. It has a positive effect on energy, growth, normal appetite, and learning capacity, and is needed for proper muscle tone of the intestines, stomach, and heart. Thiamine also acts as an antioxidant, protecting the body from the degenerative effects of aging, alcohol consumption, and smoking.

Beriberi, a nervous system disease that is rare in developed nations, is caused by a deficiency of thiamine. Other symptoms that can result from thiamine deficiency include constipation, edema, enlarged liver, fatigue, forgetfulness, gastrointestinal disturbances, heart changes, irritability, labored breathing, loss of appetite, muscle atrophy, nervousness, numbness of the hands and feet, pain and sensitivity, poor coordination, tingling sensations, weak and sore muscles, general weakness, and severe weight loss.

Benfotiamine is a fat-soluble form of the water-soluble vitamin B$_1$. Its use is reserved for cases such as alcoholic peripheral neuropathy, a disorder involving decreased nerve functioning caused by damage from excessive drinking of alcohol. It is found naturally in small quantities in roasted crushed garlic, as well as in onions, shallots, and leeks. This variant of the vitamin lasts longer in the body, yielding potentially therapeutic benefits that regular vitamin B$_1$ cannot achieve. Benfotiamine may be more effective than thiamine in controlling damage from diabetes because it is a better activator of the enzyme transketolase. This enzyme assists in keeping glucose-derived compounds out of healthy vascular (blood vessel) and nerve cells. The normal supplemental dose is 150 to 600 milligrams per day, taken under the guidance of a doctor or other qualified health care practitioner.

Sources

The richest food sources of thiamine include brown rice, egg yolks, fish, legumes, liver, peanuts, peas, pork, poultry, rice bran, sunflower seeds, wheat germ, and whole grains. Other sources include asparagus, brewer's yeast, broccoli, Brussels sprouts, dulse, kelp, most nuts, oatmeal, plums, dried prunes, raisins, spirulina, and watercress. Herbs that contain thiamine include alfalfa, bladderwrack, burdock root, catnip, cayenne, chamomile, chickweed, eyebright, fennel seed, fenugreek, hops, nettle, oat straw, parsley, peppermint, raspberry leaf, red clover, rose hips, sage, yarrow, and yellow dock.

Comments

Antibiotics, phenytoin (Dilantin, a drug used to prevent seizures), sulfa drugs, and oral contraceptives, as well as heavy alcohol or caffeine consumption, may decrease thiamine levels in the body. A high-carbohydrate diet increases the need for thiamine. Alcoholics are among those most often deficient in thiamine because the alcohol inhibits its storage. This is sometimes manifested as a disorder known as Wernicke-Korsakoff syndrome, which is characterized by memory problems, abnormal movements, confusion, drowsiness, and other symptoms. Thiamine has been helpful in treating young patients (average age, thirty-five years) with major depressive disorders who are taking antidepressants. In comparison to a placebo, adjuvant thiamine alleviated symptoms of depression faster. Importantly, improvements were observed within six weeks of initiation of treatment. Thiamine may also support heart function. Patients with chronic heart failure who took a large amount of thiamine (300 mg/day for 30 days) and were taking diuretics experienced an increased ability of the heart to pump blood. This study suggests that thiamine supplementation along with diuretic drugs has beneficial effects on cardiac function in patients with symptomatic chronic heart failure.

Vitamin B₂ (Riboflavin)

Riboflavin is necessary for red blood cell formation, antibody production, cell respiration, and growth. It alleviates eye fatigue and is important in the prevention and treatment of cataracts. It aids in the metabolism of carbohydrates, fats, and proteins. Together with vitamin A, it maintains and improves the mucous membranes in the digestive tract. Riboflavin also facilitates the use of oxygen by the tissues of the skin, nails, and hair; eliminates dandruff; and helps the absorption of iron and vitamin B_6 (pyridoxine). People over the age of sixty years are more likely to have a deficiency of riboflavin, which could lead to vitamin B_6 not functioning properly.

Consumption of adequate amounts of riboflavin is important during pregnancy, because a lack of this vitamin can damage a developing fetus even if a woman shows no signs of deficiency. Riboflavin is needed for the metabolism of the amino acid tryptophan, which is converted into niacin in the body. Carpal tunnel syndrome may benefit from a treatment program that includes riboflavin and vitamin B_6. Riboflavin may help patients who experience frequent migraine headaches. Migraine sufferers who took a proprietary blend of riboflavin, Coenzyme Q_{10}, and magnesium had fewer migraine days per month over three months (declined from 6.2 days during the baseline period to 4.4 days at the end of the treatment), and those that occurred were less severe.

Deficiency symptoms include cracks and sores at the corners of the mouth, eye disorders, inflammation of the mouth and tongue, and skin lesions, a group of symptoms collectively referred to as *ariboflavinosis*. Other possible deficiency symptoms include dermatitis, dizziness, hair loss, insomnia, light sensitivity, poor digestion, retarded growth, and slowed mental response. A low intake may impair mental and physical performance. Nearly 300 Chinese students were randomly assigned to consume a riboflavin-enriched milk or regular milk for six months. Those who got the enriched milk performed better at school, were better at sports, and overall were more confident.

Sources
High levels of vitamin B_2 are found in the following foods: cheese, egg yolks, fish, legumes, meat, milk, poultry, spinach, whole grains, and yogurt. Other sources include asparagus, avocados, broccoli, Brussels sprouts, currants, dandelion greens, dulse, kelp, leafy green vegetables, mushrooms, molasses, nuts, and watercress. Herbs that contain vitamin B_2 include alfalfa, bladderwrack, burdock root, catnip, cayenne, chamomile, chickweed, eyebright, fennel seed, fenugreek, ginseng, hops, mullein, nettle, oat straw, parsley, peppermint, raspberry leaves, red clover, rose hips, sage, and yellow dock.

Comments
Factors that increase the need for riboflavin include the use of oral contraceptives and strenuous exercise. This B vitamin is easily destroyed by light, antibiotics, and the consumption of alcohol. Taking too much riboflavin (over 50 milligrams daily) over a long period of time may lead to cataracts and retinal diseases. Taking high doses also may turn urine a deep yellow.

Vitamin B_3 (Niacin, Nicotinic Acid, Niacinamide)
Vitamin B_3 is needed for proper circulation and healthy skin. It aids in the functioning of the nervous system; in the metabolism of carbohydrates, fats, and proteins; and in the production of hydrochloric acid for the digestive system. It is involved in the normal secretion of bile and stomach fluids, and in the synthesis of sex hormones. Niacin (nicotinic acid) lowers cholesterol and

improves circulation. It is helpful for schizophrenia and other mental illnesses and also enhances memory.

Pellagra is a disease caused by niacin deficiency. Other symptoms of niacin deficiency include canker sores, dementia, depression, diarrhea, dizziness, fatigue, halitosis, headaches, indigestion, insomnia, limb pains, loss of appetite, low blood sugar, muscular weakness, skin eruptions, and inflammation.

Sources

Niacin and niacinamide are found in beef liver, brewer's yeast, broccoli, carrots, cheese, corn flour, dandelion greens, dates, eggs, fish, milk, nuts, peanuts, pork, potatoes, rabbit, tomatoes, wheat germ, and whole wheat products. Herbs that contain niacin include alfalfa, burdock root, catnip, cayenne, chamomile, chickweed, eyebright, fennel seed, hops, licorice, mullein, nettle, oat straw, parsley, peppermint, raspberry leaf, red clover, rose hips, slippery elm, and yellow dock. A cup of coffee provides about 3 milligrams of niacin.

Comments

A flush, usually harmless, may occur after you take a niacin supplement; you might develop a red rash on your skin and a tingling sensation may be experienced as well. Usually, these symptoms last only a few minutes.

There are two forms of this vitamin: niacin (or nicotinic acid) and niacinamide. In the form of niacinamide, it does not cause flushing. However, niacinamide does not have all the same properties of niacin. Specifically, it is not effective for lowering blood cholesterol.

Taking high doses of special extended-release niacin is sometimes used for cholesterol control. The intent is to lower levels of low-density lipoproteins (LDL, or "bad," cholesterol), raise levels of high-density lipoproteins (HDL, or "good," cholesterol), and reduce triglyceride levels. This type of niacin is *not* dietary niacin. A product called Niaspan, produced by Abbott Laboratories, is an extended-release type of niacin approved for cholesterol control.

Cautions
Dietary niacin should *not* be substituted for Niaspan. Taking high doses of dietary niacin (more than 500 milligrams daily) can damage the liver. People who are pregnant or who suffer from diabetes, glaucoma, gout, liver disease, or peptic ulcers should use niacin supplements with caution. Niacin can elevate blood sugar levels. People who are anxious should avoid large amounts of niacin. In one study, those who received the vitamin (100 milligrams a day) experienced more panic symptoms and seemed more fearful compared to those who didn't get niacin.

Vitamin B₅ (Pantothenic Acid)
Known as the antistress vitamin, pantothenic acid plays a role in the production of the adrenal hormones and the formation of antibodies, aids in vitamin utilization, and helps to convert fats, carbohydrates, and proteins into energy.

Pantothenic acid is required by all cells in the body and is concentrated in the organs. It is also involved in the production of neurotransmitters. This vitamin is an essential element of co-enzyme A, a vital body chemical involved in many necessary metabolic functions. Pantothenic acid is also a stamina enhancer and prevents certain forms of anemia. It is needed for normal functioning of the gastrointestinal tract and may be helpful in treating depression and anxiety. A deficiency of pantothenic acid may cause fatigue, headache, nausea, and tingling in the hands. Pantothenic acid is also needed for proper functioning of the adrenal glands.

Sources
The following foods contain pantothenic acid: avocados, beef, brewer's yeast, broccoli, eggs, fresh vegetables, kidney, legumes,

liver, lobster, milk, mushrooms, nuts, pork, royal jelly, saltwater fish, sweet potatoes, torula yeast, whole rye flour, and whole wheat.

Vitamin B$_6$ (Pyridoxine)

Pyridoxine is involved in more bodily functions than almost any other single nutrient. It affects both physical and mental health. It is beneficial if you suffer from water retention, and is necessary for the production of hydrochloric acid and the absorption of fats and protein. It also aids in maintaining sodium and potassium balance and promotes red blood cell formation.

Pyridoxine is required by the nervous system and is needed for normal brain function and for the synthesis of the nucleic acids RNA and DNA, which contain the genetic instructions for the reproduction of all cells and for normal cellular growth. It activates many enzymes and aids in the absorption of vitamin B$_{12}$, in immune system function, and in antibody production.

Vitamin B$_6$ plays a role in cancer immunity and aids in the prevention of arteriosclerosis. It inhibits the formation of a toxic chemical called homocysteine, which attacks the heart muscle and allows the deposition of cholesterol around the heart muscle. Pyridoxine acts as a mild diuretic, reducing the symptoms of premenstrual syndrome, and it may be useful in preventing calcium oxalate kidney stones as well. It is helpful in the treatment of allergies, arthritis, and asthma.

A deficiency of vitamin B$_6$ can result in anemia, convulsions, headaches, nausea, flaky skin, a sore tongue, and vomiting. Other possible signs of deficiency include acne, anorexia, arthritis, conjunctivitis, cracks or sores on the mouth and lips, depression, dizziness, fatigue, hyperirritability, impaired wound healing, inflammation of the mouth and gums, learning difficulties, impaired memory or memory loss, hair loss, hearing problems, numbness, oily facial skin, stunted growth, and tingling sensations. Carpal tunnel syndrome has been linked to a deficiency of vitamin B$_6$ as well.

Sources

All foods contain some vitamin B_6; however, the following foods have the highest amounts: brewer's yeast, carrots, chicken, eggs, fish, meat, peas, spinach, sunflower seeds, walnuts, and wheat germ. Other sources include avocado, bananas, beans, blackstrap molasses, broccoli, brown rice and other whole grains, cabbage, cantaloupe, corn, dulse (a red seaweed), plantains, potatoes, rice bran, soybeans, and tempeh. Herbs that contain vitamin B_6 include alfalfa, catnip, and oat straw.

Comments

Antidepressants, estrogen therapy, and oral contraceptives may increase the need for vitamin B_6. Diuretics and cortisone drugs block the absorption of this vitamin by the body.

Prolonged use of high doses of vitamin B_6 (over 1,000 milligrams per day) can be toxic, and may result in nerve damage and loss of coordination.

Vitamin B_{12} (Methylcobalamin)

Vitamin B_{12} is the most chemically complex of all the vitamins and is the general name for a group of essential biological compounds known as cobalamins. The cobalamins are similar to hemoglobin in the blood except that instead of iron they contain cobalt. Vitamin B_{12} comes in several forms. Not all forms are equally effective. The most effective form is *methyl*cobalamin. However, the most common form is *cyano*cobalamin, because it is easier to manufacture and is therefore less expensive.

Unfortunately, the very common and inexpensive cyanocobalamin form is difficult for the body to absorb, and the small amount that is absorbed usually fails to find its way into the cells, where it can perform its intended tasks. The liver does, however, convert a small amount of cyanocobalamin into methylcobalamin, but much larger amounts than can be converted are needed to carry out the normal functions of vitamin B_{12}. As a result, many people who take large doses of cyanocobalamin continue to be deficient in the vitamin. They often find themselves resorting to vitamin B_{12} injections, which are available from a doctor by prescription only. Vitamin B_{12} deficiency caused by malabsorption is most common in elderly people. A simple alternative is to take the methylcobalamin form in the first place, either swallowed in tablet form or sublingually. Those with severe digestive disorders may have no choice but to resort to vitamin B_{12} injections. Injections usually are administered every two to three months.

Methylcobalamin is active in the growth and protection of the nervous system. Larger quantities are especially necessary to protect against neurological deterioration as we age. One Danish study found that daily supplementation with 6 micrograms per day (the DV is 2.4 micrograms) appeared to be sufficient to correct deficiencies in women aged forty-one to seventy-five years.

Vitamin B_{12}, in the methylcobalamin form, may help prevent Parkinson's disease and slow the progression in those who already have the disease by protecting against neural toxicity caused by excess L-dopa, a probable cause of the disease. The vitamin has been shown to reverse the symptoms of such rare neurological diseases as Bell's palsy, and shows promise in the treatment of multiple sclerosis and other neurological diseases. Very few substances are known to have any impact on regenerating damaged nerves in humans. However, a 1994 study in the *Journal of Neurological Science* suggested that the methylcobalamin form of vitamin B_{12} could increase the synthesis of certain proteins that help regenerate nerves. The study showed that very high doses of methylcobalamin produced nerve regeneration in rats. No substantive human studies on nerve regeneration are known to date, but as new research is reported, it will be included in future editions of this book.

Methylcobalamin is essential in converting homocysteine into methionine, which is used to build protein. As such, it plays an important role in protein synthesis necessary for cardiovascular function. It has been found that high levels of homocysteine that have gone unconverted may be toxic to the lining of the blood vessels and may increase clotting factors, which can result in the buildup of plaque and eventually lead to heart disease and stroke. As such, vitamin B_{12} plays an important role in protein synthesis necessary for cardiovascular function.

Vitamin B_{12} is needed to prevent anemia; it aids folic acid in regulating the formation of red blood cells and helps in the utilization of iron. This vitamin is also required for proper digestion, absorption of foods, and the metabolism of carbohydrates and fats. It aids in cell formation and cellular longevity. In addition, vitamin B_{12} prevents nerve damage, maintains fertility, and promotes normal growth and development by maintaining the fatty sheaths that cover and protect nerve endings. A study reported in the *American Journal of Obstetrics and Gynecology* in 2004 found that women who gave birth to children with spina bifida had vitamin B_{12} levels that were 21 percent lower than those of mothers who had had healthy children. Vitamin B_{12} is also linked to the production of acetylcholine, a neurotransmitter that assists memory and learning. Vitamin B_{12} supplementation has been shown to enhance sleep patterns, allowing for more restful and refreshing sleep.

A vitamin B_{12} deficiency can be caused by malabsorption, which is most common in older adults and in people with digestive disorders. Deficiency can cause abnormal gait, bone loss, chronic fatigue, constipation, depression, digestive disorders, dizziness, drowsiness, enlargement of the liver, eye disorders, hallucinations, headaches (including migraines), inflammation of the tongue, irritability, labored breathing, memory loss, moodiness, nervousness, neurological damage, palpitations, pernicious anemia, ringing in the ears, and spinal cord degeneration.

Researchers caution that all patients with unexplained anemia and/or neurological symptoms, as well as patients at risk of developing low B_{12} levels like the elderly and those with intestinal disorders, should have blood levels measured. In addition, those with cognitive impairment may want to be tested for low B_{12} levels. Long-term studies that looked for benefits of B_{12} in older patients with peripheral and central nerve problems did not pan out. Widespread supplementation of B_{12} is not warranted in older individuals who are experiencing neurological problems. Thirty-four percent of patients with COPD had B_{12} deficiencies. Those who received supplements of B_{12} experienced improvements in the ability to exercise longer and harder.

Strict vegetarians must remember that they require vitamin B_{12} supplementation, as this vitamin is found almost exclusively in animal tissues. Although people who follow a strictly vegetarian diet may not see any signs of the deficiency for some time—the body can store up to five years' worth of vitamin B_{12}—signs eventually will develop. Those who have followed a vegetarian diet for a long time (more than five years) should have B_{12} blood levels measured yearly.

Sources

The largest amounts of vitamin B_{12} are found in meats, brewer's yeast, clams, eggs, herring, kidney, liver, mackerel, milk and dairy products, poultry, and seafood. Vitamin B_{12} is not found in many vegetables; it is available only from sea vegetables, such as dulse, kelp, kombu, bladderwrack, and nori, and soybeans and soy products. It is believed that bacteria present in the large intestine synthesize most B_{12}. It is also present in the herbs alfalfa and hops.

Comments

Antigout medications, anticoagulant drugs, and potassium supplements may block the absorption of vitamin B_{12} from the digestive tract. Taking vitamin B_{12} in sublingual tablets, which are dissolved under the tongue rather than swallowed, can be a good option for those who have difficulty absorbing this vitamin. *Intrinsic factor* is a protein produced in the gastrointestinal tract that is necessary for absorption of vitamin B_{12}. People who lack intrinsic factor must use a sublingual form (or injections) for absorption. A blood test called the Schilling test can be used to determine the body's ability to absorb vitamin B_{12}.

At this time there are still some health food stores that do not stock the methylcobalamin form of vitamin B_{12}. It is expected that as research results become more widely known, the methylcobalamin form will become easier to find in your local health food store or online under various brand names.

Biotin

Biotin aids in cell growth; in fatty acid production; in the metabolism of carbohydrates, fats, and proteins; and in the utilization of the other B-complex vitamins. Sufficient quantities are needed for healthy hair and skin. People with brittle nails who received a topical lacquer treatment and biotin experienced improvement in how their nails looked. Most (80 percent) had more than a 50 percent improvement on a validated questionnaire about nail appearance. One hundred milligrams of biotin daily may prevent hair loss in some men. Biotin also promotes healthy sweat glands, nerve tissue, and bone marrow. In addition, it helps to relieve muscle pain.

In infants, a condition called *seborrheic dermatitis*, or cradle cap, which is characterized by a dry, scaly scalp, may occur as a result of biotin deficiency. In adults, deficiency of this B vitamin is rare because it can be produced in the intestines from foods such as those mentioned below. However, if a deficiency does occur, it can cause anemia, depression, hair loss, high blood sugar, inflammation or pallor of the skin and mucous membranes, insomnia, loss of appetite, muscular pain, nausea, and soreness of the tongue. Biotin is showing promise for patients with progressive multiple sclerosis. Taking large amounts (100 mg, three times daily) resulted in such improvements as being less disabled and having the disease progress more slowly.

Sources

Biotin is found in avocados, brewer's yeast, cooked egg yolks, liver, meat, milk, poultry, salmon, saltwater fish, soybeans, and whole grains.

Comments

Raw egg whites contain a protein called avidin, which combines with biotin in the intestinal tract and depletes the body of this needed nutrient. Fats and oils that have been subjected to heat or exposed to the air for any length of time inhibit biotin absorption. Antibiotics, sulfa drugs, and saccharin also threaten the availability of biotin.

Choline

Choline is needed for the proper transmission of nerve impulses from the brain through the central nervous system, as well as for gallbladder regulation, liver function, and lecithin formation. It aids in hormone production and minimizes excess fat in the liver because it aids in fat and cholesterol metabolism. Without choline, brain function and memory are impaired. Choline is beneficial for disorders of the nervous system such as Parkinson's disease and tardive dyskinesia. A deficiency may result in fatty buildup in the liver, as well as in cardiac symptoms, gastric ulcers, high blood pressure, an inability to digest fats, kidney and liver impairment, and stunted growth.

Research in the last decade indicates that choline plays an important role in cardiovascular health, as well as in reproduction and fetal development. One study showed a need for choline for both prevention and treatment of arteriosclerosis and the metabolism of homocysteine. This is such an important nutrient that in 1998 it was added to the list of essential compounds. People who have a high choline intake have the lowest levels of inflammation in the body, which reduces their risk of heart disease. Postmenopausal women may have a higher need for choline because dietary choline requires estrogen to become usable by the body and estrogen levels drop with age. Also, many women have a genetic variation that limits choline availability, so it's even more important to get adequate choline from the diet.

Sources

The following foods contain significant amounts of choline: broccoli, oat bran, egg yolks, lecithin (about 13 percent choline by weight), legumes, liver, meat, milk, nuts, shrimp, soybeans, and whole-grain cereals. If you are managing your cholesterol levels, using one egg yolk for every two egg whites will help you get enough choline.

Folate

Also known as folacin, folic acid, or pteroylglutamic acid (PGA), folate is considered a brain food, and is needed for energy production and the formation of red blood cells. It also strengthens immunity by aiding in the proper formation and functioning of white blood cells. Because it functions as a coenzyme in DNA and RNA synthesis, it is important for healthy cell division and replication. It is involved in protein metabolism and has been used in the prevention and treatment of folic acid anemia. This nutrient may also help depression and anxiety, and may be effective in the treatment of uterine cervical dysplasia. People with Alzheimer's disease who received supplemental folic acid (1.25 milligrams a day) for six months had better cognition compared to a group of similar patients who did not get the supplements. Folic acid may reduce inflammation, which is associated with Alzheimer's disease.

Folate may be the most important nutrient in regulating homocysteine levels. Homocysteine is an amino acid that is naturally formed in the body as the result of the breakdown of another amino acid, methionine. In recent years, high levels of homocysteine have been found to be associated with an increased risk of atherosclerosis (hardening of the arteries due to the accumulation of fatty plaques). Normally, homocysteine is converted to other, non-harmful amino acids in the body. In order for this conversion to take place as it should, the body needs an adequate supply of folate, as well as of vitamins B_6 and B_{12}. Homocysteine levels in red blood cells have been shown to have an inverse relationship to levels of these three important

B vitamins—that is, the lower the levels of these vitamins, the higher the level of homocysteine. Folic acid may help reduce the risk of stroke. People who are taking blood-pressure-lowering medications were randomized to folic acid (0.8 milligrams a day) or none. Those getting the blood pressure drug and folic acid had a significant decrease in the development of stroke (26 percent).

Folate is very important in pregnancy. It helps to regulate embryonic and fetal nerve cell formation, which is vital for normal development. Studies have shown that a daily intake of 400 micrograms of folate in early pregnancy may prevent the vast majority of neural tube defects, such as spina bifida and anencephaly. It may also help to prevent premature birth. To be effective, this regimen must begin *before* conception and continue for at least the first three months of pregnancy; if a woman waits until she knows she is pregnant, it may be too late, because critical events in fetal development occur during the first six weeks of pregnancy—before many women know that they have conceived. In the mid-1990s, the government required that enriched grain products be fortified with folic acid. This was an attempt to achieve an across-the-board reduction in neural-tube birth defects such as spina bifida. Since the program started, there has also been a decline in stroke-related deaths that appears to be related. Researchers attribute this decline to the reduction of serum homocysteine levels in the population as a whole. However, some researchers worry that the higher folic acid intake may mask B_{12} deficiencies. If you are worried about low B_{12} (*see* B_{12}, above), consult your health care practitioner before taking folic acid supplements.

Many experts still recommend that every woman of childbearing age take a folate supplement daily as a matter of course. Folate works best when combined with vitamin B_{12} and vitamin C. Another option is to simply take a good-quality multivitamin; most have at least 400 micrograms of folic acid and these other nutrients.

A sore, red tongue is one sign of folate deficiency. Other possible signs include anemia, apathy, digestive disturbances, fatigue, graying hair, growth impairment, insomnia, labored breathing, memory problems, paranoia, weakness, and birth defects in one's offspring. Folate deficiency may be caused by inadequate consumption of fresh fruits and vegetables; consumption of only cooked or microwaved vegetables (cooking destroys folate); and malabsorption problems.

Sources
The following foods contain significant quantities of folate: asparagus, avocados, barley, beef, bran, brewer's yeast, brown rice, cheese, chicken, dates, green leafy vegetables, lamb, legumes, lentils, liver, milk, mushrooms, oranges, split peas, pork, root vegetables, salmon, tuna, wheat germ, whole grains, and whole wheat. Unlike most other nutrients, synthetic folic acid from a supplement is more bioavailable than folic acid from food. It is best to eat folate-rich foods and take a supplement, especially if you are a woman of childbearing age.

Comments
Oral contraceptives may increase the need for folate. Alcohol also can act as an enemy to folate absorption.

Cautions
Do not take high doses of folate for extended periods if you have a hormone-related cancer or seizure disorder.

Inositol
Inositol is vital for hair growth. This vitamin has a calming effect and helps to reduce cholesterol levels. It helps prevent hardening of the arteries and is important in the formation of lecithin and the metabolism of fat and cholesterol. It also helps remove fats from the liver. Deficiency can lead to arteriosclerosis, constipation, hair loss, high blood cholesterol, irritability,

mood swings, and skin eruptions. Research has also shown that high doses of inositol may help in the treatment of depression, obsessive-compulsive disorder, and anxiety disorders, without the side effects of prescription medications. Inositol coupled with alpha-lipoic acid may help insulin work better, meaning a faster removal of sugar from the blood. Postmenopausal women experienced a 20 percent drop in insulin resistance measured via HOMA, a sophisticated test to see how well insulin works in the body (lower is better).

Sources
Inositol is found in brewer's yeast, fruits, lecithin, legumes, meats, milk, unrefined molasses, raisins, vegetables, and whole grains.

Comments
Consuming large amounts of caffeine may cause a shortage of inositol in the body.

Para-Aminobenzoic Acid (PABA)
PABA is one of the basic constituents of folate and also helps in the assimilation of pantothenic acid. PABA can be converted into folate by intestinal bacteria. This antioxidant helps protect against sunburn by reducing the absorption of ultraviolet-B (UV-B) radiation. Consequently, it helps to prevent skin cancer. It also acts as a coenzyme in the breakdown and utilization of protein and assists in the formation of red blood cells.

PABA also aids in the maintenance of healthy intestinal flora. Supplementing the diet with PABA may restore gray hair to its original color if the graying was caused by stress or a nutritional deficiency. Other benefits of PABA include protection against secondhand smoke, ozone, and other air pollutants; reduced inflammation in arthritis; and enhanced flexibility.

A deficiency of PABA may lead to depression, fatigue, gastrointestinal disorders, graying of the hair, irritability, nervousness, and patchy areas of white skin.

Sources
Foods that contain PABA include kidney, liver, molasses, mushrooms, spinach, and whole grains.

Comments
Sulfa drugs may cause a deficiency of PABA.

Vitamin C (Ascorbic Acid)

Vitamin C is an antioxidant that is required for at least three hundred metabolic functions in the body, including tissue growth and repair, adrenal gland function, and healthy gums. It also aids in the production of antistress hormones and interferon, an important immune system protein, and is needed for the metabolism of folic acid, tyrosine, and phenylalanine. Studies have shown that taking vitamin C can reduce symptoms of asthma. It protects against the harmful effects of pollution, helps to prevent cancer, protects against infection, and enhances immunity. Vitamin C increases the absorption of iron. It can combine with toxic substances, such as certain heavy metals, and render them harmless so that they can be eliminated from the body.

Most people know of vitamin C and its perceived ability to prevent the common cold. But over the years there has been conflicting data on vitamin C and its effect on colds. And the data remains conflicting. A group of researchers with the Cochrane Collaboration Reviews, the largest medical literature database, looked at the effect of vitamin C and its use in the treatment of the common cold in over 11,000 people. They found that for intakes of vitamin C greater than 200 milligrams, vitamin C reduced the duration and severity of common cold symptoms but not the number of colds someone gets in a year. However, in extreme physical stress as experienced by marathon runners and skiers, vitamin C reduced the common cold risk by half. Another group of scientists found that vitamin C (when individuals used 500 milligrams per day) reduced the frequency of the common cold but did not affect the duration or severity. One study performed during the peak of cold/flu season showed that 1,000 mg of vitamin C reduced the number of colds by 36 percent and the duration if one developed by 59 percent. The participants in this study stated that they had more energy.

This vitamin also may reduce levels of low-density lipoproteins (LDL, the so-called bad cholesterol), while increasing levels of high-density lipoproteins (HDL, or "good cholesterol"), as well as lowering high blood pressure and helping to prevent atherosclerosis. People with high blood pressure, high blood sugar, or both benefited from 500 mg of vitamin C over eight weeks. Compared to a group not getting vitamin C, those who did experienced a reduction in fasting blood sugar and two markers of inflammation (i.e., C-reactive protein and interleukin-6). Vitamin C seems to be a potent anti-inflammatory agent and is likely effective because it is an antioxidant. Essential in the formation of collagen, vitamin C protects against abnormal blood clotting and bruising, may reduce the risk of cataracts, and promotes the healing of wounds and burns. It may even boost your love life by causing more of the hormone oxytocin to be released.

Vitamin C has been useful in managing *Helicobacter pylori* (commonly known as *H. pylori*). *H. pylori* is a bacteria that grows in the stomach and may result in pain, gas, and bloating. Using 1,000 milligrams of vitamin C, in combination with drugs to treat the condition, allowed for less of the drugs to be used, which resulted in a cost savings to the patients. Because vitamin C has immunomodulation and antimicrobial functions, a study has been designed for patients with the coronavirus who are in the intensive care unit. Investigators in China believe that this therapy will boost immune function and help overcome the damage to the lungs that occurs with this condition.

Vitamin C works synergistically with both vitamin E and beta-carotene—that is, when these vitamins work together, they have an effect even greater than the sum of their individual effects, and taking them together may counter the potentially adverse effects of taking these vitamins alone. Long-term users of vitamins E and C in combination seem to have higher cognitive abilities as they age, as reported by a 2003 study.

Vitamin E scavenges for dangerous free radicals in cell membranes, while vitamin C attacks free radicals in biologic fluids. These vitamins reinforce and extend each other's antioxidant activity.

Because the body cannot manufacture vitamin C, it must be obtained through the diet or in the form of supplements.

It was once thought that most of the vitamin C consumed in the diet was lost in the urine, although this idea is being challenged because initial studies apparently failed to account for the half-life, or consistent decreasing rate of elimination from the blood, of the vitamin in the original calculations.

If you require larger-than-normal amounts of vitamin C due to serious illness, such as cancer, it is more effective to take it intravenously, under the supervision of a physician, than it is to take high doses orally.

Scurvy is a disease caused by vitamin C deficiency. It is characterized by poor wound healing, soft and spongy bleeding gums, edema, extreme weakness, and "pinpoint" hemorrhages under the skin. Fortunately, this condition is rare in Western societies. More common are signs of lesser degrees of deficiency, including gums that bleed when brushed; increased susceptibility to infection, especially colds and bronchial infections; joint pains; lack of energy; poor digestion; prolonged wound healing time; a tendency to bruise easily; and tooth loss.

Sources

Vitamin C is found in berries, citrus fruits, and green vegetables. Good sources include asparagus, avocados, beet greens, black currants, broccoli, Brussels sprouts, cantaloupe, collards, dandelion greens, dulse, grapefruit, kale, lemons, mangoes, mustard greens, onions, oranges, papayas, green peas, sweet peppers, persimmons, pineapple, radishes, rose hips, spinach, strawberries, Swiss chard, tomatoes, turnip greens, and watercress. Orange juice is an excellent source of vitamin C, but *only* if it is freshly squeezed or has been processed by methods that don't involve heating or pasteurization. While freshly squeezed juice is best, frozen juices are often processed by nonthermal methods and can be good sources of vitamin C. Some so-called fruit drinks have added vitamin C, and although they are not as good a choice as real fruit juices, they are preferable to carbonated beverages that are devoid of any nutrients.

Herbs that contain vitamin C include alfalfa, burdock root, cayenne, chickweed, eyebright, fennel seed, fenugreek, hops, kelp, peppermint, mullein, nettle, oat straw, paprika, parsley, pine needle, plantain, raspberry leaf, red clover, rose hips, skullcap, violet leaves, yarrow, and yellow dock.

Comments

Alcohol, analgesics, antidepressants, anticoagulants, oral contraceptives, and steroids may reduce levels of vitamin C in the body. Smoking causes a serious depletion of vitamin C.

Diabetes medications such as chlorpropamide (Diabinese) and sulfa drugs may not be as effective if taken with vitamin C. Taking high doses of vitamin C may cause a false-negative reading in tests for blood in the stool. It is thought that for some people taking too much vitamin C may cause it to act as a pro-oxidant (creating damaging oxygen particles) rather than an antioxidant (negating the harmful effect of oxygen free radicals). For example, patients with kidney failure had increased oxidation of tissues by taking only 214 milligrams per day.

For maximum effectiveness, supplemental vitamin C should be taken in divided doses, twice daily. Esterified vitamin C (Ester-C) is an effective form of vitamin C. Recently, however, some investigators have found that Ester-C may be no more bioavailable than regular vitamin C (ascorbic acid). We will have to wait to see what is discovered in future studies. Ester-C is created by having the vitamin C react with a necessary mineral, such as calcium, magnesium, potassium, sodium, or zinc. This results in a form of the vitamin that is nonacidic and that contains vitamin C metabolites identical to those produced by the body. Esterified vitamin C enters the bloodstream and tissues four times faster than standard forms of vitamin C because it moves into the blood cells more efficiently and also stays in the body tissues longer. The levels of vitamin C in white blood cells achieved by taking esterified vitamin C are four times higher than those achieved with standard vitamin C. Further, only one-third as much is lost through excretion in the urine. A variety of manufacturers produce supplements containing Ester-C, either by itself or in combination with other valuable nutrients, including the antioxidants Pycnogenol and proanthocyanidins, and the herbs echinacea and garlic.

Cautions

If aspirin and standard vitamin C (ascorbic acid) are taken together in large doses, stomach irritation can occur, possibly leading to ulcers. If you take aspirin regularly, use an esterified form of vitamin C, and take it separately from the aspirin. With aging, vitamin C intake may decline, which is related to reduced muscle mass and potentially increased fatigue. It is possible that vitamin C may be recommended to people with sarcopenia (i.e., muscle wasting in the elderly).

If you are pregnant, do not take more than 2,000 milligrams of vitamin C daily. A developing infant may become dependent on this supplement and develop scurvy when deprived of the accustomed megadoses after birth. If you have a bruise or sprained muscle, temporarily cut back on vitamin C to less than 90 milligrams daily. Larger amounts may combine with iron produced by the injuries to cause more damage.

Avoid using chewable vitamin C supplements, because these can damage tooth enamel.

Vitamin D

Vitamin D, a fat-soluble vitamin that has properties of both a vitamin and a hormone, is required for the absorption and utilization

of calcium and phosphorus. It is necessary for growth and is especially important for the normal growth and development of bones
and teeth in children. It protects against muscle weakness and is
involved in regulation of the heartbeat. It is also important in the
prevention and treatment of breast and colon cancer, osteoarthritis, osteoporosis, and hypocalcemia; enhances immunity; and is
necessary for thyroid function and normal blood clotting.

There are several forms of vitamin D, including vitamin D_2
(ergocalciferol), which comes from food sources; vitamin D_3
(cholecalciferol), which is synthesized in the skin in response
to exposure to the sun's ultraviolet rays; and a synthetic form
identified as vitamin D_5. Of the three, vitamin D_3 is considered
the natural form of vitamin D and was thought to be the most
active. Newer data show that D_2 is as effective as D_3 in maintaining vitamin D levels in the blood.

The form of vitamin D that we get from food or supplements
is not fully active. It requires conversion by the liver, and then
by the kidneys, before it becomes fully active. This is why people
with liver or kidney disorders are at a higher risk for osteoporosis. When the skin is exposed to the sun's ultraviolet rays, a
cholesterol compound in the skin is transformed into a precursor
of vitamin D. Exposing the face and arms to the sun for fifteen
minutes three times a week is an effective way to ensure adequate amounts of vitamin D in the body.

Vitamin D has been the ignored vitamin until recently. Studies have shown that at least 40 percent of people have less-than-
optimal levels of the vitamin in their blood. As many as 70 to
80 percent of Hispanic Americans and African Americans may
be deficient in vitamin D. Those with more coloring in the skin
have a harder time absorbing vitamin D from sunlight. In addition, those who live above the 37th latitude obtain virtually no
vitamin D from sunlight between November and March.

Not getting enough vitamin D in the diet or from direct sunlight has been linked to the development of several diseases including heart disease, osteoporosis, diabetes, and cancers such

as breast and colon. As baby boomers age, the risk of osteoporosis increases. Taking more than 10 mcg (400 IU) of vitamin D has been shown to reduce the risk of fractures by 20 percent in those over sixty-five years of age. But how much is needed to optimize health is still open for debate. Some have argued that it is necessary to consume very high amounts of vitamin D—in excess of the UL for safety—in order to maintain blood levels associated with reducing the risk of disease. Before the FDA considers increasing the UL for vitamin D, more research is needed to assure that there is no risk of toxicity at the upper levels. We do not recommend exceeding the UL for vitamin D until further research has been conducted. The FDA took a different approach and doubled the daily value that should be consumed. Now we should consume 20 mcg daily (800 IU). Around Europe, people with low vitamin D levels were more likely to contract the coronavirus. The lowest levels were seen in the elderly. If COVID-19 is contracted, the severity of the disease may be mitigated with adequate blood vitamin D levels. Vitamin D helps reduce inflammation and reduces the risk of upper respiratory infections and pneumonia, which can occur with the coronavirus. It is best to determine your own blood vitamin D level so you can determine how much, if any, to take as a supplement.

Sources
Fish liver oils, fatty saltwater fish (especially mackerel), dairy products, and eggs all contain vitamin D. It is also found in butter, cod-liver oil, dandelion greens, egg yolks, halibut, liver, milk, shiitake and chanterelle mushrooms, oatmeal, oysters, pork, salmon, sardines, sweet potatoes, tuna, and vegetable oils. Herbs that contain vitamin D include alfalfa, nettle, and parsley. Vitamin D is added to some foods, including orange juice, margarine, and dairy products.

Vitamin D is also formed by the body in response to the action of sunlight on the skin. Of all the nutrients, this is one of a few that is difficult to reach the DRI from food alone and supplementation may be needed. It may make sense to take serial blood tests each year with a physical examination to see if you are getting enough vitamin D to maintain healthy levels.

Comments

Intestinal disorders and liver and gallbladder malfunctions interfere with the absorption of vitamin D. Some cholesterol-lowering drugs, antacids, mineral oil, and steroid hormones such as cortisone also interfere with absorption.

Thiazide diuretics such as chlorothiazide (Diuril) and hydrochlorothiazide (Esidrix, HydroDIURIL, Oretic) disturb the body's calcium/vitamin D ratio. Taking excessive amounts of vitamin D (over 25 mg; 1,000 IU) daily may cause a decrease in bone mass.

Cautions

Toxicity may result from taking excessive amounts of supplemental vitamin D. A seminal study reported in the prestigious *New England Journal of Medicine* showed no benefit from taking large amounts of vitamin D. In a study of more than 25,000 people followed for more than five years, taking vitamin D (50 mg; 2,000 IU) and omega-3 fatty acids (1 gram) did not reduce the risk of invasive cancer or of a variety of conditions associated with heart disease.

Vitamin E

Vitamin E is actually a family of eight antioxidant compounds. These consist of four tocopherols (alpha, beta, gamma, and delta) and four tocotrienols (also alpha through delta). The alpha-tocopherol form is the one found in the largest quantities in human blood and tissue. Small amounts of the gamma form are also found.

Alpha-tocopherol acts as an antioxidant in the human body. As an antioxidant, vitamin E prevents cell damage by inhibiting the oxidation of lipids (fats) and the formation of free radicals. It protects other fat-soluble vitamins from destruction by oxygen and aids in the utilization of vitamin A. It protects the low-density lipoproteins (LDL cholesterol) from oxidation as well. Oxidized LDL has been implicated in the development of cardiovascular disease. It is also known to inhibit blood platelet aggregation (clotting) and has other functions related to the activity of the immune system.

Vitamin E is essential for life, and Americans typically don't get enough of it from their diet. Only 8 percent of men and 2.4 percent of women consume the amount the government recommends. You at least need the DRI for vitamin E, and perhaps more. It is hard to get this nutrient from foods alone, so supplementation is recommended. We don't recommend taking unsafe doses—that is, doses in excess of the UL of safety. None of the dosages given in previous editions of this book seriously exceed the maximums (upper levels or ULs) published by the Office of Dietary Supplements at the National Institutes of Health (NIH). These upper limits were established based on the possibility of hemorrhage rather than any perceived problem with the vitamin itself.

The most common dietary form of vitamin E is the gamma-tocopherol form. However, this form is not taken up by the body in any quantity because the liver selectively incorporates alpha-tocopherol into blood lipoproteins for delivery to the tissues. About ten times more alpha-tocopherol than gamma-tocopherol is found in the blood. However, the gamma form may have some unique benefits in suppressing colon cancer, according to recent animal studies, making a sufficient amount of *dietary* vitamin E even more important to good health.

Vitamin E deficiency may result in damage to red blood cells and destruction of nerves. Signs of deficiency can include infertility (in both men and women), menstrual problems, neuromuscular impairment, shortened red blood cell life span, spontaneous abortion (miscarriage), and uterine degeneration. People with impaired balance and coordination and/or damage to the retina (pigmented retinopathy) may also be deficient. Individuals with severe malnutrition, genetic defects affecting a liver protein known as alpha-tocopherol transfer protein (alpha-TTP), or fat malabsorption problems such as those caused by cystic fibrosis, cholestatic liver disease, or Crohn's disease may have a vitamin E deficiency. True vitamin E deficiency is rare, but low intake (lower than required) is relatively common. One study showed that 27 to 41 percent of people studied had blood levels of alpha-tocopherol less than 20 micromoles per liter (μmoles/L), the level below which there appears to be an increased risk for cardiovascular disease. Low levels of vitamin E in the body have been linked to both bowel cancer and breast cancer.

The d-alpha-tocopherol form of vitamin E is the most potent and is the one we recommend. Also, natural sources of vitamin E are better than synthetic vitamin E because natural vitamin E is more available for use by the body than the synthetic form. Synthetic vitamin E is only 67 percent as active as the natural form. Read labels closely. The natural form of vitamin E is listed as *d-alpha-tocopherol, rrr-alpha-tocopherol, d-alpha-tocopherol acetate*, or *d-alpha-tocopherol succinate*. The synthetic form is listed as *dl-alpha-tocopherol* or *all-rac alpha-tocopherol* (watch out for the *l* after the *d*). The synthetic form costs only about half as much as the natural form, but it has significantly less activity, or potency. Some vitamin manufacturers have been known to mix 10 percent natural and 90 percent synthetic vitamin E, then label the product *natural*. Your responsibility is to check the label and make sure it says *100 percent potency* or *100 percent natural vitamin E*.

If you cannot absorb fat, there is a special water-soluble form of vitamin E available from various suppliers.

Sources

Vitamin E is found in the following food sources: avocados, cold-pressed vegetable oils (olive, soybean, corn, canola, safflower, and sunflower), dark green leafy vegetables, fortified cereals, legumes, nuts (almonds, hazelnuts, peanuts), seeds, and whole

THE VITAMIN E CONTROVERSY

A common complaint among consumers of nutritional information is that researchers are always changing their minds about what is good for you. The problem is that two different studies using the same nutrient have the potential to produce contradictory data. This is because nutrients are consumed in varying amounts, making it almost impossible to determine the exact intake of a single compound. Moreover, the only way to completely isolate a nutrient for study would be to remove it entirely, and this would risk making the person ill. Vitamin E serves as a perfect example of these challenges and why there is often conflicting data among nutritional research studies. In 2004, a group of researchers reported that consuming vitamin E in supplement form in excess of 90 mg (200 IU) per day actually increased the chances of dying. Previous studies, and these were numerous, had been fairly unanimous in their findings that 180 mg (400 IU) of vitamin E actually reduced the risk of heart disease and prostate cancer. How is it possible that researchers came up with such different conclusions about the same vitamin? First, in the 2004 study, participants were rarely given vitamin E on its own. Usually it was given with beta-carotene and vitamin C. Other studies have shown that beta-carotene increases the risk of death in smokers. So some of the increased risk of death attributed to vitamin E was likely related to smokers who took both nutrients. Second, the study included all forms of vitamin E. Sometimes vitamin E was given as alpha-tocopherol and sometimes as mixed tocopherols, and since each has distinct biological effects, they cannot be lumped together. This is an important point, echoed over the past several years. Vitamin E in the form of tocotrienols have a greater antioxidant and anti-inflammatory effect than vitamin E in the tocopherol form. In the future, different forms of vitamin E will likely be identified that reduce cancer risk and support healthy bones, eyes, the heart, and the nervous system. Third, because most participants were over sixty and a majority had preexisting conditions, such as heart disease, the study's application to younger, healthy adults may be limited.

grains. Significant quantities of this vitamin are also found in brown rice, cornmeal, dulse, eggs, kelp, desiccated liver, milk, oatmeal, organ meats, soybeans, sweet potatoes, watercress, wheat, and wheat germ. Herbs that contain vitamin E include alfalfa, bladderwrack, dandelion, dong quai, flaxseed, nettle, oat straw, raspberry leaf, and rose hips.

Comments

The body needs zinc in order to maintain the proper level of vitamin E in the blood. Vitamin E that has oxidized a free radical can be revitalized by vitamin C and enabled to battle additional free radicals, according to Lester Packer, PhD, who was a noted researcher and professor of molecular and cell biology at the University of California–Berkeley. Adding vitamin E to fats and oils prevents them from becoming rancid. The oxidation of fats is a key factor in the formation of plaque adhering to blood vessel walls.

If you take both vitamin E and iron supplements, take them at different times of the day. Inorganic forms of iron (such as ferrous sulfate) destroy vitamin E. Organic iron (ferrous gluconate or ferrous fumarate) leaves vitamin E intact.

Cautions

If you are taking an anticoagulant medication (blood thinner), do not take more than 90 milligrams (200 IU) of vitamin E daily. If you suffer from diabetes, rheumatic heart disease, or an overactive thyroid, do not take more than the recommended dose. If you have high blood pressure, start with a small amount, such as 45 milligrams (100 IU), and increase slowly to the desired amount. If you have retinitis pigmentosa that is *not* associated with vitamin E deficiency, do not take any supplemental vitamin E.

Vitamin K

Vitamin K is needed for the production of prothrombin, which is necessary for blood clotting. It is also essential for bone formation and repair; it is necessary for the synthesis of osteocalcin, the protein in bone tissue on which calcium crystallizes. Consequently, it may help prevent osteoporosis. In addition, it may protect the vascular system by preventing calcification in the arteries. The liver is a very efficient extractor of vitamin K, which it uses to make clotting factors for the blood. Investigators from the Netherlands have argued that the current DRIs may be insufficient to meet the needs of other tissues in the body. The recommendations were based on the amount of vitamin K needed to clot blood, and other tissues do not have enough. The problem becomes more acute in those over forty years of age.

Vitamin K plays an important role in the intestines and aids in converting glucose into glycogen for storage in the liver, promoting healthy liver function. It may increase resistance to infection in children and help prevent cancers that target the inner linings of the organs. It aids in promoting longevity. A deficiency of this vitamin can cause abnormal and/or internal bleeding.

There are three forms of vitamin K. The first is vitamin K_1 (phylloquinone or phytonadione), which comes from plants and makes up your dietary vitamin K. The second is vitamin K_2, a family of substances called menaquinones, which are made by intestinal bacteria and also found in butter, cow liver, chicken, egg yolks, fermented soybean products, and some cheeses. Third, there is vitamin K_3 (menadione), which is a synthetic substance.

Sources
Vitamin K_1 is found in some foods, including asparagus, blackstrap molasses, broccoli, Brussels sprouts, cabbage, cauliflower, chicken, dark green leafy vegetables, egg yolks, leaf lettuce, liver, oatmeal, oats, rye, safflower oil, soybeans, wheat, and yogurt. Herbs that can supply vitamin K_1 include alfalfa, green tea, kelp, nettle, oat straw, and shepherd's purse. However, the majority of

the body's supply of this vitamin is synthesized by the "friendly" bacteria normally present in the intestines, which comes as a result of consuming soluble fiber.

Comments

Antibiotics increase the need for dietary or supplemental vitamin K. Because bacteria in the intestines synthesize vitamin K, taking antibiotics—which kill the bacteria—interferes with this process. Antibiotics also interfere with the absorption of vitamin K. Vitamin K deficiency can be caused by any of the following:

- A poor or restricted diet lacking in fiber.

- Crohn's disease, ulcerative colitis.

- Liver disease that interferes with vitamin K storage.

- The use of antibiotics, cholesterol-lowering drugs, mineral oil, aspirin, and/or blood thinners.

Low levels of vitamin K are associated with insulin release and glucose regulation problems, and may lead to low bone density in women. Supplementing the diet with this vitamin enhances the bone-building process by attracting calcium to the bone. Supplemental vitamin K also reduces the amount of calcium in the urine and frees up more calcium to be used by the bone-building process.

Cautions

Do not take large doses of synthetic vitamin K during the last few weeks of pregnancy. It can result in a toxic reaction in the newborn. If you are taking anticoagulant (blood-thinning) drugs, consult with your health care provider before taking any supplemental vitamin K, as it can interfere with the action of these medications. Megadoses of this vitamin can accumulate in the body and cause flushing and sweating.

Bioflavonoids

Although bioflavonoids are not true vitamins in the strictest sense, they are sometimes referred to as vitamin P. Bioflavonoids are essential for the absorption of vitamin C, and the two should be taken together. There are many different bioflavonoids, including citrin, eriodictyol, flavones, hesperetin, hesperidin, quercetin, quercitrin, and rutin. The human body cannot produce bioflavonoids, so they must be supplied in the diet.

Bioflavonoids are used extensively in the treatment of athletic injuries because they relieve pain, bumps, and bruises. They also reduce pain located in the legs or across the back, and lessen symptoms associated with prolonged bleeding and low serum calcium. Bioflavonoids act synergistically with vitamin C to protect and preserve the structure of capillaries. In addition, bioflavonoids have an antibacterial effect and promote circulation, stimulate bile production, lower cholesterol levels, and treat and prevent cataracts. When taken with vitamin C, bioflavonoids also reduce the symptoms of oral herpes.

Quercetin, a bioflavonoid available in supplement form, may effectively treat and prevent asthma symptoms. Activated Quercetin from Source Naturals is a good source of quercetin. It also contains two other ingredients that increase its efficacy: bromelain, an enzyme from pineapple, and vitamin C, in the nonacidic form of magnesium ascorbate. Bromelain and quercetin are synergists and should be taken in conjunction to enhance absorption.

Sources

Peppers, buckwheat, black currants, and the white material just beneath the peel of citrus fruits contain bioflavonoids. Sources of bioflavonoids include apricots, blackberries, cherries, grapefruit, grapes, lemons, oranges, plums, and prunes. Herbs that contain bioflavonoids include chervil, elderberries, hawthorn berry, rose hips, and shepherd's purse.

Comments
Extremely high doses of bioflavonoids may cause diarrhea.

Coenzyme Q$_{10}$
Coenzyme Q$_{10}$ is a vitamin-like substance found in all parts of the body, the action of which resembles that of vitamin E. It may be an even more powerful antioxidant. It is also called ubiquinone. There are ten common substances designated coenzyme Qs, but coenzyme Q$_{10}$ is the only one found in human tissue. This substance plays a critical role in the production of energy in every cell of the body. It aids circulation, stimulates the immune system, increases tissue oxygenation, and has vital antiaging effects. Deficiencies of coenzyme Q$_{10}$ have been linked to periodontal disease, diabetes, and muscular dystrophy.

Research has revealed that supplemental coenzyme Q$_{10}$ has the ability to counter histamine and therefore is beneficial for people with allergies, asthma, or respiratory disease. Many people also use it when taking cholesterol-lowering drugs in the statin family to reduce leg cramps. Medical literature does not support this practice, but coenzyme Q$_{10}$ is not harmful and there is enough anecdotal information that it may relieve cramping, so it can't hurt to try it.

Coenzyme Q$_{10}$ is used by many health care professionals to treat anomalies of mental function, such as those associated with schizophrenia and Alzheimer's disease. It is also beneficial in fighting obesity, candidiasis, multiple sclerosis, and diabetes. Other conditions—such as heart disease, migraines, and Parkinson's disease—are related to a defect in the body's ability to turn food into energy, and coenzyme Q$_{10}$ may help. Autism is thought to be caused in part by oxidative stress, and coenzyme Q$_{10}$ may be beneficial. Children with autism spectrum disorders who took 60 mg daily experienced a reduction in oxidative stress in the blood and improvements in sleep and gastrointestinal symptoms.

Coenzyme Q_{10} appears to be a giant step forward in the treatment and prevention of cardiovascular disease. A six-year study conducted by scientists at the University of Texas found that people being treated for congestive heart failure who took coenzyme Q_{10} in addition to conventional therapy had a 75 percent chance of survival after three years, compared with a 25 percent survival rate for those using conventional therapy alone. In a similar study by the University of Texas and the Center for Adult Diseases in Japan, coenzyme Q_{10} was shown to be able to lower high blood pressure without medication or dietary changes. For patients over sixty-five years of age receiving kidney dialysis three times each week, coenzyme Q_{10} reduced a marker of oxidative stress (F_2-isoprostane). After four months, those taking 1,200 mg of coenzyme Q_{10}, but not those taking 600 mg, experienced this reduction in oxidative stress.

In addition to its use in fighting cardiovascular disease, coenzyme Q_{10} has been shown to be effective in reducing mortality in experimental animals afflicted with tumors and leukemia. Some doctors give their patients coenzyme Q_{10} to reduce the side effects of cancer chemotherapy.

Coenzyme Q_{10} is widely used in Japan. More than 12 million people in that country are reportedly taking it at the direction of their physicians for treatment of heart disease (it strengthens the heart muscle) and high blood pressure, and also to enhance the immune system. Research in Japan has shown that coenzyme Q_{10} also protects the stomach lining and duodenum, and may help heal duodenal ulcers.

The amount of coenzyme Q_{10} present in the body declines with age, so it should be supplemented in the diet, especially by people who are over the age of fifty. Nature's Plus and Carlson Labs both make soft gel capsules of coenzyme Q_{10} in dosage levels up to 300 milligrams. Oil-based forms are best.

Sources

Mackerel, salmon, and sardines contain the largest amounts of coenzyme Q_{10}. It is also found in beef, peanuts, and spinach. People consume about 10 to 15 milligrams a day, mainly from meat and fish. Vegetarians should be aware that their intake may be less than optimal and should consider supplementation.

Comments

Coenzyme Q_{10} is oil soluble and is best absorbed when taken with oily or fatty foods, such as fish. Be cautious when purchasing coenzyme Q_{10}. Not all products offer it in its purest form. Its natural color is dark bright yellow to orange, and it has very little taste in the powdered form. It should be kept away from heat and light. Pure coenzyme Q_{10} is perishable and deteriorates in temperatures above 115°F. A liquid or oil form is preferable.

Minerals

INTRODUCTION

Every living cell on this planet depends on minerals for proper function and structure. Minerals are needed for the proper composition of body fluids, the formation of blood and bone, the maintenance of healthy nerve function, and the regulation of muscle tone, including that of the muscles of the cardiovascular system. Like vitamins, minerals function as coenzymes, enabling the body to perform its functions, including energy production, growth, and healing. Because all enzyme activities involve minerals, minerals are essential for the proper utilization of vitamins and other nutrients.

The human body, as with all of nature, must maintain its proper chemical balance. This balance depends on the levels of different minerals in the body and especially the ratios of certain mineral levels to one another. The level of each mineral in the body has an effect on every other one, so if one is out of balance, all mineral levels are affected. If not corrected, this can start a chain reaction of imbalances that leads to illness.

Minerals are naturally occurring elements found in the earth. Rock formations are made up of mineral salts. Rock and stone are gradually broken down into tiny fragments by erosion, a process that can take literally millions of years.

The resulting dust and sand accumulate, forming the basis of soil. The soil is teeming with microbes that utilize these tiny crystals of mineral salts, which are then passed from the soil to plants. Herbivorous animals eat the plants. We obtain these minerals by consuming plants or herbivorous animals.

Nutritionally, minerals belong to two groups: bulk minerals (also called macrominerals) and trace minerals (microminerals).

Bulk minerals include calcium, magnesium, sodium, potassium, and phosphorus. These are needed in larger amounts than trace minerals. Although only minute quantities of trace minerals are needed, they are nevertheless important for good health. Trace minerals include boron, chromium, copper, germanium, iodine, iron, manganese, molybdenum, selenium, silicon, sulfur, vanadium, and zinc.

Because minerals are stored primarily in the body's bone and muscle tissue, it is possible to develop mineral toxicity if extremely large quantities are consumed. Such situations are rare, however, because toxic levels of minerals generally accumulate only if massive amounts are ingested for a prolonged period of time.

WHAT'S ON THE SHELVES

As with vitamins, it can be difficult, if not impossible, to obtain the amounts of minerals needed for optimum health through diet alone. Mineral supplements can help you to make sure you are getting all the minerals your body requires.

Minerals are often found in multivitamin formulas. Minerals also are sold as single supplements. These are available in tablet, capsule, powder, and liquid forms. Some are available in chelated form, which means that the minerals are bonded to protein molecules that transport them to the bloodstream and enhance their absorption. When mineral supplements are taken with a meal, they are usually automatically chelated in the stomach during digestion. There is some controversy over which mineral supplements are best, but we prefer the chelated preparations. Our experience with the various chelated formulas available has shown that, in general, arginate forms of minerals make the most effective supplements.

Once a mineral is absorbed, it must be carried by the blood to the cells and then transported across the cell membranes in a form that can be utilized by the cells. After minerals enter the body, they compete with one another for absorption. For example, too much zinc can deplete the body of copper; excessive calcium intake can affect magnesium absorption (and vice versa). Consequently, supplemental minerals should always be taken in balanced amounts. Otherwise, they will not be effective and may even be harmful. The absorption of minerals can also be affected by the use of fiber supplements. Fiber decreases the body's absorption of minerals. Therefore, supplemental fiber and minerals should be taken at different times.

THE ABCS OF MINERALS

Boron

Boron is needed in trace amounts for healthy bones and muscle growth because it assists in the production of natural steroid compounds within the body. It is also necessary for the metabolism of calcium, phosphorus, and magnesium.

Boron enhances brain function, promotes alertness, and plays a role in how the body utilizes energy from fats and sugars. Most people are not deficient in boron. However, elderly people usually benefit from taking a supplement of 2 to 3 milligrams daily because they have greater problems with calcium absorption. Boron deficiency accentuates vitamin D deficiency.

Boron helps to prevent postmenopausal osteoporosis and build muscle. New research indicates that taking supplemental boron can shrink prostate tumor size, can lower blood levels of prostate-specific antigen (PSA, a marker for prostate cancer), and may help prevent prostate cancer. Boron alleviates joint discomfort by reducing levels of both COX-2 and LOX enzymes and helps to preserve cognitive function. Studies have shown that in areas of the world where the level of boron in the soil is low, there are a greater number of people suffering from arthritis. A study conducted by the U.S. Department of Agriculture indicated that within eight days of supplementing their daily diet with 3 milligrams of boron, a test group of postmenopausal women lost 40 percent less calcium, one-third less magnesium, and slightly less phosphorus through their urine than they had before beginning boron supplementation. Boron may exert anti-inflammatory properties and be helpful for women with painful menstrual cycles. University students consumed 10 mg per day of boron two days before the onset of their periods and three days while menstruating. When this group was compared to a placebo group, there was no difference in pain between the two, but after the use of boron was completed (two menstrual cycles), the severity and duration of pain was lower.

Sources
Boron is found naturally in apples, carrots, grapes, dark green leafy vegetables, raw nuts, pears, and whole grains.

Cautions
Do not take more than 3 to 6 milligrams of supplemental boron daily unless it is prescribed by a health care professional. Boron is toxic in high doses (15 milligrams or more daily for adults, less for children) but is not carcinogenic or mutagenic. Many supplements for bone health contain 3 milligrams of boron. If you are also using a multivitamin/multimineral supplement, be sure that your total intake through diet and supplements does not exceed 20 milligrams.

Calcium

Calcium is vital for the formation of strong bones and teeth and for the maintenance of healthy gums. It is also important in the maintenance of a regular heartbeat and in the transmission of nerve impulses. Calcium lowers cholesterol levels and helps prevent cardiovascular disease. It is needed for muscular growth and contraction, and for the prevention of muscle cramps. It may increase the rate of bone growth and bone mineral density in children. Calcium from dairy products or supplements has been shown to promote weight loss, especially in terms of fat loss. However, these findings are not universally accepted. Supplemental calcium of 500 mg daily helped improve bone mass in postmenopausal women aged fifty to seventy-five. Even for women who did not regularly engage in physical activity, supplemental calcium reduced the loss of bone mass in the spine and hips. Exercise has a protective effect against bone loss, but supplemental calcium seemed to help preserve the bones even without it. A combination of calcium and vitamin D was shown to promote weight loss in a group of obese women. Women were assigned to a weight loss diet, and some were prescribed supplements of weekly vitamin D of 1,250 mcg (50,000 IU) and daily calcium of 1,200 mg. They were all deficient in vitamin D at the start of the study. After three months, these women experienced significant weight loss and reduction of waist circumference.

This important mineral is also essential in blood clotting and helps prevent cancer. It may lower blood pressure and prevent the bone loss associated with osteoporosis as well. Calcium provides energy and participates in the protein structuring of RNA and DNA. It is also involved in the activation of several enzymes, including lipase, which breaks down fats for utilization by the body. In addition, calcium maintains proper cell membrane permeability, aids in neuromuscular activity, helps keep the skin healthy, and protects against the development of preeclampsia during pregnancy, the number one cause of maternal death. If high blood pressure develops due to pregnancy, it can be reduced by calcium intake.

Calcium protects the bones and teeth from lead by inhibiting absorption of this toxic metal. If there is a calcium deficiency, lead can be absorbed by the body and deposited in the teeth and bones.

Calcium deficiency can lead to the following problems: aching joints, brittle nails, eczema, elevated blood cholesterol, heart palpitations, hypertension (high blood pressure), insomnia, muscle cramps, nervousness, numbness in the arms and/or legs, a pasty complexion, rheumatoid arthritis, rickets, and tooth decay. Deficiencies of calcium are also associated with cognitive impairment, convulsions, depression, delusions, and hyperactivity.

Sources
Calcium is found in dairy foods, salmon (with bones), sardines, seafood, and dark green leafy vegetables. Other food sources include almonds, asparagus, blackstrap molasses, brewer's yeast, broccoli, buttermilk, cabbage, carob, cheese, collards, dandelion greens, dulse, figs, filberts, goat's milk, kale, kelp, milk, mustard greens, oats, prunes, sesame seeds, soybeans, tofu, turnip greens, watercress, whey, and yogurt.

Herbs that contain calcium include alfalfa, burdock root, cayenne, chamomile, chickweed, chicory, dandelion, eyebright, fennel seed, fenugreek, flaxseed, hops, kelp, lemongrass, mullein, nettle, oat straw, paprika, parsley, peppermint, plantain, raspberry leaves, red clover, rose hips, shepherd's purse, violet leaves, yarrow, and yellow dock. The amount of calcium in these herbs is so small, however, that they should not be considered as contributing to dietary intake.

Comments
The amino acid lysine is needed for calcium absorption. Food sources of lysine include cheese, eggs, fish, lima beans, milk, potatoes, red meat, soy products, and brewer's yeast. Lysine is also available in supplement form.

Female athletes and menopausal women need greater amounts of calcium than other women because their estrogen levels are lower. Estrogen protects the skeletal system by promoting the deposition of calcium in bone.

Heavy exercising hinders calcium uptake, but moderate exercise promotes it. Insufficient vitamin D intake or the ingestion of excessive amounts of phosphorus and magnesium also hinders the uptake of calcium.

If you are taking medication for osteoporosis, a supplement containing vitamin D and calcium is required to help the medicine work properly. Other types of prescription medicines, such as steroids and anticonvulsants (antiseizure drugs), interfere with bone metabolism, and taking supplemental calcium will help with that.

If calcium is taken with iron, they bind together, preventing the optimal absorption of both minerals. It is therefore best to take calcium and iron at different times. Too much calcium can interfere with the absorption of zinc, and excess zinc can interfere with calcium absorption (especially if calcium intake is low). For most people, the best ratio between supplemental calcium and zinc is up to 2,500 milligrams of calcium with 50 milligrams of zinc daily. A hair analysis can determine the levels of these and other minerals in the body.

A diet that is high in protein, fat, and/or sugar affects calcium uptake. The average American diet of meats, refined grains, and soft drinks (which are high in phosphorus) leads to increased excretion of calcium. Consuming alcoholic beverages, coffee, junk foods, excess salt, and/or white flour also leads to the loss of calcium by the body. A diet based on foods such as vegetables, fruits, and whole grains, which contain significant amounts of calcium but lower amounts of phosphorus, is preferable.

Oxalic acid (found in almonds, beet greens, cashews, chard, cocoa, rhubarb, soybeans, and spinach) interferes with calcium absorption by binding with it in the intestines and producing insoluble salts that cannot be absorbed. The normal consumption of foods containing oxalic acid should not pose a problem, but overindulgence in these foods inhibits the absorption of calcium. Oxalic acid can also combine with calcium to form calcium oxalate kidney stones. Studies have shown, however, that taking magnesium and potassium supplements can prevent the formation of this type of stone.

Calcium supplements are more effective when taken in smaller doses spread throughout the day and before bedtime. This mineral works *less* effectively when taken in a single mega-dose. Most experts agree that no more than 500 milligrams should be taken at one time, as this is the maximum amount the body can absorb in one dose. However, because calcium also promotes a sound sleep when taken at night, and because a high-fiber diet can interfere with calcium absorption, some recommend taking a single dose at bedtime. The National Academy of Sciences recommends an intake of at least 1,000 to 1,300 milligrams of calcium per day, particularly for those who have or are at risk of developing osteoporosis. Because the body is more likely to absorb a higher percentage of the calcium when taken in smaller doses, we recommend taking 1,500 to 2,000 milligrams in divided doses with food throughout the day.

Some vitamin companies use a compound called D_1-calcium phosphate in their products. This form of calcium is insoluble and interferes with the absorption of the nutrients in a multinutrient supplement. Antacids such as Tums are *not* recommended as a source of calcium. While they do contain calcium, if taken in quantities sufficient to serve as a source of this mineral, they could neutralize the stomach acid needed for calcium absorption. Additionally, a significant percentage (estimates range from 20 to 40 percent) of people over the age of sixty may have a condition called *atrophic gastritis*. This is a chronic inflammation of the stomach, and it reduces the ability to break down the calcium carbonate contained in Tums. People under sixty are more likely to have an overproduction of acid; in that case, calcium carbonate could neutralize some of the excess and reduce the associated symptoms of belching, gas, and bloating.

Since the amount of calcium required per day is large, some people find it difficult to swallow the pills. Chewable versions are available; these are ideal for children who do not meet calcium needs from dairy products. It is best to match the percentage Daily Value for calcium and vitamin D. For example, a good product would have 50 percent DV for calcium and vitamin D in a single unit. Then you can take two or more depending upon your need.

Cautions

Calcium may interfere with the effects of verapamil (Calan, Isoptin, Verelan), a calcium channel blocker sometimes prescribed for heart problems and high blood pressure.

Calcium can also interfere with the effectiveness of tetracycline, thyroid hormone, certain anticonvulsants, and steroids. Consult your health care provider before taking supplemental calcium if you must take any of these drugs.

Phenobarbital and diuretics may cause a deficiency of calcium. Although several major studies have shown that added calcium in the diet does not appear to increase the risk for either a first or a repeat attack of kidney stones, persons with a history of kidney stones or kidney disease should not take calcium supplements except on the advice of a physician. The maximum safe dosage of supplemental calcium is now placed at 2,500 milligrams per day.

Newer data has shown that calcium from dairy and supplements increases the risk of prostate cancer. Men in the United States who consumed more than 2½ servings a day of dairy products (about 600 milligrams) had a 32 percent increase in prostate cancer. Studies done in Europe found a relationship between dairy product consumption and the nonaggressive form of prostate cancer but not the aggressive form. The low-fat dairy products were more harmful than those with more fat or than calcium-containing foods that are not dairy products. Dairy products may also lead to an increased risk when used in conjunction with a high-protein diet.

Chromium

Because it is involved in the metabolism of glucose, chromium (sometimes also called glucose tolerance factor, or GTF) is needed for energy. It is also vital in the synthesis of cholesterol, fats, and proteins. This essential mineral maintains stable blood sugar levels through proper insulin utilization and can be helpful both for people with diabetes and those with hypoglycemia. Studies have shown that low plasma chromium levels can be an indication of coronary artery disease. Additional chromium is needed during pregnancy because the developing fetus increases demand for this mineral. Chromium supplements can help an expectant mother maintain healthy blood sugar levels during pregnancy.

The average American diet is chromium deficient. Only one in ten Americans has an adequate amount of chromium in his or her diet. There are five main reasons for this: The form of chromium in many foods is not easily absorbed (only 0.4 to 2.5 percent of dietary chromium is absorbed); not enough foods containing chromium are consumed; much of the chromium content is lost during processing; many people do not like the foods that are the best sources of chromium; and high quantities of sugar in the diet cause a loss of chromium from the body. Researchers estimate that two out of every three Americans have glucose regulation issues including hypoglycemia, pre-hypoglycemia, or diabetes. The ability to maintain normal blood sugar levels is jeopardized by the lack of chromium in our soil and water supply and by a diet high in refined white sugar, flour, and junk foods. A number of human and animal studies have found that chromium supplements can improve insulin sensitivity and blood sugar control in the face of insulin resistance, elevated blood glucose levels, impaired glucose tolerance, and diabetes.

A deficiency of chromium can lead to anxiety, fatigue, glucose intolerance (particularly in people with diabetes), inadequate metabolism of amino acids, and an increased risk of arteriosclerosis. Excessive intake (the level depends upon individual tolerance) can lead to chromium toxicity, which has been associated with dermatitis, gastrointestinal ulcers, and kidney and liver impairment. No toxicities have been reported, and thus chromium does not have an Upper Limit of Safety (UL). (*See* the chart on page 24 for this book's recommended chromium intake.) As depicted in the movie *Erin Brockovich*, people can become ill from chromium, but it is important to note that this was a different form of the mineral. The form that is obtained through diet is called divalent, and the one that is toxic is hexavalent.

Supplemental chromium is best absorbed by the body when it is taken in a form called *chromium picolinate* (chromium chelated with picolinate, a naturally occurring amino acid metabolite). Picolinate enables chromium to readily enter into the body's cells, where the mineral can then help insulin do its job much more effectively.

Chromium picolinate has been used successfully to control blood cholesterol and blood glucose levels. The NIH funded a study to look at the benefits of chromium picolinate for patients with diabetes and heart disease. Preliminary data shows it lowers blood sugar and cholesterol. It also promotes the loss of fat and an increase in lean muscle tissue. Studies show it may increase longevity and help to fight osteoporosis. In addition, when combined with biotin, chromium picolinate reduces insulin resistance and reduces "bad" (LDL) cholesterol in patients with type 2 diabetes. Chromium was of benefit to people with a binge-eating disorder. In those given a high dose (1,000 mcg) or lower dose of 600 mcg of chromium picolinate, blood sugar was lowered, body weight went down, and the urge to eat was reduced.

Chromium polynicotinate (chromium bonded to niacin) is an effective form of this mineral as well.

Sources

Chromium is found in the following food sources: beef, beer, brewer's yeast, brown rice, cheese, turkey, fish, and whole grains. It may also be found in apples, bananas, dried beans, blackstrap molasses, broccoli, calf liver, chicken, corn and corn oil, dairy products, dried liver, dulse, eggs, green beans, mushrooms, and potatoes. Herbs that contain chromium include catnip, licorice, nettle, oat straw, red clover, sarsaparilla, wild yam, and yarrow.

Comments

Active, athletic individuals—people who engage in vigorous aerobic activities and consume higher amounts of carbohydrates than the general population—have higher chromium requirements than nonathletes. Chromium levels start to decrease as we age, starting in our early forties.

Some smaller studies have confirmed that added chromium in the diet can reduce total body fat and increase the percentage of muscle.

Cautions

If you have insulin-dependent diabetes, you should not use chromium unless your health care practitioner prescribes it. Chromium supplements can make insulin function more effectively and, in effect, reduce insulin requirements. People with diabetes therefore have to monitor their blood sugar levels very carefully when using chromium. Chromium requirements differ from person to person; consult your health care provider to determine the correct amount of this mineral for you. One study showed that in people with poorly controlled type 2 diabetes, blood sugar and hemoglobin A1c went down after four months of receiving 600 mcg daily of chromium picolinate. Longer-term studies are needed to confirm the use of chromium in glucose management.

Some people experience light-headedness or a slight skin rash when taking chromium. If you feel light-headed, stop taking the supplement and consult your health care provider. If you develop a rash, either try switching brands or discontinue use.

Copper

Among its many functions, copper aids in the formation of bone, hemoglobin, and red blood cells, and works in balance with zinc and vitamin C to form elastin, an important skin protein. It is involved in the healing process, energy production, hair and skin coloring, and taste sensitivity.

This mineral is also needed for healthy nerves and joints. One of the early signs of copper deficiency is osteoporosis.

Copper is essential for the formation of collagen, one of the fundamental proteins making up bones, skin, and connective tissue. Other possible signs of copper deficiency include anemia, baldness, diarrhea, general weakness, impaired respiratory function, and skin sores. A lack of copper can also lead to increased blood fat levels.

Excessive intake of copper can lead to toxicity, which has been associated with depression, irritability, nausea and vomiting, nervousness, and joint and muscle pain. Ingesting a quantity as small as 10 milligrams usually causes nausea. A dose of 60 milligrams generally results in vomiting, and just 3.5 grams (3,500 milligrams) can be fatal. Children can be affected at much smaller dosage levels.

Sources
Besides its use in cookware and plumbing, copper is also widely distributed in foods. Food sources include almonds, avocados, barley, beans, beets, blackstrap molasses, broccoli, garlic, lentils, liver, mushrooms, nuts, oats, oranges, pecans, radishes, raisins, salmon, seafood, soybeans, and green leafy vegetables.

Comments
The level of copper in the body is related to the levels of zinc and vitamin C. Copper levels are reduced if large amounts of zinc or vitamin C are consumed. If copper intake is too high, levels of vitamin C and zinc drop.

The consumption of high amounts of fructose (fruit sugar) can make a copper deficiency significantly worse. In a study conducted by the U.S. Department of Agriculture, people who obtained 20 percent of their daily calories from fructose showed decreased levels of red blood cell superoxide dismutase (SOD), a copper-dependent enzyme critical to antioxidant protection within the red blood cells.

Cautions

Excessive copper in the body can promote destruction of eye tissue through oxidation. Persons with eye problems should be especially careful to balance their intake of copper with that of iron, zinc, and calcium. In one study, elderly individuals who consumed a high-fat diet, one rich in saturated fat and trans fat, and had high copper intakes (greater than 1.6 milligrams per day) seemed to experience greater cognitive impairment compared to those who ate a diet low in these fats or a diet lower in copper (0.88 mg per day) with high amounts of these dietary fats. In this study, it was best to get copper from foods rather than supplements.

Germanium

Germanium improves cellular oxygenation but is not an essential nutrient. It helps to fight pain, keep the immune system functioning properly, and rid the body of toxins and poisons. Researchers have shown that consuming foods containing organic germanium is an effective way to increase tissue oxygenation, because, like hemoglobin, germanium acts as a carrier of oxygen to the cells. A Japanese scientist, Kazuhiko Asai, found that an intake of 100 to 300 milligrams of germanium per day improved many illnesses, including rheumatoid arthritis, food allergies, elevated cholesterol, candidiasis, chronic viral infections, cancer, and AIDS.

Sources

Germanium is found in all organic material, of both plant and animal origin. The following foods contain the greatest concentrations of germanium: broccoli, celery, garlic, shiitake mushrooms, milk, onions, rhubarb, sauerkraut, tomato juice, and the herbs aloe vera, comfrey, ginseng, and suma.

Comments

Germanium is best obtained through the diet.

Cautions

Although it is rare, some individuals may have a toxic reaction to this mineral if they take it in excessive amounts. People have been known to develop kidney problems, and there have been some deaths associated with germanium. Speak to a health care professional before using it, particularly if you have kidney problems.

Iodine

Needed only in trace amounts, iodine helps to metabolize excess fat and is important for physical and mental development. It is also needed for a healthy thyroid gland and for the prevention of goiter, a grossly swollen gland rarely seen these days. Certain parts of the country have little or no iodine in the soil, and isolated agrarian cultural groups that refrained from using iodized salt and cattle feed were subject to this disorder. Iodine deficiency in children may result in mental retardation. In addition, iodine deficiency has been linked to breast cancer and is associated with fatigue, neonatal hypothyroidism, and weight gain. People following the Paleo diet may develop iodine deficiency. This diet can produce weight loss but eliminates the two major sources of iodine in the diet—table salt and dairy products. The people in this study followed the diet for two years, showing that the risk of iodine deficiency is possible.

Excessive iodine intake (sometimes as little as 750 micrograms daily) may inhibit the secretion of thyroid hormone and can produce a metallic taste and sores in the mouth, swollen salivary glands, diarrhea, and vomiting. If you have any problem with your thyroid, speak with your physician about iodine. In most cases, however, the small risk of chronic iodine excess is far outweighed by the hazards of a low-iodine diet. It is especially important for women of childbearing age and children to get adequate amounts of iodine.

Sources

Foods that are high in iodine include dairy products (from cattle fed iodine-supplemented feed and salt licks), iodized salt, seafood, saltwater fish, and kelp. It may also be found in asparagus, dulse, garlic, lima beans, mushrooms, sea salt (which provides nature's own balance of minerals), sesame seeds, soybeans, spinach (*see* COMMENTS, below), summer squash, Swiss chard, turkey, and turnip greens. Most fruits and vegetables grown near the coasts contain more iodine than those grown inland.

Comments
Some foods block the uptake of iodine into the thyroid gland when eaten raw in large amounts. These include Brussels sprouts, cabbage, cauliflower, kale, peaches, pears, spinach, and turnips. If you have an underactive thyroid, you should limit your consumption of these foods.

Iron
Perhaps the most important of iron's functions in the body is the production of hemoglobin and myoglobin (the form of hemoglobin found in muscle tissue), and the oxygenation of red blood cells. Iron is the mineral found in the largest amounts in the blood. It is essential for many enzymes, including catalase, and is important for growth. Iron is also required for a healthy immune system and for energy production.

Iron deficiency is most often caused by insufficient intake. However, it may result from intestinal bleeding, a diet high in phosphorus, poor digestion, long-term illness, ulcers, prolonged use of antacids, excessive coffee or tea consumption, and other causes. Menstruating women may become iron deficient, especially if they have heavy or prolonged periods and/or short menstrual cycles. In some cases, a deficiency of vitamin B_6 (pyridoxine) or vitamin B_{12} can be the underlying cause of anemia. Strenuous exercise and heavy perspiration also deplete iron from the body. Strict vegetarians are susceptible to iron deficiency and should have regular blood tests to check iron levels. Elite athletes may benefit from supplemental iron. One group of male endurance athletes received 24 milligrams of iron a day and another group got nothing; both engaged in sessions of running on a treadmill over three consecutive days. Those who received the modest doses of iron experienced an increase in hepcidin levels, which indicated better iron absorption.

Iron deficiency symptoms include anemia, brittle hair, difficulty swallowing, digestive disturbances, dizziness, fatigue, fragile bones, hair loss, inflammation of the tissues of the mouth, nails that are spoon-shaped or that have ridges running lengthwise, nervousness, obesity, pallor, and slowed mental reactions. Iron deficiency is present in 30 to 83 percent of people with heart disease. In a retrospective review, only a few were screened (158 out of 10,000) and even fewer were treated with intravenous iron (23 people total). Iron supplementation has been shown to improve heart function and quality of life.

Because iron is stored in the body, excessive iron intake can also cause problems. Too much iron in the tissues and organs leads to the production of free radicals and increases the need for vitamin E. High levels of iron were once thought to be associated with heart disease and cancer. Newer data indicates that having high iron stores does not seem to predict who will get cancer but may predict who will get heart disease. However, ferritin, a protein in the body that binds to iron, was associated with an increased risk of cancer in women when the level was greater than 160 micrograms per liter.

The buildup of iron in the tissues has been associated with a rare disease known as hemochromatosis, a hereditary disorder of iron metabolism that is found mostly in men and postmenopausal women and that causes excessive absorption of iron from both foods and supplements, leading to bronze skin pigmentation, arthritis, cirrhosis of the liver, diabetes, and heart disorders.

Sources

Iron is found in eggs, fish, liver, meat, poultry, green leafy vegetables, whole grains, and enriched breads and cereals. Other food sources with lesser amounts include almonds, avocados, beets, blackstrap molasses, brewer's yeast, dates, dulse, kelp, kidney and lima beans, lentils, millet, peaches, pears, dried prunes, pumpkins, raisins, rice and wheat bran, sesame seeds, soybeans, and watercress. Herbs that contain very small amounts of iron include alfalfa, burdock root, catnip, cayenne, chamomile, chickweed, chicory, dandelion, dong quai, eyebright, fennel seed, fenugreek, kelp, lemongrass, licorice, milk thistle seed, mullein, nettle, oat straw, paprika, parsley, peppermint, plantain, raspberry leaf, rose hips, sarsaparilla, shepherd's purse, uva ursi, and yellow dock. Foods are distinguished between heme iron (only from animal sources) and non-heme sources. The heme iron foods present iron in a form that is more readily absorbed into the body.

Comments

Unless you are diagnosed as anemic, are menstruating, or are of childbearing age, you should not take iron supplements. If you take a multivitamin and mineral supplement, choose a product that does not contain iron. Be sure to read labels. Some products contain iron below the DRI and should be avoided by everyone; the amount in these products is too low if you are anemic or require iron and too high if you don't need more. If you do need to take iron supplements, do not take them at the same time as vitamin E, and choose an organic form of iron such as ferrous gluconate or ferrous fumarate. Inorganic forms of iron, such as ferrous sulfate, can oxidize vitamin E. The RDA for iron is 8 milligrams per day for adult men, 12 milligrams a day for male children above age ten, and 18 milligrams per day for adult women and girls over eleven years of age (27 milligrams for pregnant women). Combining vitamin E with iron was shown to be beneficial to the microbiome. Iron therapy induces inflammation, which can be mitigated by vitamin E, thereby improving the GI tract. An increase in the genus *Roseburia* (phylum Firmicutes), a butyrate producer, was observed.

There must be sufficient hydrochloric acid (HCl) present in the stomach in order for iron to be absorbed. Copper, manganese, molybdenum, vitamin A, and the B-complex vitamins are also needed for complete iron absorption. Taking vitamin C can increase iron absorption by as much as 30 percent.

Taking calcium with meals can inhibit the absorption of iron from dietary sources. If you are iron deficient, take calcium supplements at bedtime or at other times when you are not consuming foods containing iron. Excessive amounts of zinc and vitamin E can also interfere with iron absorption. The utilization of iron may be impaired by rheumatoid arthritis and cancer. These diseases can result in anemia despite adequate amounts of iron stored in the liver, spleen, and bone marrow. Iron deficiency is more prevalent in people with candidiasis or chronic herpes infections.

Cautions

Do not take iron supplements if you have an infection. Because bacteria require iron for growth, the body "hides" iron in the liver and other storage sites when an infection is present. Taking extra iron at such times encourages the proliferation of bacteria in the body. Iron may cause constipation.

Magnesium

Magnesium is a vital catalyst in enzyme activity, especially the activity of those enzymes involved in energy production. It also assists in calcium and potassium uptake. A deficiency of magnesium interferes with the transmission of nerve and muscle impulses, causing irritability and nervousness. Supplementing the diet with magnesium can help prevent depression, dizziness, muscle weakness and twitching, and premenstrual syndrome (PMS), and also aids in maintaining the body's proper pH balance and normal body temperature.

Magnesium is necessary to prevent the calcification of soft tissue. This essential mineral protects the arterial linings from stress caused by sudden blood pressure changes and plays a role in the formation of bone and in carbohydrate and mineral metabolism. With vitamin B$_6$ (pyridoxine), magnesium helps to reduce and dissolve calcium phosphate kidney stones and may prevent calcium oxalate kidney stones. Research has shown that magnesium may help prevent cardiovascular disease, osteoporosis, and certain forms of cancer, and it may reduce cholesterol levels. It is effective in preventing premature labor and convulsions in pregnant women.

Studies have shown that taking magnesium supplements during pregnancy has a dramatic effect in reducing birth defects. According to a study reported in the *Journal of the American Medical Association* (*JAMA*), there was a 70 percent lower incidence of mental retardation in the children of mothers who had taken magnesium supplements during pregnancy. The incidence of cerebral palsy was 90 percent lower.

Possible manifestations of magnesium deficiency include confusion, insomnia, irritability, poor digestion, rapid heartbeat, seizures, and tantrums; often, a magnesium deficiency can be synonymous with diabetes. Magnesium deficiencies are at the root of many cardiovascular problems. It is possible that magnesium is related to depression. People diagnosed with mild or moderate depression took 248 mg of elemental magnesium as magnesium chloride. After only two weeks, the participants reported feeling happier; this did not occur in the control group. The participants stated that they found the magnesium easy to take. It offered good results quickly and had no major side effects.

Magnesium deficiency may be a major cause of fatal cardiac arrhythmia, hypertension, and sudden cardiac arrest, as well as asthma, chronic fatigue and chronic pain syndromes, depression, insomnia, irritable bowel syndrome, and pulmonary disorders. Research has also shown that magnesium deficiency may contribute to the formation of kidney stones. To test for magnesium deficiency, a procedure called an intracellular (mononuclear cell) magnesium screen should be performed. This is a more sensitive test than the typical serum magnesium screen and can detect a deficiency with more accuracy. Magnesium screening should be a routine test, as a low magnesium level makes nearly every disease worse. It is particularly important for individuals who have or who are considered at risk for developing cardiovascular disease. Muscle biopsies give a better picture of your magnesium status than blood tests do.

Sources
Magnesium is found in most foods, especially dairy products, fish, meat, and seafood. Other rich food sources include apples, apricots, avocados, bananas, black-eyed peas, blackstrap molasses, brewer's yeast, brown rice, cantaloupe, dulse, figs, garlic, grapefruit, green leafy vegetables, kelp, lemons, lima beans, millet, nuts, peaches, potatoes, salmon, sesame seeds, soybeans, tofu, torula yeast, watercress, wheat, and whole grains. Herbs that contain magnesium include alfalfa, bladderwrack, catnip, cayenne, chamomile, chickweed, dandelion, eyebright, fennel seed, fenugreek, hops, lemongrass, licorice, mullein, nettle, oat straw, paprika, parsley, peppermint, raspberry leaf, red clover, sage, shepherd's purse, yarrow, and yellow dock.

Comments
The consumption of alcohol, the use of diuretics, diarrhea, the presence of fluoride, and high levels of zinc and vitamin D all increase the body's need for magnesium. The consumption of large amounts of fats, cod-liver oil, calcium, vitamin D, and protein decrease magnesium absorption. Fat-soluble vitamins also hinder the absorption of magnesium, as do foods high in oxalic acid, such as almonds, chard, cocoa, rhubarb, spinach, and tea.

Manganese
Minute quantities of manganese are needed for protein and fat metabolism, healthy nerves, a healthy immune system, and blood sugar regulation. Manganese is used in energy production and is required for normal bone growth and for reproduc-

tion. In addition, it is used in the formation of cartilage and synovial (lubricating) fluid in the joints. It is also necessary for the synthesis of bone.

Manganese is essential for people with iron-deficiency anemia and is needed for the utilization of vitamin B₁ (thiamine) and vitamin E. Manganese works well with the B-complex vitamins to give an overall feeling of well-being. It aids in the formation of mother's milk and is a key element in the production of enzymes needed to oxidize fats and to metabolize purines, including the antioxidant enzyme superoxide dismutase (SOD). In a study involving more than 1,000 elderly men, high manganese intake was shown to increase markers of inflammation. The authors acknowledge a need for manganese but observe that too much may have an inflammatory effect in the body.

A deficiency of manganese (which is extremely rare) may lead to atherosclerosis, confusion, convulsions, eye problems, hearing problems, heart disorders, high cholesterol levels, hypertension, irritability, memory loss, muscle contractions, pancreatic damage, profuse perspiration, rapid pulse, teeth grinding, tremors, and a tendency toward breast ailments.

Sources

The largest quantities of manganese are found in avocados, nuts and seeds, seaweed, spinach, and whole grains. This mineral may also be found in blueberries, egg yolks, legumes, dried peas, pineapples, and green leafy vegetables. Herbs that contain manganese include alfalfa, burdock root, catnip, chamomile, chickweed, dandelion, eyebright, fennel seed, fenugreek, ginseng, hops, lemongrass, mullein, parsley, peppermint, raspberry, red clover, rose hips, wild yam, yarrow, and yellow dock.

Molybdenum

This essential mineral is required in extremely small amounts for nitrogen metabolism. It aids in the final stages of the conversion of purines to uric acid. It promotes normal cell function, aids in the activation of certain enzymes, and is a component of the metabolic enzyme xanthine oxidase.

Molybdenum is found in the liver, bones, and kidneys. It supports bone growth and strengthening of the teeth. A low intake is associated with mouth and gum disorders and cancer. A molybdenum deficiency may cause impotence in older men. People whose diets are high in refined and processed foods are at risk for deficiency.

Sources
This trace mineral is found in beans, beef liver, cereal grains, dark green leafy vegetables, legumes, and peas.

Comments
Heat and moisture can change the action of supplemental molybdenum. A high intake of sulfur may decrease molybdenum levels. Excess amounts of molybdenum (more than 15 milligrams daily) may interfere with copper metabolism.

Cautions
Do not take more than 15 milligrams of molybdenum daily. Higher doses may lead to the development of gout.

Phosphorus
Phosphorus is needed for blood clotting, bone and tooth formation, cell growth, contraction of the heart muscle, normal heart rhythm, and kidney function. It also assists the body in the utilization of vitamins and the conversion of food to energy. A proper balance of magnesium, calcium, and phosphorus should be maintained at all times. If one of these minerals is present in either excessive or insufficient amounts, this will have adverse effects on the body. When 500 mg of phosphorus was taken with a 648-calorie meal high in carbohydrates, increased energy expenditure was noted in both lean and obese males, and in lean

males, there was an increase in fat burning. The combination offers a potential regimen to promote weight loss.

Deficiencies of phosphorus are rare, but can lead to such symptoms as anxiety, bone pain, fatigue, irregular breathing, irritability, numbness, skin sensitivity, trembling, weakness, and weight changes.

Sources

Phosphorus deficiency is rare because this mineral is found in most foods, especially processed cooked foods and carbonated soft drinks. Significant amounts of phosphorus are contained in asparagus; bran; brewer's yeast; corn; dairy products; eggs; fish; dried fruit; garlic; legumes; nuts; sesame, sunflower, and pumpkin seeds; meats; poultry; salmon; and whole grains.

Comments

Excessive amounts of phosphorus interfere with calcium uptake. A diet high in processed cooked foods and junk food such as carbonated beverages is a common culprit. Vitamin D increases the effectiveness of phosphorus.

Potassium

This mineral is important for a healthy nervous system and a regular heart rhythm. It helps prevent stroke, aids in proper muscle contraction, and works with sodium to control the body's water balance. Potassium is important for chemical reactions within the cells and aids in maintaining stable blood pressure and in transmitting electrochemical impulses. A 1997 review of earlier studies showed that low potassium intake might be a significant factor in the development of high blood pressure. A high intake of potassium protects several body systems, including cardiovascular, renal, and skeletal. The potassium in fruits and vegetables contains organic salts such as malate and citrate, which neutralize the acid urine that can cause kidney stones. Potassium also regulates the transfer of nutrients through cell membranes. This function of potassium has been shown to decrease with age, which may account for some of the circulatory damage, lethargy, and weakness experienced by older people. Together with magnesium, potassium can help prevent calcium oxalate kidney stones.

In one study, healthy individuals with normal blood pressure experienced lower blood pressure from both potassium chloride and potassium citrate. The levels were still normal, but on the lower side of normal, which is desirable. The amount of potassium given in this study was the equivalent of what is found in five half-cup servings of fruits and vegetables. Anyone with high blood pressure would benefit from lowered blood pressure to reduce heart disease risk. In a carefully controlled study in people with high blood pressure, a diet high in salt increased blood pressure and a diet high in potassium lowered it. In each case, subjects received capsules of only 3 grams of added sodium or potassium per day, and the lowering of blood pressure occurred after four weeks in those taking potassium. In another study, consumption of low-sodium, high-potassium, nutrient-rich foods resulted in the lowering of blood pressure after eight weeks. The hypertensive participants in this study consumed three dry packaged meals that needed to be reconstituted with water. The decrease in blood pressure was similar to that obtained by drugs, and unlike drugs, the dietary intervention had no side effects. Some have proposed that consuming a diet that has a potassium-to-sodium ratio of more than 1 is important to help control blood pressure.

Signs of potassium deficiency include abnormally dry skin, acne, chills, cognitive impairment, constipation, depression, diarrhea, diminished reflex function, edema, nervousness, insatiable thirst, fluctuations in heartbeat, glucose intolerance, growth impairment, high cholesterol levels, insomnia, low blood pressure, muscular fatigue and weakness, nausea and vomiting, periodic headaches, proteinuria (protein in the urine), respiratory distress, and salt retention.

Sources

Food sources of potassium include dairy foods, fish, fruit, legumes, meat, poultry, vegetables, and whole grains. High amounts are found in apricots, avocados, bananas, lima beans, blackstrap molasses, brewer's yeast, brown rice, dates, dulse, figs, dried fruit, garlic, nuts, potatoes, raisins, spinach, torula yeast, wheat bran, winter squash, yams, and yogurt. Herbs that contain potassium include catnip, hops, nettle, plantain, red clover, sage, and skullcap. In general, if it is grown in the ground—for example, fruits and vegetables—it is rich in potassium. In addition, these foods are very low in sodium. It is desirable to consume 2.5 to 3.5 grams of potassium per day from your diet.

Comments

Kidney disorders, diarrhea, and the use of diuretics or laxatives all disrupt potassium levels. Tobacco and caffeine reduce potassium absorption. Using large amounts of licorice over long periods can deplete the body's potassium supply.

Potassium is needed for hormone secretion. The secretion of stress hormones causes a decrease in the potassium-to-sodium ratio both inside and outside the cells. As a result, stress increases the body's potassium requirements.

Too much potassium from supplements could be harmful. Check with your health care professional before using potassium supplements.

Selenium

Selenium's principal function is to inhibit the oxidation of lipids (fats) as a component of the enzyme glutathione peroxidase. It is a vital antioxidant, especially when combined with vitamin E. It protects the immune system by preventing the formation of free radicals that can damage the body. (*See* ANTIOXIDANTS later in this book.) It plays a vital role in regulating the effects of thyroid hormone on fat metabolism.

Selenium has also been found to function as a preventive against the formation of certain types of tumors. One study found that men who took 200 micrograms of selenium daily over a ten-year period had roughly half the risk of developing lung, prostate, and colorectal cancer as compared with men who did not. Selenium supplementation of 200 micrograms a day reduced inflammation, demonstrated by lowered C-reactive protein levels. Selenium also lowered cholesterol and blood sugar levels in people with Alzheimer's disease. Another group of people with Alzheimer's disease got the selenium and a blend of probiotics. That group experienced improvements in blood measures of lowered oxidation, better blood cholesterol and blood sugar levels, and improved cognitive function.

Selenium and vitamin E act synergistically to aid in the production of antibodies and to help maintain a healthy heart and liver. This trace element is needed for pancreatic function and tissue elasticity. When combined with vitamin E and zinc, it may also provide relief from an enlarged prostate. Selenium supplementation has been found to protect the liver in people with alcoholic cirrhosis. Studies conducted at the University of Miami indicate that taking supplemental selenium may enhance the survival of people with AIDS by increasing both red and white blood cell counts. It has shown promise in the treatment of arthritis, cardiovascular disease, male infertility, cataracts, AIDS, and high blood pressure. For very sick patients in the intensive care unit, selenium appears to reduce mortality rates. In one study, the death rate was 14 percent lower in those getting a high dose of selenium (1,000 micrograms a day). Selenium is incorporated into over twenty-five proteins, called selenoproteins, that play pivotal roles in a number of bodily activities, from activating thyroid hormones to regenerating vitamin C.

Selenium deficiency has been linked to cancer and heart disease. It has also been associated with exhaustion, growth impairment, high cholesterol levels, infections, liver impairment, pancreatic insufficiency, and sterility. There is some thought that selenium deficiency might be linked to a host of viral outbreaks, from new strains of influenza to Ebola, wrought by the rapidly mutating virus's interaction with selenium-deficient hosts in places like Africa and China where there is little or no selenium in the soil.

Some have found selenium to be related to cognitive function. One study found that lower selenium content in fingernails was related to poorer cognitive function in a group of elderly Chinese. This finding supports the hypothesis that a lifelong low selenium level is associated with lower cognition.

Sources

Selenium can be found in meat and grains, depending on the selenium content of the soil where the food is raised. Because New Zealand soils are low in selenium, cattle and sheep raised there have suffered a breakdown of muscle tissue, including the heart muscle. However, human intake of selenium there is adequate because of imported Australian wheat. The soil of much American farmland is low in selenium, resulting in selenium-deficient produce.

Selenium can be found in Brazil nuts (the only truly concentrated natural source), brewer's yeast, broccoli, brown rice, chicken, dairy products, dulse, eggs, garlic, kelp, liver, molasses, onions, salmon, seafood, torula yeast, tuna, vegetables, wheat germ, and whole grains. Herbs that contain selenium include alfalfa, burdock root, catnip, cayenne, chamomile, chickweed, fennel seed, fenugreek, garlic, ginseng, hawthorn berry, hops, lemongrass, milk thistle, nettle, oat straw, parsley, peppermint, raspberry leaf, rose hips, sarsaparilla, uva ursi, yarrow, and yellow dock.

Comments

The typical dietary intake of selenium is 80 to 150 micrograms. Taking up to 200 micrograms per day is considered safe for most people. This is half the maximum allowable dose.

Cautions

Symptoms of selenosis (excessively high selenium levels) can include arthritis, brittle nails, garlicky breath, gastrointestinal disorders, hair loss, irritability, liver and kidney impairment, a metallic taste in the mouth, pallor, skin eruptions, tooth loss, and yellowish skin. Unless your health care provider prescribes it, do *not* take more than 400 micrograms daily. One ounce of Brazil nuts can contain as much as 544 micrograms of selenium. If you take supplemental selenium, do not consume Brazil nuts. If you are pregnant, you should *not* take more than 400 micrograms of supplemental selenium daily, nor should you consume Brazil nuts.

Silicon

Silicon is the second most abundant element on the planet (oxygen is the first). It is necessary for the formation of collagen for bones and connective tissue; for healthy nails, skin, and hair; and for calcium absorption in the early stages of bone formation. It is needed to maintain flexible arteries and plays a major role in preventing cardiovascular disease. Silicon counteracts the effects of aluminum on the body and is important in the prevention of Alzheimer's disease and osteoporosis. It stimulates the immune system and inhibits the aging process in tissues. Silicon levels decrease with aging, so elderly people need larger amounts. A seven-year study of French women showed that higher silicon intakes, primarily from drinking water, appeared to be protective against developing Alzheimer's disease.

Sources

Foods that contain silicon include alfalfa, beets, brown rice, rice bran, rice hulls, whole and rolled oats, bell peppers, soybeans, leafy green vegetables, and whole grains.

Comments

Silicon is most commonly found in the form of silica, a compound of silicon and oxygen also known as silicon dioxide (SiO_2). One form of silicon, called silicic acid (actually, orthosilicic acid, or OSA), appears to be extremely absorbable and useful as a silicon transport agent in the body. Two good sources of silicon are Body Essential Silica Gel from NatureWorks and JarroSil from Jarrow Formulas. The minerals boron, calcium, magnesium, manganese, and potassium are needed for the efficient utilization of silicon.

Sodium

Sodium is necessary for maintaining proper water balance and blood pH. It is also needed for stomach, nerve, and muscle function. Most people consume too much sodium, which can lead to high blood pressure. The main regimen recommended for high blood pressure is called the DASH (Dietary Approaches to Stop Hypertension) diet, one rich in fruits, vegetables, low-fat dairy, and low in saturated fats and cholesterol. Restricting salt intake in addition to following the DASH diet resulted in lower blood pressure levels than simply following the DASH diet alone, according to a study involving more than 400 hypertensive individuals. Although sodium deficiency is rare—most people have adequate (if not excessive) levels of sodium in their bodies—it can occur. This condition is most likely to affect people who take diuretics for high blood pressure, especially if they simultaneously adhere to low-sodium diets.

Some experts estimate that as many as 20 percent of elderly people who take diuretics may be deficient in sodium. In some cases of disorders such as fibromyalgia, studies have shown that moderate amounts of sodium may be needed as well (natural sea salt is recommended). Symptoms of sodium deficiency can include abdominal cramps, anorexia, confusion, dehydration, depression, dizziness, fatigue, flatulence, hallucinations, headache, heart palpitations, an impaired sense of taste, lethargy, low blood pressure, memory impairment, muscular weakness, nausea and vomiting, poor coordination, recurrent infections, seizures, and weight loss. Excessive sodium intake can result in edema, high blood pressure, potassium deficiency, and liver and kidney disease.

Sources

Virtually all foods contain some sodium, but those that are processed (i.e., in a package rather than being fresh) have more.

Comments

A proper balance of potassium and sodium is necessary for good health. Because most people consume too much sodium, they typically need more potassium as well. An imbalance between sodium and potassium can lead to heart disease. If you sweat excessively from exercise or heat, you will need to make sure to replace salt lost in perspiration through foods or beverages with added salt.

Sulfur

An acid-forming mineral that is part of the chemical structure of the amino acids methionine, cysteine, taurine, and glutathione, sulfur disinfects the blood, helps the body to resist bacteria, and protects the protoplasm of cells. It aids in necessary oxidation reactions in the body, stimulates bile secretion, and protects against toxic substances. Because of its ability to protect against the harmful effects of radiation and pollution, sulfur slows the aging process. Found in all body tissues, it is needed for the synthesis of collagen, a principal protein that gives the skin its structural integrity.

Sources

Brussels sprouts, dried beans, cabbage, eggs, fish, garlic, kale, meats, onions, soybeans, turnips, and wheat germ contain sulfur, as do the amino acids cysteine, cystine, and methionine. Sulfur is also available in tablet and powder forms. Methylsufonylmethane (MSM) is a good form of sulfur.

Comments

Moisture and heat may destroy or change the action of sulfur in the body. Sulfur is one of the key substances that makes garlic the "king of herbs."

Vanadium

Vanadium is needed for cellular metabolism and for the formation of bones and teeth. It plays a role in growth and reproduction and inhibits cholesterol synthesis. Vanadium has been shown to have the ability to improve insulin utilization, resulting in improved glucose tolerance. A vanadium deficiency may be linked to cardiovascular and kidney disease, impaired reproductive ability, and increased infant mortality. Vanadium is not easily absorbed. Athletes may require more of this trace mineral than nonathletes.

Sources

Vanadium is found in dill, fish, olives, meat, radishes, snap beans, vegetable oils, and whole grains.

Comments

There may be an interaction between vanadium and chromium. If you take supplemental chromium and vanadium, take them at different times. Tobacco use decreases the uptake of vanadium.

Zinc

This essential mineral is important in prostate gland function and the growth of the reproductive organs. Zinc may help prevent acne and regulate the activity of oil glands. It is required for protein synthesis and collagen formation and promotes a healthy immune system and the healing of wounds. Zinc also enhances acuity of taste and smell. It protects the liver from chemical damage and is vital for bone formation. It is a constituent of insulin and many vital enzymes, including the antioxidant enzyme superoxide dismutase (SOD). It also helps to fight and prevent the formation of free radicals in other ways. A form of zinc called zinc monomethionine (zinc bound with the amino acid methionine), sold under the trade name OptiZinc, has been found to have antioxidant activity comparable to that of vitamin C, vitamin E, and beta-carotene. Zinc lozenges have been reported to be effective in relieving symptoms of the common cold and reducing the duration of colds.

Sufficient intake and absorption of zinc are needed to maintain the proper concentration of vitamin E in the blood. In addition, zinc increases the absorption of vitamin A. For optimum health, a proper 1-to-10 balance between copper and zinc levels should be maintained.

A deficiency of zinc may result in the loss of the senses of taste and smell. It can also cause fingernails to become thin, peel, and develop white spots. Other possible signs of zinc deficiency include acne, delayed sexual maturation, fatigue, growth impairment, hair loss, high cholesterol levels, impaired night vision, impotence, increased susceptibility to infection, infertility, memory impairment, a propensity to diabetes, prostate trouble, recurrent colds and flu, skin lesions, and slow wound healing.

Sources

Zinc is found in the following food sources: beef, brewer's yeast, dairy products, dulse, egg yolks, fish, kelp, lamb, legumes, lima beans, liver, meats, mushrooms, oysters, pecans, poultry, pumpkin seeds, sardines, seafood, soy lecithin, soybeans, sunflower seeds, torula yeast, and whole grains. Herbs that contain zinc include alfalfa, burdock root, cayenne, chamomile, chickweed, dandelion, eyebright, fennel seed, hops, milk thistle, mullein, nettle, parsley, rose hips, sage, sarsaparilla, skullcap, and wild yam.

Comments

Zinc levels may be lowered by diarrhea, kidney disease, cirrhosis of the liver, diabetes, or the consumption of fiber, which causes zinc to be excreted through the intestinal tract. A significant amount of zinc is lost through perspiration.

The consumption of hard water also can upset zinc levels. Compounds called phytates that are found in grains and legumes bind with zinc so that it cannot be absorbed.

If you take both zinc and iron supplements, take them at different times. If these two minerals are taken together, they interfere with each other's activity.

Cautions

Do not take a total of more than 40 milligrams of zinc daily. While daily doses less than 40 milligrams enhance the immune response, doses of more than 40 milligrams can depress the immune system.

Air

INTRODUCTION

Air is what we breathe. It is made up almost entirely of nitrogen, oxygen, argon, carbon dioxide, some water vapor, and tiny amounts of inert gases such as krypton, neon, and helium. The part essential for life is oxygen, which makes up about 21 percent of the air. The nitrogen component is basically 78 percent, and argon is less than 1 percent. The remaining gases are found in very small quantities, measured as parts per million.

Water vapor can exist in varying amounts (0 to 5 percent) in any given location, depending on the air temperature and other factors. Suffice it to say that as the air temperature rises, its ability to hold water vapor increases.

Nonstandard components can include particulates, chemical vapors, methane, sulfur dioxide, oxides of nitrogen, ammonia, and carbon monoxide, among others. Levels of these compounds can vary from place to place and are collectively called *air pollution*.

AIR POLLUTION—WHAT IS IT?

Air pollution is basically contamination of the air caused by the discharge of harmful substances. It can cause immediate health problems, such as burning eyes and nose, an itchy irritated throat, and/or breathing difficulties. Over long periods, exposure to some of the chemicals and particulates found in polluted air can cause cancer, birth defects, brain and nerve damage, and injury to the lungs and breathing passages. Dust and particulates from smokestacks, and especially from diesel exhaust, are suspected of increasing the number of deaths from heart attacks by affecting the heart's ability to maintain its rhythm. The very young and the very old suffer the most from the effects of air pollution, but the duration of the exposure and the concentration of the chemical pollutants are important. Certain contaminants can, at high levels, cause severe injury or even death in short order.

Air pollution also causes damage to the environment and to the infrastructure. Trees, lakes, crops, and animals (both wild and domestic) are affected, as are buildings, bridges, monuments, and other man-made structures. Air pollution almost certainly has thinned the protective ozone layer above the earth, allowing dangerous radiation from the sun's rays to cause cancers, birth defects, and other injuries to humans throughout the world.

Smog is a type of large-scale air pollution caused by chemical reactions in the air between different pollutants from vehicle exhaust and industrial sources. Smog can have a different specific cause depending on location, wind, and weather, but the effect is essentially the same. Smog becomes a real problem when a phenomenon known as a *temperature inversion*, or a *thermal inversion*, occurs. That is, the air near the ground is cooler than the air above, which holds down the pollution so it can't disperse. Cities surrounded by mountains, such as Los Angeles, are particularly prone to this phenomenon. If the inversion happens in the winter, it traps mostly particulates and carbon monoxide. If it happens in the summer, expect smog.

Indoor air pollution, including secondhand smoke, is almost as big a problem as outdoor air pollution. In the United States, most people now spend between 80 and 90 percent of their time indoors. It sounds unbelievable until you actually do the math. We live in sealed buildings, our kids go to school in sealed buildings, and we commute in air-conditioned cars to work in sealed offices. It's no wonder that indoor pollution has such an effect on our health. And the effect may be even more serious in northern climates, where the weather keeps people indoors in the winter. Defective air-handling equipment, faulty air-conditioning and building design, poor maintenance of air-conditioning and heating systems, plus gas emissions from carpeting, paints, paneling, computers, copying machines, plastic furniture—all contribute to an ever-growing problem. The coronavirus spreads more easily indoors than out. Exposure relates to how close someone is to the infected person and how long they are in contact. To reduce the risk of developing COVID-19, practice social distancing, use masks, wash hands, clean household surfaces with a disinfectant, and avoid crowded spaces.

THE MAJOR POLLUTANTS

There are thousands of potential air pollutants. Some of the major ones are as follows.

Carbon Monoxide

Carbon monoxide (CO) is colorless, odorless, and poisonous. After it is inhaled, the carbon monoxide molecules enter the bloodstream via the lungs. They bind with the red blood cells, preventing them from picking up oxygen. Because the cells throughout the body are then starved of oxygen, serious problems result. Low concentrations cause dizziness, headaches, and fatigue. Exposure to high concentrations is usually fatal.

Carbon monoxide is created for the most part by automobile engines as a product of incomplete combustion, although even a wood-burning stove emits plenty of the gas. At-home kits are available to test the levels at home.

Carbon Dioxide

Carbon dioxide (CO_2) is a greenhouse gas that is normally found in the atmosphere. As we use oxygen, we generate carbon dioxide, which is exhaled with each breath. Luckily for us, plants that use photosynthesis need this carbon dioxide to live. They take it in, use it, and excrete oxygen. This has been a good relationship. At present, the concentration in the air is around 360 parts per million (ppm). This varies with location and season (it's a bit higher in the summer). This so-called natural concentration has been trending upward for the last 11,000 years, since the end of the last ice age. About the time the ice sheets began to retreat, the concentration of CO_2 in the air was around 200 ppm.

The oceans hold most of the CO_2 on the planet—at least fifty times more than is in the air and ten times more than in all the plant and soil sources. Circulation patterns, or megacurrents, transport the CO_2 up and down in the oceans—most of the CO_2 is held in deep, cold waters—and there is a constant interchange of CO_2 between the oceans and the atmosphere. As the oceans have warmed up, they are giving up their CO_2 to the air. By the late 1700s, the atmospheric CO_2 level was up to 280 ppm, by 1960 it was up to 315 ppm, and today it is approximately 390 ppm. Over the past fifty years, atmospheric CO_2 has been increasing by about 1 ppm per year, which is an indicator not only of the natural processes taking place but also the rapid increase in the burning of fossil fuels.

Why is this important? Because CO_2 is a greenhouse gas, the more of it there is in the atmosphere, the warmer the climate will become.

Chlorofluorocarbons (CFCs)

These CFCs, used widely in industry and especially as a refrigerant in air-conditioning systems, are commonly known as *freon*. There are several commercial forms of freon; all are greenhouse gases. The latest form of freon being used extensively is designated R134. An older form, R12, was used as a solvent and in air conditioners through the 1990s (and is still used in some countries). When released into the atmosphere, all forms of freon eventually rise into the stratosphere. Through reaction with other atmospheric chemicals, freon has reduced the amount of ozone (O_3). This ozone layer is a protective shield against harmful solar ultraviolet (UV) radiation. Increased skin cancers and other related problems caused by an increased level of UV radiation at the earth's surface have been the result.

In addition, the reduction in the ozone layer has lowered the temperature of the stratosphere, and the temperature differential between it and the troposphere (the layer closest to the ground) has caused an increase in both stratospheric and surface wind speeds and thus has the potential for altering the climate.

In a vicious cycle, the lowered stratospheric temperature can further reduce the ozone layer, because as the temperature drops, the amount of ozone naturally decreases.

Hazardous Air Pollutants (HAPs)

This is a general class of chemicals that can cause serious health and environmental effects. Health effects can include cancer, birth defects, nervous system disorders, respiratory problems, and even death at high concentrations. There are literally thousands of these chemicals, and almost 200 of them have been positively identified as potential hazards. Most are produced in chemical plants for industrial use or as intermediate products used to manufacture other chemicals.

Examples of these chemicals are acrolein, formaldehyde, acetaldehyde, beryllium, and arsenic, among others. The greatest hazard still comes from diesel emissions.

Lead

Lead is a highly toxic metal that produces a number of problems, especially neurological disorders in young children. Lead has been phased out of gasoline and consumer products, but there are still quantities of lead in the environment as lead paint and lead piping, and lead-contaminated dust and soil from years of lead emission is still a problem. Luckily, the number of children with elevated blood levels of lead has dropped significantly. More information on lead can be obtained from the National Lead Information Center (NLIC) at https://www.epa.gov/lead/forms/lead-hotline-national-lead-information-center.

Ozone (O_3)

Ozone is beneficial only if it remains in the stratosphere, where a layer of it shields us from ultraviolet radiation. This form of oxygen, having three atoms rather than two, is toxic and can damage our health, the environment, trees, and crops. It is also corrosive to many materials. Normally, the health problems most experienced by ozone exposure include respiratory tract irritation, chest pain, coughing, increased susceptibility to lung infections, and an inability to catch one's breath. Ozone at ground level comes from the oxidation of organic compounds given up naturally by vegetation, auto emissions, electrical discharges (brush-type motors, generators, and lightning), and the burning of coal.

Oxides of Nitrogen (NO_x)

There are several significant oxides of nitrogen (the subscript x denotes any number of oxygen atoms) that affect air pollution. These nitrogen compounds react with many volatile organic compounds, both man-made and natural, to form what we call smog. Smog causes breathing difficulties, coughing, and general respiratory system distress. One by-product is acid rain, which kills vegetation and sterilizes lakes. The burning of fossil fuels, either gasoline in automobiles or coal and oil in power plants, predominantly produces these oxides of nitrogen. As energy demands increase, we can expect NO_x emissions to increase, and consequently more ozone and smog will be created.

Particulate Matter

The term *particulate matter* refers to any type of solid material in the air in the form of dust, smoke, or vapor, which can remain suspended for a long time. Breathing in these microscopic particles is one of the major causes of lung damage and respiratory disease. Particles from diesel engines have been rated as the most hazardous pollutant in an entire arsenal of pollutants, simply on the basis of tonnage emitted. Nobody is exempt. People in urban areas are subjected to heavy traffic and industrial pollution. Farmers who don't have to contend with heavy traffic nevertheless work amid clouds of soil dust, chemical vapors, fertilizer, and flour and grain dust. Industrial processes, mining, road construction, and any number of other modern activities contribute to the problem. New evidence suggests that as many as 50,000 Americans may die each year from inhaling these microscopic specks. The World Health Organization has estimated that deaths worldwide could be as high as 2.8 million annually. People with existing respiratory problems are naturally more prone to feel the effects when air quality is bad.

Many others have been dying from sudden heart failure, which may be caused by abnormalities in the heart rhythm in response to changing demands. When the air is thick with dust and soot, the heart is less able to adjust its rhythm. These pollutants also reduce lung capacity, depending on the particulate level: the greater the particle density, the less the lung capacity. Smaller particles appear to be more hazardous than larger ones.

Particulates also pick up hitchhikers, such as toxic metals, acidic aerosols, and other particles of different chemical composition than themselves. Particles of dust from the sub-Saharan region of Africa have reached all the way into Arizona and Texas, causing asthma problems for people there and all throughout the Caribbean basin.

Sulfur Dioxide (SO_2)

Sulfur dioxide is a pungent toxic gas produced by the burning of coal, usually in power plants. More than 65 percent, or 13 million tons a year, comes from our electric utilities. This takes into account the large number of domestic power plants that have installed scrubbers. Worldwide, the problem is almost out of control. Coal-fired power plants in China and other areas of Asia are not even equipped with rudimentary stack scrubbers. A few other industrial processes, including some paper mills and smelters, also produce SO_2 (from the odor, people generally know where they are). Like the oxides of nitrogen, sulfur dioxide is a major contributor to acid rain and smog. Corrosive acids (such as sulfurous acid and sulfuric acid) formed in the air can rain down to cause massive damage to wildlife, vegetation, streams, rivers, and lakes. Lung problems are caused by breathing sulfur dioxide, including permanent lung damage from long-term exposure (or exposure for shorter times at higher doses).

Volatile Organic Compounds (VOCs)

There are many volatile organic compounds. Volatile chemicals form vapors easily at normal room temperature. Many of the VOCs we find in the air are natural, excreted as part of natural processes by vegetation. Others are not found in nature and are escapees from a petrochemical plant (a source site) or somewhere downstream where the chemical is being utilized. An example is gasoline. Vapor can escape right at the refinery, during transfer to storage, during delivery to the distributor and gas station, or right at the pump when it is being pumped into the gas tank.

Other VOCs include benzene, one of the most prevalent chemicals known. Solvents such as toluene, xylene, and perchloroethylene are VOCs, as are a host of other products. VOCs are also released as combustion products, such as during the burning of coal, natural gas, oil, and even wood. Vehicle emissions are a major source of VOCs, as are vapors from industrial glues, solvents, paints, and many other consumer products.

Water

INTRODUCTION

Human beings can survive without food for thirty to forty days—about five weeks—but without water, life would end in three to five days. The average person's body is composed of approximately 70 percent water, although the water content varies considerably from person to person and even from one body part to another. The body's water supply is responsible for and involved in nearly every bodily process, including digestion, absorption, circulation, and excretion. Water is also the primary transporter of nutrients throughout the body and so is necessary for all building functions in the body. Water helps maintain normal body temperature and is essential for carrying waste material out of the body. Therefore, replacing the water that is continually being lost through sweating and elimination is very important.

A drop in the body's water content causes a decline in blood volume. The lowering of blood volume in turn triggers the hypothalamus, which is the brain's thirst center, to send out the demand for a drink. This causes a slight rise in the concentration of sodium in the blood. These changes quickly trigger a sensation of thirst. Unfortunately, people often consume only enough liquid to quench a dry or parched throat—not enough to cover all of their water loss.

As a result, they can become dehydrated. As we age, the sense of thirst becomes dulled. At the same time, we have a lower percentage of reserve body water than we had when we were younger. This is why it is important to drink water even when you do not feel thirsty. Drinking water can also help control overeating, as thirst is sometimes mistaken for hunger.

Quality water is beneficial for virtually all disorders known to humankind. Bowel and bladder problems, as well as headaches, can be reduced by drinking water. If not enough water is consumed, toxins can build up in the system, causing headaches. Water flushes out these toxins.

Anxiety attacks, food intolerances, "acid stomach" and heartburn, muscle pains, colitis pain, hot flashes, and many other discomforts and disorders can be eased quickly by drinking a full glass of water. Chronic fatigue syndrome (CFS) is another disorder that necessitates consuming plenty of quality water daily to flush out toxins and other substances that contribute to muscle aches and extreme fatigue.

Without adequate water, we would poison ourselves with our own metabolic wastes. The kidneys remove waste products, such as uric acid, urea, and lactic acid, all of which must be dissolved in water. If there is not enough water available to remove these substances effectively, they may cause damage to the kidneys. Digestion and metabolism also rely on water for certain enzymatic and chemical reactions in the body. Water carries nutrients and oxygen to cells through the blood and is involved in the regulation of body temperature through perspiration. Water is especially important for people who have musculoskeletal problems such as arthritis, or who are athletic, as it lubricates the joints. Because lung tissue must be moist to facilitate oxygen intake and carbon dioxide excretion, water is essential for breathing. Approximately one pint of liquid is lost each day through exhaling. If you do not take in enough water to maintain fluid balance, every bodily function can be impaired. And the more active you are, the more water you must consume in order to keep your body's water level in balance.

Inadequate water consumption may contribute to excess body fat; poor muscle tone; digestive problems; poor functioning of many organs, including the brain; joint and muscle soreness; and, paradoxically, water retention. Consuming plenty of quality water can slow the aging process, and can prevent or improve arthritis, kidney stones, constipation, arteriosclerosis, obesity, glaucoma, cataracts, diabetes, hypoglycemia, and many other diseases. It is not expensive, and you should feel a difference quickly, but you must drink about ten full glasses of quality water (80 ounces) daily.

Obtaining quality water would seem to be an easy matter. However, due to the numerous types of classifications water is given, the average consumer can easily be confused about what is available. This section offers a guide to understanding what the most commonly used classifications of water mean and how these different kinds of water may help or harm the body.

TAP WATER

Water that comes out of household taps or faucets is generally obtained either from surface water or from groundwater. Surface water is water that has run off from ponds, creeks, streams, rivers, and lakes, and is collected in reservoirs. Groundwater is water that has filtered through the ground to the water table and is extracted by means of a well. Approximately half of the tap water in the United States comes from lakes, rivers, or other surface sources. Underground aquifers and municipal wells provide 35 percent of tap water, and the remaining 15 percent comes from private wells.

The Safety of Tap Water

Most people assume that when they turn on the kitchen tap, they are getting clean, safe, healthy drinking water. Unfortunately, this often is not the case. Regardless of the original source of tap water, it is vulnerable to a number of different types of impurities and may be full of harmful chemicals and inorganic minerals that the body cannot use.

Some undesirable substances found in water—including radon, fluoride, and arsenic, as well as iron, lead, copper, and other heavy metals—can occur naturally. Other contaminants, such as fertilizers, asbestos, cyanides, herbicides, pesticides, and industrial chemicals, may leach into groundwater through the soil, or into any tap water from plumbing pipes. Many of these chemicals have been linked to cancer and other disorders. Water can also contain biological contaminants, including viruses, bacteria, and parasites.

Still other substances—including chlorine, fluorides, carbon, lime, phosphates, soda ash, and aluminum sulfate—are intentionally added to public water supplies to kill bacteria, adjust pH, and eliminate cloudiness, among other things. Even if the levels of individual substances in water are well within "allowable" limits, the total of all contaminants present may still be harmful to your health. And private wells may not be regulated at all, except at the local level.

The greatest concerns about water quality today focus on chlorine, arsenic, atrazine and other compounds known as triazenes, perchlorate, organophosphate pesticides, trihalomethanes, lead, herbicides such as acetochlor, and parasites. Chlorine has long been added to public water supplies to kill disease-causing bacteria. However, the levels of chlorine in drinking water today can be quite high, and some by-products of chlorine are known carcinogens. As a result, the U.S. Environmental Protection Agency (EPA) is considering steps to reduce the level of chlorine in drinking water but is facing opposition from industry groups.

Pesticides pose a risk in any area where the tap water is extracted from an underground source. These chemicals are suspected of causing, or at least contributing to, an increased incidence of cancer, especially breast cancer. The pesticide problem is a particular concern in areas where agriculture is (or was) a major part of the economy. These chemicals are persistent. Residues from pesticides used decades ago may still be present in water coming out of the tap today and may pose a risk to health.

Long considered a problem limited to developing countries, the presence of bacteria and parasites in drinking water—especially a parasite called *Cryptosporidium*—is becoming a serious problem in the United States. In April 1993, as many as 370,000 people in and around Milwaukee, Wisconsin, were stricken by the parasite *Cryptosporidium parvum* from the city's water supply. Thousands suffered from severe diarrhea, and up to 100 deaths were attributed to the outbreak. These "unacceptable" levels of cryptosporidia, most likely from agricultural runoff, forced users of the public water system to boil their tap water before using it. The same organism has created controversy over the safety of the water in New York City; many people with weakened immune systems have charged that cryptosporidia in the city water have made them sick, even though local officials insist that the water is safe to drink. For people with HIV or AIDS, cryptosporidia can be lethal.

The chlorine added to water to kill bacteria is not effective at killing these parasites. Like *cryptosporidiosis*, *giardiasis* is caused by an intestinal parasite and can be contracted through drinking water. And like cryptosporidia, *Giardia* resists the effects of chlorine (outbreaks have occurred in areas where the water is routinely treated with chlorine) and poses a more serious problem for people with diminished immune response. Indeed, because of increasing concern over the danger contaminated drinking water poses for people with compromised immune systems, the U.S. Centers for Disease Control and Prevention (CDC) and the EPA have issued suggestions that immune-compromised individuals boil tap water for at least one minute before use, use an appropriate filtration system, or buy quality bottled drinking water.

The biggest problem is that even when municipalities comply with EPA regulations, the regulations themselves are weak and have been written in such a way that it is relatively easy to comply. For instance, according to studies, there is no safe level for arsenic in drinking water per se. The EPA sets its limits based on the risk of developing cancer as 1 in every 10,000 people. This still may represent too great a risk for some people. Average levels of arsenic in drinking water are around 5 parts per billion (ppb). In 2002, the EPA upgraded the standard for arsenic from 50 to 10 ppb (the lower the amount, the better the standard). The National Academy of Sciences has found that even at 10 ppb, the lifetime risk of developing life-threatening cancer is 1 in 333. This is thirty times higher than the EPA's own standard for what it says is acceptable risk. The good news about drinking city water is that the contaminants are published on the EPA website. With bottled water, you need to contact the manufacturer to get such information. The risk of getting sick may be lower with public water because more people become exposed and word gets out faster.

Whatever the source of your water, it is important to know some warning signs of bad water. Watch for cloudiness or murkiness in water. Chlorination can cause some cloudiness, but it usually clears if the water is left to stand, whereas bacterial or sedimentary cloudiness will remain. Foaming may be caused by bacterial contamination, by floating particles of sediment, or by soaps or detergents. Bacteria can be destroyed by boiling water for at least five minutes, while sediment should settle out if you let the water stand for several hours. Strange smells or tastes in water that was previously fine could mean chemical contamination. However, many toxic hazards that work their way into water do not change its taste, smell, or appearance. Fear of contracting the coronavirus from tap water seems unfounded. According to the Environmental Protection Agency (EPA), the COVID-19 virus has not been detected in supplies of drinking water. Based on current evidence, the risk to water supplies is low. Americans can continue to use and drink water from their tap as usual. The EPA also advises that you put only toilet paper, not disinfecting wipes or other items, into the toilet.

Hard Versus Soft Water

Hard water, found in various parts of the country, contains relatively high concentrations of the minerals calcium and magnesium. The presence of these minerals prevents soap from lathering and results in a filmy sediment being deposited on hair, clothing, pipes, dishes, washtubs, and anything else that comes into regular contact with the water. It also affects the taste. Hard water can be annoying, and though some studies have shown that deaths from heart disease may be lower in areas where the drinking water is hard, we believe that the calcium found in hard water is not good for the heart, arteries, or bones. Hard water deposits its calcium and other minerals on the *outside* of these structures, while it is the calcium and magnesium found *within* these structures that are beneficial to the body.

Soft water can be naturally soft or it may be hard water that has been treated to remove the calcium and magnesium. Standard water-softening systems work by using pressure to pass the water through exchange media to exchange "hard" calcium and magnesium ions for "soft" sodium or potassium ions. Most use either sodium chloride or potassium chloride for this purpose. The primary benefit of softening is in improved cleaning properties for the water and less mineral buildup inside household pipes and equipment. One potentially serious problem with artificially softened water is that it is more likely than hard water to dissolve the lining of pipes. This poses an especially significant threat if pipes are made of lead. Another threat comes from certain plastic and galvanized pipes, which contain cadmium, a toxic heavy metal. These types of pipes are rarely used in construction today, but they may be present in older buildings that have not undergone extensive renovation. But leaching from pipes can be a problem with today's copper pipes as well. Dangerous levels of copper, iron, zinc, and arsenic can leach into softened water from copper pipes. Another potential problem with artificially softened water is of concern to people with kidney failure. People with kidney failure must restrict their intake of potassium.

Potassium-based water-softening systems can therefore pose a danger to such individuals.

Fluoridation

For many years now, controversy has raged over whether fluoride should be added to drinking water. As early as 1961, as recorded in the *Congressional Record*, fluoride was exposed as a lethal poison in our nation's water supply.

Proponents say that fluoride occurs naturally and helps develop and maintain strong bones and teeth. Opponents of fluoridation contend that when fluoridated water is consumed regularly, toxic levels of fluorine, the poisonous substance from which fluoride is derived, build up in the body, causing irreparable harm to the immune system. The Delaney Congressional Investigation Committee, the government body charged with monitoring additives and other substances in the food supply, has stated "fluoridation is mass medication without parallel in the history of medicine." Meanwhile, no convincing scientific proof has ever been generated that fluoridated water makes for stronger bones and teeth. It is known, however, that chronic fluoride use can result in health problems, including osteoporosis and osteomalacia, and can also damage teeth and leave them mottled. But this occurs only with very high doses. Fluorine is never found in elemental form in nature because it is so reactive. Numerous compounds of fluorine can, however, exist. These are notoriously toxic compounds, so much so that they are used in rat poison and insecticides. The naturally occurring form of fluoride, calcium fluoride, is not toxic— but this form of fluoride is not used to fluoridate water. Sodium fluoride (NaF) is added to city water supplies in the proportion of about one part per million to help prevent tooth decay. Sodium fluoride (NaF), stannous fluoride (SnF_2), and sodium monofluorophosphate (Na_2PO_3F) are also added to toothpaste, also to help prevent tooth decay.

Today, more than half the cities in the United States fluoridate their water supplies. In fact, in many states it is required.

Although many ailments and disorders—including Down syndrome, mottled teeth, and cancer—have been linked to fluoridated water, fluoridation has become the standard rather than the exception.

Individuals have different levels of tolerance for toxins such as fluoride. In addition, many water sources have levels of fluoride higher than one part per million, the level generally recognized as safe and originally set as the acceptable limit by the EPA. After the EPA learned that water in many towns had natural fluoride levels much higher than this, the permissible fluoride limit was raised—quadrupled, in fact—to four parts per million. And this is in addition to fluoride encountered from other sources. Since so many local water supplies are fluoridated, there is a good chance that virtually any packaged food product made with water, such as soft drinks and reconstituted juices, contains fluoride. It is easy to see how many Americans may be ingesting excessive amounts of this potentially toxic substance.

If your tap water contains fluoride and you wish to remove it, you can use a reverse osmosis, distillation, or activated alumina filtration system to eliminate almost all of the fluoride from your water.

Water Analysis

Not all drinking water contains significant amounts of toxic substances. Some places rate higher in water safety than others. In addition, not all cities and towns process their water supplies the same way. Some do nothing at all to their water. Others add chemicals to the water to kill bacteria. Still others filter their water. It is up to the individual to find out how local drinking water is treated and to determine how safe the water coming out of the tap is.

The EPA has defined pure water as "bacteriologically safe" water, and it recommends—but does not require—that tap water have a pH between 6.5 and 8.5. This allows for a great deal of leeway in what passes as acceptable water. If you are con-

MTBE AND
DRINKING WATER

Since 1979, methyl tertiary-butyl ether (MTBE) has been added to gasoline to increase its oxygen content. It took the place of lead as an octane enhancer and was supposed to reduce the problems of both smog and carbon monoxide in the atmosphere. The Clean Air Act of 1990 required the use of reformulated gasoline, or RFG, in certain parts of the country, with the goal of reducing air pollution in those areas. RFG accounts for some 30 percent of gasoline sold in the United States, and MTBE is now added to over 80 percent of RFG fuel.

According to a disturbing report aired on the CBS television program *60 Minutes* on January 16, 2000, this measure to improve air quality has ironically given Americans yet another reason to be concerned about the safety of their drinking water supply. MTBE has been seeping into all our water supplies, both surface and underground, at an alarming rate. It has been found in storm water in 592 samples collected in sixteen cities between 1991 and 1995. The primary sources of the MTBE that ends up in water systems are leaking gasoline tanks, and reservoirs, drinking water lakes, and rivers where gasoline-powered recreational watercraft are permitted. Less than a tenth of a gallon (roughly 12 ounces) of MTBE is capable of contaminating 13 million gallons of drinking water. It is estimated that more than 1 million gallons of fuel are deposited, unburned, into the water supply each year as a result of recreational boating.

Few long-term studies have been done on this chemical, but what little research there is indicates that MTBE is a likely human carcinogen and immune-system depressant. Certainly, tests on rats have provided evidence that MTBE is a cancer-causing agent. To date, drinking water supplies in the states of California, New York, Maine, Pennsylvania, Connecticut, and Rhode Island have been closed down due to contamination by MTBE (boiling drinking water does not help purge it of this agent). MTBE-contaminated tap water can cause problems even if you do not drink it. This chemical can also be absorbed through the skin when showering and can be inhaled as a vapor in the air. Possible effects of inhaling MTBE include headaches, burning of the nose and throat, dizziness, nausea, asthma, and respiratory problems. The possible effects on wildlife have not yet been documented.

If you have a private well, your local health department may be able to tell you if MTBE has been found in your area. To get your water tested, call the EPA's Safe Drinking Water Hotline at 800-426-4791 or go to https://www.epa.gov/ground-water-and-drinking-water/safe-drinking-water-information.

The EPA still has not made a determination on the continued use of MTBE.

cerned about the safety of the water coming out of your tap, you can contact your local water officials or local health department, which may test your tap water free of charge. In some cases, you may have to contact your state's water supply or health department. Typically, however, these agencies test the water only for bacteria levels, not for toxic substances. Therefore, you might want to contact a commercial laboratory or local state university laboratory to test your water for its chemical content. If you find that your tap water is unacceptable either because of its taste or because of its toxic chemical content, you may choose to use one of the alternative water supplies described in this section.

The Water Quality Association is prepared to answer questions about the various types of water and methods of water treatment. In addition, the EPA operates the toll-free Safe Drinking Water Hotline, which can help you to locate an office or laboratory in your area that does certified water testing. There are also a number of laboratories that will send a self-addressed container for you to fill and return by mail for testing. Results are usually available in two to three weeks.

To help you understand the results of water testing, you should obtain information on the EPA's Recommended Maximum Contaminant Levels. This and other water quality information is available from NSF International at www.nsf.org or 800-426-4791.

Improving Tap Water

Tap water can be improved in several ways. Heating tap water to a rolling boil and keeping it there for three to five minutes will kill bacteria and parasites. However, most people find boiling their drinking water too impractical and time-consuming. In addition, this procedure has the effect of concentrating whatever lead is present in the water, and the water must then be refrigerated if it is to be used for drinking. The taste of chlorinated tap water can be improved by keeping the water in an uncovered pitcher for several hours to allow the chlorine taste and odor to dissipate.

Water can also be aerated in a blender to remove chlorine and other chemicals. Nevertheless, neither of these last two methods will improve the quality of the water—only the taste.

Filtration is a means by which contaminants in water are removed, rendering the water cleaner and better tasting. There are many different ways in which water can be filtered.

Nature filters water as the water runs through streams and as it seeps down through the soil and rocks to the water table. As water passes through the earth or over the rocks in a stream, the bacteria in the water leach into the rocks and are replaced with minerals such as calcium and magnesium.

There are also man-made ways of filtering water. There are three basic types of filter available:

- Absorbent types, which use materials such as carbon to pick up impurities.

- Microfiltration systems, which run water through filters with tiny pores to catch and eliminate contaminants (the filter may be made of any of a number of different materials).

- Special media such as ion-exchange resins that are designed to remove heavy metals.

Filters are often arranged in series so that the filtering media that are most effective for specific types of contaminants can be used. The primary advantages of filters are relatively low cost and ease of use.

Water filtration systems vary in effectiveness. Two types that are considered good are reverse osmosis and ceramic filtration systems. In reverse osmosis filtering, the water is forced through a semipermeable membrane, while charged particles and larger molecules are repelled. It is the best system for treating water that is brackish (high in salt), high in nitrates, and loaded with inorganic heavy metals such as iron and lead. However, no filter can remove absolutely all contaminants. Each pore of even the finest filter is large enough for some viruses to permeate. To remove parasites such as cryptosporidia, the EPA and CDC recommend purchasing a filter that has an NSF rating for parasite reduction *and* that has an absolute pore size of one micron or smaller (a micron is 1×10^{-6} meter).

Other water treatment systems that remove various contaminants include distillers and ultraviolet treatment units. The latter are used to kill bacteria and viruses in water. Each treatment method has its advantages and disadvantages (*see* HOME WATER TREATMENT METHODS, later in this book). Costs can vary from under fifty dollars for faucet-mounted units to many thousands of dollars for whole-house reverse osmosis systems. Using a combination of methods can result in the best overall quality drinking water. Even the quality and taste of distilled water can be improved by passing the water through a charcoal/carbon filter as a final step.

Before you purchase a water treatment unit, contact NSF International or the Water Quality Association. These nonprofit testing and certification organizations verify manufacturers' claims and certify that the materials used are nontoxic and structurally sound. They conduct periodic unannounced audits of the products they certify to ensure that the products still comply with standards.

BOTTLED WATER

Because of concerns over the safety and health effects of tap water, many people today are turning to bottled water. Bottled water is usually classified by its source (spring, spa, geyser, public water supply, etc.), by its mineral content (containing at least 250 parts per million of dissolved solids), and/or by the type of treatment it has undergone (deionized, steam-distilled, etc.). Because there is a lot of overlap, some water falls into more than one classification. In addition, most states have no rules governing appropriate labeling, so some bottled water claims may be misleading or incorrect. The biggest problem with bottled water is its threat to the environment from the improper disposal of the bottles. Only 20 percent of Americans recycle bottles. Americans drink 18 gallons of bottled water per capita. This equals 144 16-ounce bottles per person per year, which mostly goes to the garbage or incinerator. Incineration causes toxic by-products such as chloride gas and ash, containing heavy metals. Energy is needed to transport these empty bottles as well. If you use bottled water, buy it in bulk and transfer water to reusable containers.

While the EPA is charged with the regulation of public water supplies, it is the FDA that has responsibility for overseeing the quality and safety of bottled drinking water. There has been concern over the possible leaching of plastic particles into the water that comes in plastic bottles. Researchers from the Harvard School of Public Health found that people who drank from clear plastic polycarbonate bottles had an increase in bisphenol A (BPA) of 69 percent. BPA is used to make reusable hard plastic—such as those used in watercooler bottles—more durable. The harder the bottle, the more BPA in it. BPA is used in hundreds of everyday products. The health effects on adults are not well understood, though a large human study linked BPA concentrations in people's urine to an increased prevalence of diabetes, heart disease, and liver toxicity. For adults, most BPA is flushed from the body in a matter of hours. The real risk in terms of developing these diseases actually comes from what we eat and drink, not the BPA in the containers.

The FDA defined the terms used to describe bottled drinking waters in specific requirements in April 1997, making the choices for the consumer somewhat clearer than in the past. In 2001, the FDA adopted the EPA's MCLs and maximum residual disinfectant levels (MRDLs) for four disinfection by-products (bromate, chlorite, haloacetic acids, and total trihalomethanes) and for three disinfectants (chloramine, chlorine, and chlorine dioxide), respectively, as allowable levels in its standard of quality regulations for bottled waters.

The FDA regulations for bottled water allow for the various terms that have been defined to be used with one another if bottled water meets more than one definition, so it is possible for some water labels to include a number of different terms.

All the terms that are legally necessary to describe bottled drinking water are discussed in the paragraphs that follow. Any term you find on a label that is *not* defined or included here is a marketing slogan added to entice the consumer to buy the product. It can mean anything that the manufacturer of the product says it means.

Artesian Water
Artesian water, or artesian well water, is water drawn from a well where the water is brought to the surface by natural pressure or flow.

Bottled Water
Bottled water, or bottled drinking water, is water that is intended for human consumption and that is sealed in bottles or other containers with no added ingredients except for optional antimicrobial agents. These must be identified on the label. If bottled water comes from a community water system or from a municipal source, this information must appear on the label. About 25 percent of bottled waters now sold come from the same water supplies that flow into some areas' household taps.

HOME WATER TREATMENT METHODS

TREATMENT TYPE	CONFIGURATIONS	HOW IT WORKS	WHAT IT DOES
Activated Carbon	Faucet-Mounted Pour-Through Countertop Under Sink Whole House	Water is filtered through a carbon trap that absorbs the contaminants.	Reduces levels of chlorine, herbicides, lead, hydrogen sulfide, and VOCs (volatile organic compounds). Also improves color and reduces turbidity.
Carbon Filtration	Faucet-Mounted Under Sink or Counter	Water is passed through charcoal granules or a solid block of charcoal that captures contaminants. When carbon is used up or plugged, cartridge is replaced.	Reduces levels of chlorine, organic chemicals, and pesticides. Improves taste and odor.
Distillation	Countertop Freestanding Whole House	Raises water temperature to boiling, leaving contaminants behind. Pure condensate is collected.	Reduces levels of arsenic, cadmium, chromium, iron, lead, giardia cysts, nitrates, and sulfates. Reduces turbidity.

TREATMENT TYPE	CONFIGURATIONS	HOW IT WORKS	WHAT IT DOES
Reverse Osmosis	Countertop Under Sink Whole House	Forces pressurized water through a semipermeable membrane and sends improved water to a holding tank.	Reduces levels of arsenic, cadmium, iron, chlorine, lead, giardia cysts, nitrates, sulfates, and radium. Reduces color and turbidity.
Water Softener	Whole House	Replaces calcium and magnesium with sodium to "soften" the water.	Reduces levels of calcium, magnesium, iron, and radium.

Deionized or Demineralized Water

When the electric charge of a molecule of water has been neutralized by the addition or removal of electrons, the resulting water is called *deionized* or *demineralized*. The deionization process removes nitrates and the minerals calcium and magnesium, in addition to the heavy metals cadmium, barium, lead, mercury, and some forms of radium.

Groundwater

This is water that comes from underground, in the water table, that is under pressure equal to or greater than atmospheric pressure, and that does not come into contact with surface water. Groundwater must be pumped mechanically for bottling.

Mineral Water

Mineral water is water containing not less than 250 parts per million total dissolved solids (TDS), originating from a geologically and physically protected underground water source or spring that has been tapped at the spring opening or through a bore-hole. Mineral water is distinguished from other types of water by constant levels and relative proportions of minerals and trace elements at its source, allowing for seasonal variations. No minerals may be added to this water. If the TDS content of mineral water is below 500 parts per million, the water may be labeled *low mineral content.* If it is greater than 1,500 parts per million, the label *high mineral content* may be used.

Depending on where the source is, the minerals the water contains will vary. If you are suffering from a deficiency of certain minerals and are drinking mineral water for therapeutic reasons, you must be aware of which minerals are in the particular brand of water you drink. If you are drinking mineral water containing minerals that you do not lack, you could be doing yourself more harm than good.

Most mineral waters are carbonated. However, some sparkling waters, such as club soda, are called mineral waters because the manufacturer added bicarbonates, citrates, and sodium phosphates to filtered or distilled tap water.

Natural Spring Water

The term *natural spring water* on a bottled water label doesn't tell you where the water came from, only that the mineral content of the water has not been altered. It may or may not have been filtered or otherwise treated. While the number of gallons of "natural spring water" flowing through watercoolers and from bottles has more than doubled in recent years, the meaning of these words on a label has been firmly defined only since the final changes in the FDA bottled drinking water regulations have been in place.

Spring water is water that comes from an underground formation from which water flows naturally to the surface of the earth. It must be collected at the spring or through a borehole tapping the underground formation that feeds the spring. To meet the definition of *spring,* there must be natural force bringing the water to the surface opening. The location of the spring must be identified on the label of any water labeled as spring water.

If you use a watercooler for bottled spring water, you should be sure to clean the cooler once a month to destroy bacteria. Run a 50-50 mixture of hydrogen peroxide and baking soda through the reservoir and spigots; then remove the residue by rinsing the cooler with four or more gallons of tap water.

Sparkling Water

This is bottled water that contains the same amount of carbon dioxide that it had at emergence from the water source. It can be a healthful alternative to soda and alcoholic beverages, but if it is loaded with fructose and other sweeteners, it may be no better than soda pop. Read labels before you buy. Soda water, seltzer water, and tonic water are *not* considered bottled waters. They are regulated separately, may contain sugar and calories, and are considered soft drinks.

Understanding where the carbonation in sparkling water comes from isn't always easy. So-called naturally sparkling water must get its carbonation from the same source as the water. If water is labeled *carbonated natural water,* that means the carbonation came from a source other than the one that supplied the water. That doesn't mean the water is of poor quality. It can still be called natural because its mineral content is the same as when it came from the ground, even though it has been carbonated from a separate source. People suffering from intestinal disorders or ulcers should avoid drinking carbonated water because it may be irritating to the gastrointestinal tract.

Steam-Distilled Water

Distillation involves vaporizing water by boiling it. The steam rises, leaving behind most of the bacteria, viruses, chemicals, minerals, and pollutants from the water. The steam is then moved into a condensing chamber, where it is cooled and condensed to become distilled water.

Once consumed, steam-distilled water leaches inorganic minerals rejected by the cells and tissues out of the body.

We believe that only steam-distilled or reverse-osmosis-filtered water should be consumed. This water should be used not only for drinking but also for cooking, because foods such as pasta, rice, and beans can absorb chemicals found in unpurified water.

Flavor can be added to distilled water by adding 1 to 2 tablespoons of raw apple cider vinegar (obtained from a health food store) per gallon of distilled water. Vinegar is an excellent solvent and aids in digestion. Lemon juice is another good flavoring agent, one that has cleansing properties as well. For added minerals, you can add mineral drops to steam-distilled water. ConcenTrace from Trace Minerals Research is a good product for this purpose. Add 1¼ teaspoons of mineral drops to every 5 gallons of water.

Amino Acids

INTRODUCTION

Amino acids are the chemical units, or building blocks, as they are popularly known, that make up proteins. They also are the end products of protein digestion, or *hydrolysis*.

Amino acids contain about 16 percent nitrogen. Chemically, this is what distinguishes them from the other two basic nutrients, sugars and fatty acids, which do not contain nitrogen.

To understand how vital amino acids are, you must understand how essential proteins are to life. It is protein that provides the structure for all living things. Every living organism, from the largest animal to the tiniest microbe, is composed of protein. In its various forms, protein participates in the vital chemical processes that sustain life.

Proteins are a necessary part of every living cell in the body. Next to water, protein makes up the greatest portion of our body weight. In the human body, protein substances make up the muscles, ligaments, tendons, organs, glands, nails, hair, and many vital body fluids, and are essential for the growth of bones. The enzymes and hormones that catalyze and regulate all bodily processes are proteins. Proteins help to regulate the body's water balance and maintain the proper internal pH. They assist in the exchange of nutrients between the intercellular fluids and the tissues, blood, and lymph. A deficiency of protein can upset the body's fluid balance, causing edema. Proteins form the structural basis of chromosomes, through which genetic information is passed from parents to offspring. The genetic "code" contained in each cell's DNA is actually information for how to make that cell's proteins.

Proteins are chains of amino acids linked together by what are called *peptide bonds*. Each individual type of protein is composed of a specific group of amino acids in a specific chemical arrangement. It is the particular amino acids present and the way in which they are linked together in sequence that gives the proteins that make up the various tissues their unique functions and characters. Each protein in the body is tailored for a specific need; proteins are not interchangeable.

The proteins that make up the human body are not obtained directly from the diet. Rather, dietary protein is broken down into its constituent amino acids, which the body then uses to build the specific proteins it needs. Thus, it is the amino acids rather than protein that are the essential nutrients.

In addition to those that combine to form the body's proteins, there are other amino acids that are important in metabolic functions. Some, such as citrulline, glutathione, ornithine, and taurine, can be similar to (or by-products of) the protein-building amino acids. Some act as neurotransmitters or as precursors of neurotransmitters, the chemicals that carry information from one nerve cell to another. Certain amino acids are thus necessary for the brain to receive and send messages. Unlike many other substances, neurotransmitters are able to pass through the *blood-brain barrier.* This is a kind of defensive shield designed to protect the brain from toxins and foreign invaders that may be circulating in the bloodstream. The endothelial cells that make up the walls of the capillaries in the brain are much more tightly meshed together than are those of capillaries elsewhere in the body. This prevents many substances, especially water-based substances, from diffusing through the capillary walls into brain tissue. Because certain amino acids can pass through this barrier, they can be used by the brain to communicate with nerve cells elsewhere in the body.

Amino acids also enable vitamins and minerals to perform their jobs properly. Even if vitamins and minerals are absorbed and assimilated by the body, they cannot be effective unless the necessary amino acids are present. For example, low levels of the amino acid tyrosine may lead to iron deficiency. Deficiency and/or impaired metabolism of the amino acids methionine and taurine has been linked to allergies and autoimmune disorders. Many elderly people suffer from depression or neurological problems that may be associated with deficiencies of the amino acids tyrosine, tryptophan, phenylalanine, and histidine, and also of the *branched-chain amino acids*—valine, isoleucine, and leucine.

These are amino acids that can be used to provide energy directly to muscle tissue. High doses of branched-chain amino acids have been used in hospitals to treat people suffering from trauma and infection. Some people are born with an inability to metabolize the branched-chain amino acids. This potentially life-threatening condition, branched-chain ketoaciduria (often referred to as *maple syrup urine disease* because keto acids released into the urine cause it to smell like maple syrup), can result in neurological damage and necessitates a special diet, including a synthetic infant formula that does not contain leucine, isoleucine, or valine.

There are approximately twenty-eight commonly known amino acids that are combined in various ways to create the hundreds of different types of proteins present in all living things. In the human body, the liver produces about 80 percent of the amino acids needed. The remaining 20 percent must be obtained from the diet. These are called the *essential amino acids*. The essential amino acids that must enter the body through diet are histidine, isoleucine, leucine, lysine, methionine, phenylalanine, threonine, tryptophan, and valine. Although infants need to obtain histidine from their diet, most adult bodies can make enough. The *nonessential amino acids*, which can be manufactured in the body from other amino acids obtained from dietary sources, include alanine, arginine, asparagine, aspartic acid, citrulline, cysteine, cystine,

gamma-aminobutyric acid, glutamic acid, glutamine, glycine, ornithine, proline, serine, taurine, and tyrosine.

The fact that they are termed *nonessential* does not mean
that they are not necessary, only that they need not be obtained
through the diet because the body can manufacture them as
needed. Nonessential amino acids can indeed become essential
under certain conditions. For instance, the nonessential amino
acids cysteine and tyrosine are made from the essential amino
acids methionine and phenylalanine. If methionine and phenylalanine are not available in sufficient quantities, cysteine and
tyrosine then become essential in the diet. Also, in times of
stress such as an illness, both arginine and glutamine are considered to be "conditionally essential." Hospitalized patients have
benefited from amino acid supplements of each to enhance the
functioning of their immune systems. Arginine is popular with
bodybuilders, who claim they feel a rush of blood flow, which
helps them lift heavier weights.

The processes of assembling amino acids to make proteins
and of breaking down proteins into individual amino acids for
the body's use are continuous ones. When we need more enzyme proteins, the body produces more enzyme proteins; when
we need more cells, the body produces more proteins for cells.
These different types of proteins are produced as the need
arises. Should the body become depleted of its reserves of any
of the essential amino acids, it would not be able to produce the
proteins that require those amino acids. An inadequate supply
of even one essential amino acid can hinder the synthesis, and
reduce the body levels, of necessary proteins. This can result in
negative nitrogen balance, an unhealthy condition in which the
body excretes more nitrogen than it assimilates. Further, *all* of
the essential amino acids must be present simultaneously in the
diet in order for the other amino acids to be utilized—otherwise,
the body remains in negative nitrogen balance. A lack of vital
proteins in the body can cause problems ranging from indigestion to depression to stunted growth.

How could such a situation occur? More easily than you might think. Many factors can contribute to deficiencies of essential amino acids, even if you eat a well-balanced diet that contains enough protein. Impaired absorption, infection, trauma, stress, drug use, age, and imbalances of other nutrients can all affect the availability of essential amino acids in the body. Insufficient intake of vitamins and minerals, especially vitamin C, can interfere with the absorption of amino acids in the lower part of the small intestines. Vitamin B_6 is needed also, for the transport of amino acids in the body.

If your diet is not properly balanced—that is, if it fails to supply adequate amounts of the essential amino acids—sooner or later, this will become apparent as some type of physical disorder. When the brain senses the lack of any of the essential amino acids, it immediately sends a signal to the muscles to release some of their tissue. Human muscle is rich in essential amino acids, so it can support the vital organs like the liver and heart during times of poor intake. Sometimes in the case of cancer patients who are unable to eat, a massive muscle wasting called cachexia will occur. This condition can be reversed with food, but it takes a long time.

This does not mean, however, that eating a diet containing enormous amounts of protein is the answer. In fact, it is unhealthy to consume a diet that is deficient in protein or one that contains too much. Excess protein puts undue stress on the kidneys and the liver, which are faced with processing the waste products of protein metabolism. Nearly half of the amino acids in dietary protein are transformed into glucose by the liver and utilized to provide needed energy to the cells. This process results in a waste product, ammonia. Ammonia is toxic to the body, so the body protects itself by having the liver turn the ammonia into a much less toxic compound, urea, which is then carried through the bloodstream, filtered out by the kidneys, and excreted.

As long as protein intake is not too great and the liver is working properly, ammonia is neutralized almost as soon as it is produced, so it does no harm. However, if there is too much ammonia for the liver to cope with—as a result of too much protein consumption, poor digestion, and/or a defect in liver function—toxic levels may accumulate.

Strenuous exercise also tends to promote the accumulation of excess ammonia. This may put a person at risk for serious health problems, including encephalopathy (brain disease) or hepatic coma. Abnormally high levels of urea can also cause problems, including inflamed kidneys and back pain. (*See* NUTRITION, DIET, AND WELLNESS earlier in this book.)

It is possible to take supplements containing amino acids, both essential and nonessential. For certain disorders, taking supplements of specific amino acids can be very beneficial. When you take a specific amino acid or amino acid combination, it supports the metabolic pathway involved in your particular illness. Vegetarians, especially vegans, would be wise to take a formula containing all of the essential amino acids to ensure that their protein requirements are met.

WHAT'S ON THE SHELVES

Supplemental amino acids are available in combination with various multivitamin formulas, as protein mixtures, in a wide variety of food supplements, and in a number of amino acid formulas. They can be purchased as capsules, tablets, liquids, and powders. Most amino acid supplements are derived from animal protein, yeast protein, or vegetable protein. Crystalline free-form amino acids are generally extracted from a variety of grain products. Brown rice bran is a prime source, although cold-pressed yeast and milk proteins are also used.

Free-form means the amino acid is in its purest form. Free-form amino acids need no digestion and are absorbed directly into the bloodstream. These white crystalline amino acids are stable at room temperature and decompose when heated to temperatures of 350°F to 660°F (180°C to 350°C). They are rapidly absorbed and do not come from potentially allergenic food sources. For best results, choose encapsulated powders or powder.

When choosing amino acid supplements, look for products that contain USP (U.S. Pharmacopeia) pharmaceutical-grade L-crystalline amino acids. A good company is Ajinomoto. It manufactures amino acids for intravenous use as well as orally for the public. Most of the amino acids (except for glycine) can appear in two forms, the chemical structure of one being the mirror image of the other. These are called the D- and L- forms—for example, D-cystine and L-cystine. The D stands for *dextro* (Latin for right) and the L for *levo* (Latin for left); these terms denote the direction of the rotation of the spiral that is the chemical structure of the molecule. Proteins in animal and plant tissue are made from the L- form of amino acids (with the exception of phenylalanine, which is also used in the form of DL-phenylalanine, a mixture of the D- and L- forms). Thus, with respect to supplements of amino acids, products containing the L- forms of amino acids are considered to be more compatible with human biochemistry.

Each amino acid has specific functions in the body. The many functions and possible symptoms of deficiency of twenty-eight amino acids and related compounds are described below. When taking amino acids individually for healing purposes, take them on an empty stomach to avoid making them compete for absorption with the amino acids present in foods. When taking individual amino acids, it is best to take them in the morning or between meals, with small amounts of vitamin B_6 and vitamin C to enhance absorption.

When taking an amino acid complex that includes all of the essential amino acids, it is best to take it a half hour away from a meal, either before or after. If you are taking individual amino acids, it is wise also to take a full amino acid complex, including both essential and nonessential amino acids, at a different time. This is the best way to assure you have adequate amounts of all the necessary amino acids.

Be aware that individual amino acids should not be taken for long periods of time. A good rule to follow is to alternate the individual amino acids that fit your needs and back them up with an amino acid complex, taking the supplements for two months and then discontinuing them for two months. Moderation is the key. Some amino acids have potentially toxic effects when taken in high doses (over 6,000 milligrams per day) and may cause neurological damage. These include aspartic acid, glutamic acid, homocysteine, serine, and tryptophan. Cysteine can be toxic if taken in amounts over 1,000 milligrams per day. Do not give supplemental amino acids to a child. Also, don't take doses of any amino acid in excess of the amount recommended unless specifically directed to do so by your health care provider.

Some recommended amino acid products include the following:

- A/G-Pro from Miller Pharmacal Group, a complete amino acid and mineral supplement.

- Anabolic Amino Balance and Muscle Octane from Anabol Naturals. Anabolic Amino Balance is a complex of twenty-three free-form amino acids. Muscle Octane is a blend of free-form branched-chain amino acids (L-leucine, L-valine, and L-isoleucine). Anabol Naturals also produces free-form single amino acids.

- Super Daily Amino Blend from Carlson Laboratories, a complex containing twenty amino acids, both essential and nonessential.

THE ABCS OF AMINO ACIDS

Alanine
Alanine plays a major role in the transfer of nitrogen from peripheral tissue to the liver. It aids in the metabolism of glucose, a simple carbohydrate that the body uses for energy.

Alanine also guards against the buildup of toxic substances that are released in the muscle cells when muscle protein is broken down to meet energy needs quickly, such as happens with aerobic exercise. Epstein-Barr virus and chronic fatigue syndrome have been associated with excessive alanine levels and low levels of tyrosine and phenylalanine. One form of alanine, beta-alanine, is a constituent of pantothenic acid (vitamin B_5) and coenzyme A, a vital catalyst in the body.

Research has found that for people with insulin-dependent diabetes, taking an oral dose of L-alanine can be more effective than a conventional bedtime snack in preventing nighttime hypoglycemia.

Arginine

Arginine retards the growth of tumors and cancer by enhancing immune function. It increases the size and activity of the thymus gland, which manufactures T lymphocytes (T cells), crucial components of the immune system. Arginine may therefore benefit those suffering from AIDS and malignant diseases that suppress the immune system. It is also good for liver disorders such as cirrhosis of the liver and fatty liver; it aids in liver detoxification by neutralizing ammonia. It may also reduce the effects of chronic alcohol toxicity.

Seminal fluid contains arginine. Studies suggest that sexual maturity may be delayed by arginine deficiency; conversely, arginine is useful in treating sterility in men. It is found in high concentrations in the skin and connective tissues, making it helpful for the healing and repair of damaged tissue.

Arginine is important for muscle metabolism. It helps to maintain a proper nitrogen balance by acting as a vehicle for transportation and storage, and aiding in the excretion, of excess nitrogen. Studies have shown that it also reduces nitrogen losses in people who have undergone surgery and improves the function of cells in lymphatic tissue. This amino acid aids in weight loss because it facilitates an increase in muscle mass and a reduction of body fat. It is also involved in a variety of enzymes and hormones. It aids in stimulating the pancreas to release insulin, is a component of the pituitary hormone vasopressin, and assists in the release of growth hormones. Because arginine is a component of collagen and aids in building new bone and tendon cells, it can be good for arthritis and connective tissue disorders. Arginine has also been shown to improve sports performance, as demonstrated by increasing VO_2 max—the maximum amount of oxygen a person can utilize during exercise.

Scar tissue that forms during wound healing is made up of collagen, which is rich in arginine. A variety of functions, including insulin production, glucose tolerance, and liver lipid metabolism, are impaired if the body is deficient in arginine.

This amino acid can be produced in the body; however, in newborn infants, production may not occur quickly enough to keep up with requirements. It is therefore deemed essential early in life. Foods high in arginine include carob, chocolate, coconut, dairy products, gelatin, meat, oats, peanuts, soybeans, walnuts, white flour, wheat, and wheat germ. Eating watermelon can increase plasma arginine levels because watermelon is rich in citrulline, which is a precursor to arginine. Some people who engage in strength-training activities might want to increase nitric oxide levels to increase blood flow and enhance performance. One study showed that taking 3 grams of arginine a day with a protein supplement slightly increased nitric oxide production and did not cause harm.

People with viral infections such as herpes should *not* take supplemental arginine and should avoid foods rich in arginine and low in the amino acid lysine, as this appears to promote the growth of certain viruses. Pregnant and lactating women should avoid L-arginine supplements. Persons with schizophrenia should avoid amounts over 30 milligrams daily. Long-term use, especially of high doses, is not recommended. One study found that several weeks of large doses might result in thickening and coarsening of the skin.

Asparagine

Asparagine, created from another amino acid, aspartic acid, is needed to maintain balance in the central nervous system; it prevents you from being either overly nervous or overly calm. As it is converted back into aspartic acid, asparagine releases energy that brain and nervous system cells use for metabolism. It promotes the process by which one amino acid is transformed into another in the liver.

Aspartic Acid

Because aspartic acid increases stamina, it is good for fatigue and depression, and plays a vital role in metabolism. Chronic fatigue syndrome may result from low levels of aspartic acid, because this leads to lowered cellular energy. In proper balance, aspartic acid is beneficial for neural and brain disorders; it has been found in increased levels in persons with epilepsy and in decreased levels in people with some types of depression. It is good for athletes and helps to protect the liver by aiding in the removal of excess ammonia. Aspartic acid was thought to increase testosterone levels in nonathletic males, but this did not appear to happen in a group of fit men. Giving well-trained men 6 grams daily of aspartic acid had no effect on blood testosterone levels.

Aspartic acid combines with other amino acids to form molecules that absorb toxins and remove them from the bloodstream. It also helps to move certain minerals across the intestinal lining and into the blood and cells, aids cell function, and aids the function of RNA and DNA, which are the carriers of genetic information. It enhances the production of immunoglobulins and antibodies (immune system proteins). Plant protein, especially that found in sprouting seeds, contains an abundance of aspartic acid. The artificial sweetener aspartame is made from aspartic acid and phenylalanine, another amino acid.

Carnitine

Carnitine is not an amino acid in the strictest sense (it is actually a substance related to the B vitamins). However, because it has a chemical structure similar to that of amino acids, it is usually considered together with them.

Unlike true amino acids, carnitine is not used for protein synthesis or as a neurotransmitter. Its main function in the body is to help transport long-chain fatty acids, which are burned within the cells, mainly in the mitochondria, to provide energy. This is a major source of energy for the muscles. Carnitine thus increases the use of fat as an energy source. This prevents fatty buildup, especially in the heart, liver, and skeletal muscles. Carnitine may be useful in treating chronic fatigue syndrome (CFS), because a disturbance in the function of the mitochondria (the site of energy production within the cells) may be a factor in fatigue. Studies have shown decreased carnitine levels in many people with CFS.

Carnitine reduces the health risks posed by poor fat metabolism associated with diabetes; inhibits alcohol-induced fatty liver; and lessens the risk of heart disorders.

Studies have shown that damage to the heart from cardiac surgery can be reduced by treatment with carnitine. According to *The American Journal of Cardiology,* one study showed that propionyl-L-carnitine, a carnitine derivative, helps to ease the severe pain of intermittent claudication, a condition in which a blocked artery in the thigh decreases the supply of blood and oxygen to leg muscles, causing pain, especially with physical activity. Carnitine has the ability to lower blood triglyceride levels, aid in weight loss, improve the motility of sperm, and improve muscle strength in people with neuromuscular disorders. It may be useful in treating Alzheimer's disease. Conversely, carnitine deficiency may be a contributor to certain types of muscular dystrophy, and it has been shown that these disorders lead to losses of carnitine in the urine. People with such conditions need greater-than-normal amounts of carnitine. Carnitine has also been shown to reduce fatigue, which is common in many diseases. In studies, people with celiac disease (an autoimmune disorder of the small intestine) and people with cancer had more energy with carnitine supplementation.

Carnitine also enhances the effectiveness of the antioxidant vitamins E and C. It works with antioxidants to help slow the aging process by promoting the synthesis of carnitine acetyltransferase, an enzyme in the mitochondria of brain cells that is vital for the production of cellular energy there. Supplemental carnitine has been shown to reduce damage to the bad cholesterol, LDL, in patients with type 2 diabetes. This shows that carnitine is effective at limiting the oxidative stress that is common in diabetes and many other conditions.

The body can manufacture carnitine if sufficient amounts of iron, vitamin B_1 (thiamine), vitamin B_6 (pyridoxine), and the amino acids lysine and methionine are available. The synthesis of carnitine also depends on the presence of adequate levels of vitamin C. Inadequate intake of any of these nutrients can result in a carnitine deficiency. Carnitine can also be obtained from food, primarily meats and other foods of animal origin. Omnivores have a different pattern of microbes in the intestine compared to vegetarians or lacto-vegetarians. Dietary carnitine, obtained from meat, has been shown to promote the production of trimethylamine N-oxide (TMAO), which is associated with an increased risk of heart disease and blood clots.

Many cases of carnitine deficiency have been identified as partly genetic in origin, resulting from an inherited defect in carnitine synthesis. Possible symptoms of deficiency include confusion, heart pain, muscle weakness, and obesity.

Because of their generally greater muscle mass, men need more carnitine than do women. Vegetarians are more likely than nonvegetarians to be deficient in carnitine because it is not found in vegetable protein. Moreover, neither methionine nor lysine, two of the key constituents from which the body makes carnitine, are obtainable from vegetable sources in sufficient amounts. To ensure adequate production of carnitine, vegetarians should take supplements or should eat grains, such as corn-meal, that have been fortified with lysine.

Supplemental carnitine is available in different forms, including D-carnitine, L-carnitine, and DL-carnitine. DL-carnitine is not recommended, as it may cause toxicity.

Acetyl-L-carnitine (ALC), a carnitine derivative produced naturally in the body, is involved in carbohydrate and protein metabolism and in the transport of fats into the mitochondria. It increases levels of carnitine in tissues and even surpasses the metabolic potency of carnitine. ALC has become one of the most studied compounds for its antiaging effects, particularly with regard to degeneration of the brain and nervous system. Several major studies have shown that daily supplementation with ALC significantly slows the progression of Alzheimer's disease, resulting in less deterioration in memory, attention and language, and spatial abilities.

It also can be used to treat other cognitive disorders, as well as depression. ALC provides numerous other benefits to many of the body's systems. It helps to limit damage caused by oxygen starvation, enhance the immune system, protect against oxidative stress, stimulate the antioxidant activity of certain enzymes, protect membranes, slow cerebral aging, prevent nerve disease associated with diabetes and sciatica, modulate hormonal changes caused by physical stress, and increase the performance-enhancing benefits of branched-chain amino acids.

Total brain levels of ALC (and carnitine) decline with age. In most of the studies of ALC done with humans, subjects took 500 to 2,500 milligrams daily, in divided doses. No toxic or serious side effects have been reported.

Carnosine

L-carnosine is a dipeptide composed of two bonded amino acids—alanine and histidine. It is found naturally in the body, particularly in brain tissue, the heart, skin, muscles, kidneys, and stomach. Carnosine levels in the body decline with age. This compound has the ability to help prevent glycosylation, the cross-linking of proteins with sugars to form advanced glycosylation end products, or AGEs. This effect may be beneficial for combating diabetes, kidney failure, neuropathy, and aging in general.

To date, no serious side effects have been noted in trials. The normal oral dose is 100 to 500 milligrams daily (with occasional breaks). Avoid megadosing. This is the oral form, not the eye-drop form used in Russia for cataract treatment (that is N-alpha-acetylcarnosine).

Citrulline

The body makes citrulline from another amino acid, ornithine. Citrulline promotes energy, stimulates the immune system, is metabolized to form L-arginine, and detoxifies ammonia, which damages living cells. Citrulline is found primarily in the liver. It is helpful in treating fatigue.

Cysteine and Cystine

These two amino acids are closely related; each molecule of cystine consists of two molecules of cysteine joined together.

Cysteine is very unstable and is easily converted to L-cystine; however, each form is capable of converting into the other as needed. Both are sulfur-containing amino acids that aid in the formation of skin and are important in detoxification.

Cysteine is present in alpha-keratin, the chief protein constituent of the fingernails, toenails, skin, and hair. Cysteine aids in the production of collagen and promotes the proper elasticity and texture of the skin. It is also found in a variety of other proteins in the body, including several of the digestive enzymes.

Cysteine helps to detoxify harmful toxins and protect the body from radiation damage. It is one of the best destroyers of free radicals, and works best when taken with selenium and vitamin E. Cysteine is also a precursor to glutathione, a substance that detoxifies the liver by binding with potentially harmful substances there. It helps to protect the liver and brain from damage due to alcohol, drugs, and toxic compounds in cigarette smoke.

Since cysteine is more soluble than cystine, it is used more readily in the body and is usually best for treating most illnesses. This amino acid is formed from L-methionine in the body. Vitamin B_6, vitamin B_{12}, and folate are necessary for cysteine synthesis, which may not take place as it should in the presence of chronic disease. Therefore, people with chronic illnesses may need higher-than-normal doses of cysteine, as much as 1,000 milligrams three times daily for a month at a time.

Supplementation with L-cysteine is recommended in the treatment of rheumatoid arthritis, hardening of the arteries, and mutagenic disorders such as cancer. It promotes healing after surgery and severe burns, chelates heavy metals, and binds with soluble iron, aiding in iron absorption. This amino acid also promotes the burning of fat and the building of muscle. Because of its ability to break down mucus in the respiratory tract, L-cysteine is often beneficial in the treatment of bronchitis, emphysema, and tuberculosis. It promotes healing from respiratory disorders and plays an important role in the activity of white blood cells, which fight disease.

Cystine or the N-acetyl form of cysteine (N-acetylcysteine, or NAC) may be used in place of L-cysteine. NAC aids in preventing side effects from chemotherapy and radiation therapy. Because it increases glutathione levels in the lungs, kidneys, liver, and bone marrow, it has an antiaging effect on the body—reducing the accumulation of age spots, for example. NAC has been shown to be more effective at boosting glutathione levels than supplements of cystine or even of glutathione itself. NAC was thought to help children with autism. In a six-month study where children got 500 milligrams of NAC or a placebo, no benefits were observed in behavior or communication.

People who have diabetes should be cautious about taking supplemental cysteine because it is capable of inactivating insulin. Persons with cystinuria, a rare genetic condition that leads to the formation of cystine kidney stones, should also not take cysteine.

Gamma-Aminobutyric Acid

Gamma-aminobutyric acid (GABA) is an amino acid that acts as a neurotransmitter in the central nervous system. It is essential for brain metabolism, aiding in proper brain function. GABA is formed in the body from another amino acid, glutamic acid. Its function is to decrease neuron activity and inhibit nerve cells from overfiring. Together with niacinamide and inositol, it prevents anxiety- and stress-related messages from reaching the motor centers of the brain by occupying their receptor sites.

GABA can be taken to calm the body in much the same way as diazepam (Valium), chlordiazepoxide (Librium), and other tranquilizers, but without the fear of addiction. It has been used in the treatment of epilepsy and hypertension.

GABA is good for depressed sex drive because of its ability as a relaxant. It is also useful for enlarged prostate glands, probably because it plays a role in the mechanism regulating the release of sex hormones. GABA is effective in treating attention deficit disorder and may reduce cravings for alcohol. It is also thought to promote growth hormone secretion.

Too much GABA, however, can cause increased anxiety, shortness of breath, numbness around the mouth, and tingling in the extremities. Further, abnormal levels of GABA unbalance the brain's message delivery system and may cause seizures.

Glutamic Acid

Glutamic acid is an excitatory neurotransmitter that increases the firing of neurons in the central nervous system. It is a major excitatory neurotransmitter in the brain and spinal cord. It is converted into either glutamine or GABA.

This amino acid is important in the metabolism of sugars and fats, and aids in the transportation of potassium into the spinal fluid and across the blood-brain barrier. Although it does not pass the blood-brain barrier as readily as glutamine does, it is found at high levels in the blood and may infiltrate the brain in small amounts. The brain can use glutamic acid as fuel. Glutamic acid can detoxify ammonia by picking up nitrogen atoms, in the process creating another amino acid, glutamine. The conversion of glutamic acid into glutamine is the only means by which ammonia in the brain can be detoxified.

Glutamic acid helps to correct personality disorders and is useful in treating childhood behavioral disorders. It is used in the treatment of epilepsy, mental retardation, muscular dystrophy, ulcers, and hypoglycemic coma, a complication of insulin treatment for diabetes. It is a component of folate (folic acid), a B vitamin that helps the body break down amino acids. Because one of its salts is monosodium glutamate (MSG), glutamic acid should be avoided by anyone who is allergic to MSG.

Glutamine

Glutamine is the most abundant free amino acid found in the muscles of the body. Because it can readily pass the blood-brain barrier, it is known as brain fuel. In the brain, glutamine is converted into glutamic acid—which is essential for cerebral function—and vice versa. It also increases the amount of GABA, which is needed to sustain proper brain function and mental activity. It assists in maintaining the proper acid/alkaline balance in the body and is the basis of the building blocks for the synthesis of RNA and DNA. It promotes mental ability and the maintenance of a healthy digestive tract.

When an amino acid is broken down, nitrogen is released. The body needs nitrogen, but free nitrogen can form ammonia, which is especially toxic to brain tissues. The liver can convert nitrogen into urea, which is excreted in the urine, or nitrogen may attach itself to glutamic acid. This process forms glutamine. Glutamine is unique among the amino acids in that each molecule contains not one nitrogen atom but two. Thus, its creation helps to clear ammonia from the tissues, especially brain tissue, and it can transfer nitrogen from one place to another.

Glutamine is found in large amounts in the muscles and is readily available when needed for the synthesis of skeletal muscle proteins. Because this amino acid helps to build and maintain muscle, supplemental glutamine is useful for dieters and bodybuilders. More important, it helps to prevent the kind of muscle wasting that can accompany prolonged bed rest or diseases such as cancer and AIDS. This is because stress and injury (including surgical trauma) cause the muscles to release glutamine into the bloodstream. In addition, glutamine helps strengthen the lining of the intestinal tract, so that nutrients are more efficiently absorbed. This is important for wasting diseases such as cancer.

In fact, during times of stress, as much as a third of the glutamine present in the muscles may be released. As a result, stress and/or illness can lead to the loss of skeletal muscle. If enough glutamine is available, however, this can be prevented.

Supplemental L-glutamine can be helpful in the treatment of arthritis, autoimmune diseases, fibrosis, intestinal disorders, peptic ulcers, connective tissue diseases such as polymyositis and scleroderma, and tissue damage due to radiation treatment for cancer. L-glutamine can enhance mental functioning and has been used to treat a range of problems, including developmental disabilities, epilepsy, fatigue, impotence, depression, schizophrenia, and senility.

It preserves glutathione in the liver and protects that organ from the effects of acetaminophen overdose. It enhances antioxidant protection. L-glutamine decreases sugar cravings and the desire for alcohol and thus is useful for recovering alcoholics.

Many plant and animal substances contain glutamine, but cooking easily destroys it. If eaten raw, spinach and parsley are good sources. Supplemental glutamine must be kept absolutely dry or the powder will degrade into ammonia and pyroglutamic acid. Glutamine should *not* be taken by persons with cirrhosis of the liver, kidney problems, Reye's syndrome, or any type of disorder that can result in an accumulation of ammonia in the blood. For such individuals, taking supplemental glutamine may only cause further damage to the body. Be aware that although the names sound similar, glutamine, glutamic acid (also sometimes called glutamate), glutathione, gluten, and monosodium glutamate are all different substances.

Glutathione

Like carnitine, glutathione is not technically one of the amino acids. It is a compound classified as a tripeptide, and the body produces it from the amino acids cysteine, glutamic acid, and glycine. Because of its close relationship to these amino acids, however, it is usually considered together with them.

Glutathione is a powerful antioxidant produced in the liver. The largest stores of glutathione are found in the liver, where it detoxifies harmful compounds so that they can be excreted through the bile. Some glutathione is released from the liver directly into the bloodstream, where it helps to maintain the integrity of red blood cells and to protect white blood cells. Glutathione is also found in the lungs and the intestinal tract. It is needed for carbohydrate metabolism and appears to exert anti-aging effects, aiding in the breakdown of oxidized fats that may contribute to atherosclerosis.

It can mitigate some of the damage caused by tobacco smoke because it modifies the harmful effects of aldehydes, chemicals present in cigarette smoke that damage cells and molecules, and it may protect the liver from alcohol-induced damage. Glutathione likely works as an antioxidant when ingested as a supplement. Taking a low dose (250 milligrams a day) or a larger dose (1,000 milligrams a day) for six months increased blood glutathione levels and improved markers of immune function.

A deficiency of glutathione affects the nervous system first, causing such symptoms as lack of coordination, mental disorders, tremors, and difficulty maintaining balance. These problems are believed to be due to the development of lesions in the brain. A study sponsored in part by the National Cancer Institute found that people with HIV disease who had low glutathione levels had a lower survival rate over a three-year period than those whose glutathione levels were normal. As we age, glutathione levels decline, although it is not known whether this is because we use it more rapidly or produce less of it to begin with. Unfortunately, if not corrected, the lack of glutathione in turn accelerates the aging process.

Supplemental glutathione is expensive, and the effectiveness of oral formulas is questionable. To raise glutathione levels, it is better to supply the body with the raw materials it uses to make this compound: cysteine, glutamic acid, and glycine. The N-acetyl form of cysteine, N-acetylcysteine (NAC), is considered particularly effective for this purpose.

Glycine

Glycine retards muscle degeneration by supplying additional creatine, a compound that is present in muscle tissue and is utilized in the construction of DNA and RNA. It improves glycogen storage, thus freeing up glucose for energy needs. It is essential for the synthesis of nucleic acids, bile acids, and other nonessential amino acids in the body.

Glycine is used in many gastric antacid agents. Because high concentrations of glycine are found in the skin and connective tissues, it is useful for repairing damaged tissues and promoting healing.

Glycine is necessary for central nervous system function and a healthy prostate. It functions as an inhibitory neurotransmitter and as such can help prevent epileptic seizures. It has been used in the treatment of manic (bipolar) depression and can also be effective for hyperactivity.

Having too much of this amino acid in the body can cause fatigue, but having the proper amount produces more energy. If necessary, glycine can be converted into the amino acid serine in the body.

Histidine

Histidine is an essential amino acid that is significant in the growth and repair of tissues. It is important for the maintenance of the myelin sheaths, which protect nerve cells, and is needed for the production of both red and white blood cells. Histidine also protects the body from radiation damage, helps lower blood pressure, aids in removing heavy metals from the system, and may help in the prevention of AIDS.

Histidine levels that are too high may lead to stress and even psychological disorders such as anxiety and schizophrenia; people with schizophrenia have been found to have high levels of histidine in their bodies. Inadequate levels of histidine may contribute to rheumatoid arthritis and may be associated with nerve deafness. Methionine has the ability to lower histidine levels. Histidine looks promising for treating obesity because it can reduce inflammation, which leads to weight loss. Obese women who took 4 grams of histidine daily for twelve weeks experienced a reduction in body mass index (BMI), waist circumference, and markers of inflammation.

Histamine, an important immune system chemical, is derived from histidine. Histamine aids in sexual arousal.

Because the availability of histidine influences histamine production, taking supplemental histidine—together with vitamins B_3 (niacin) and B_6 (pyridoxine), which are required for the transformation from histidine to histamine—may help improve sexual functioning and pleasure.

Because histamine also stimulates the secretion of gastric juices, histidine may be helpful for people with indigestion resulting from a lack of stomach acid.

Persons with manic (bipolar) depression should not take supplemental histidine unless a deficiency has been identified. Natural sources of histidine include rice, wheat, and rye.

Homocysteine

Homocysteine is an amino acid that is produced in the body in the course of methionine metabolism. This amino acid has been the focus of increasing attention because high levels of homocysteine in the blood are associated with an increased risk of cardiovascular disease. In individuals with Parkinson's disease, high levels of homocysteine were associated with cognitive decline. Treatment with vitamins B_{12}, B_6, and folate (folic acid) may help maintain cognitive function despite the progression of this disease.

Further, it is known that homocysteine has a toxic effect on cells lining the arteries, makes the blood more prone to clotting, and promotes the oxidation of low-density lipoproteins (LDL, the so-called bad cholesterol), which makes it more likely that cholesterol will be deposited as plaque in the blood vessels.

Like other amino acids, homocysteine does perform a necessary function in the body. It is then usually broken down quickly into the amino acid cysteine and other important compounds, including adenosine triphosphate (ATP, an important source of cellular energy) and S-adenosylmethionine (SAMe). However, a genetic defect or, more commonly, deficiencies of vitamins B_6 and B_{12} and folate can prevent homocysteine from converting rapidly enough. As a result, high levels of the amino acid accumulate in the body, damaging cell membranes and blood vessels, and increasing the risk of cardiovascular disease, particularly atherosclerosis. Vitamins B_6 and B_{12} and folate work together to facilitate the breakdown of homocysteine, and thus help protect against heart disease.

Isoleucine

Isoleucine, one of the essential amino acids, is needed for hemoglobin formation and also stabilizes and regulates blood sugar and energy levels. It is metabolized in muscle tissue. It is one of the three branched-chain amino acids. These amino acids are valuable for athletes because they enhance energy, increase endurance, and aid in the healing and repair of muscle tissue.

Isoleucine has been found to be deficient in people suffering from many different mental and physical disorders. A deficiency of isoleucine can lead to symptoms similar to those of hypoglycemia.

Food sources of isoleucine include almonds, cashews, chicken, chickpeas, eggs, fish, lentils, liver, meat, rye, most seeds, and soy protein. It is also available in supplemental form. Supplemental L-isoleucine should always be taken with a correct balance of the other two branched-chain amino acids, L-leucine and L-valine—approximately 2 milligrams of leucine for each milligram of valine and isoleucine. Combination supplements that provide all three of the branched-chain amino acids are available and may be more convenient to use.

Leucine

Leucine is an essential amino acid and one of the branched-chain amino acids (the others are isoleucine and valine). These work together to protect muscle and act as fuel. Leucine plus other dietary proteins fosters muscle growth even without the other two branched-chain amino acids. They promote the healing of bones, skin, and muscle tissue, and are recommended for those recovering from surgery. Leucine-enriched protein may help prevent muscle loss in older people. One study showed that only a small amount of protein containing 3 grams of leucine was as good as a greater amount of protein to add muscle in response to exercise in elderly women. Leucine also lowers elevated blood sugar levels and aids in increasing growth hormone production.

Natural sources of leucine include brown rice, beans, meat, nuts, soy flour, and whole wheat. Supplemental L-leucine must be taken in balance with L-isoleucine and L-valine (*see* ISOLEUCINE earlier in this section), and it should be taken in moderation, or symptoms of hypoglycemia may result. An excessively high intake of leucine may also contribute to pellagra and may increase the amount of ammonia present in the body.

Lysine

Lysine is an essential amino acid that is a necessary building block for all protein. It is needed for proper growth and bone development in children; it helps calcium absorption and maintains a proper nitrogen balance in adults. This amino acid aids in the production of antibodies, hormones, and enzymes, and helps in collagen formation and tissue repair. Because it helps to build muscle protein, it is good for those recovering from surgery and sports injuries. It also lowers high serum triglyceride levels.

Another very useful ability of this amino acid is its capacity for fighting cold sores and herpesviruses. Taking supplemental L-lysine, together with vitamin C with bioflavonoids, can effectively fight and/or prevent herpes outbreaks, especially if foods containing the amino acid arginine are avoided. Supplemental L-lysine also may decrease acute alcohol intoxication.

Lysine is an essential amino acid, and so cannot be manufactured in the body. It is therefore vital that adequate amounts be included in the diet. Deficiencies can result in anemia, bloodshot eyes, enzyme disorders, hair loss, an inability to concentrate, irritability, lack of energy, poor appetite, reproductive disorders, retarded growth, and weight loss. Food sources of lysine include cheese, eggs, fish, lima beans, milk, potatoes, red meat, soy products, and yeast.

Methionine

Methionine is an essential amino acid that assists in the breakdown of fats, thus helping to prevent a buildup of fat in the liver and arteries that might obstruct blood flow to the brain, heart, and kidneys. The synthesis of the amino acids cysteine and taurine may depend on the availability of methionine. This amino acid helps the digestive system; helps to detoxify harmful agents such as lead and other heavy metals; helps diminish muscle weakness, prevent brittle hair, and protect against radiation; and is beneficial for people with osteoporosis or chemical allergies. It is useful also in the treatment of rheumatic fever and toxemia of pregnancy.

Methionine is a powerful antioxidant. It is a good source of sulfur, which inactivates free radicals and helps prevent skin and nail problems. It is also good for people with Gilbert's syndrome, an anomaly of liver function, and is required for the synthesis of nucleic acids, collagen, and proteins found in every cell of the body. It is beneficial for women who take oral contraceptives because it promotes the excretion of estrogen. It reduces the level of histamine in the body, which can be useful for people with schizophrenia, whose histamine levels are typically higher than normal. Some have proposed that methionine is a pro-aging amino acid. Over four weeks of following an alternate day fasting diet, blood methionine levels went down, suggesting that this diet plan may slow the aging process. Methionine is essential, so removing it entirely from the diet is not advised.

As levels of toxic substances in the body increase, the need for methionine increases. The body can convert methionine into the amino acid cysteine, a precursor of glutathione. Methionine thus protects glutathione; it helps to prevent glutathione depletion if the body is overloaded with toxins. Since glutathione is a key neutralizer of toxins in the liver, this protects the liver from the damaging effects of toxic compounds.

An essential amino acid, methionine is not synthesized in the body and so must be obtained from food sources or from dietary supplements. Good food sources of methionine include beans, eggs, fish, garlic, lentils, meat, onions, soybeans, seeds, and yogurt. Because the body uses methionine to derive a brain food called choline, it is wise to supplement the diet with choline or lecithin (which is high in choline) to ensure that the supply of methionine is not depleted.

Ornithine

Ornithine helps to prompt the release of growth hormone, which promotes the metabolism of excess body fat. This effect is enhanced if ornithine is combined with arginine and carnitine. Ornithine is necessary for proper immune system and liver function. This amino acid also detoxifies ammonia and aids in liver regeneration. High concentrations of ornithine are found in the skin and connective tissue, making it useful for promoting healing and repairing damaged tissues. In animals, ornithine has been shown to mitigate stress and promote sleep. In a study of individuals who reported feeling stressed, supplementation with 400 milligrams of ornithine for 8 weeks resulted in decreased levels of the stress hormone cortisol and better sleep.

Ornithine is synthesized in the body from arginine, and in turn serves as the precursor of citrulline, proline, and glutamic acid. Children, pregnant women, nursing mothers, or anyone with a history of schizophrenia should not take supplemental L-ornithine, unless they are specifically directed to do so by a physician.

Phenylalanine

Phenylalanine is an essential amino acid. Because it can cross the blood-brain barrier, it can have a direct effect on brain chemistry. Once in the body, phenylalanine can be converted into another amino acid, tyrosine, which in turn is used to synthesize two key neurotransmitters that promote alertness: dopamine and norepinephrine. Because of its relationship to the action of the central nervous system, this amino acid can elevate mood, decrease pain, aid in memory and learning, and suppress the appetite. It can be used to treat arthritis, depression, menstrual cramps, migraines, obesity, Parkinson's disease, and schizophrenia.

Phenylalanine is available in three different forms, designated L-, D-, and DL-. The L- form is the most common type and is the form in which phenylalanine is incorporated into the body's proteins. The D- form acts as a painkiller. The DL- form is a combination of the D- and the L-. Like the D- form, it is effective for controlling pain, especially the pain of arthritis; like the L- form, it functions as a building block for proteins, increases mental alertness, suppresses the appetite, and helps people with Parkinson's disease. It has been used to alleviate the symptoms of premenstrual syndrome (PMS) and various types of chronic pain.

Supplemental phenylalanine, as well as products containing aspartame (an artificial sweetener made from phenylalanine and another amino acid, aspartic acid), should *not* be taken by pregnant women or by people who suffer from anxiety attacks, diabetes, high blood pressure, phenylketonuria (PKU), or preexisting pigmented melanoma, a type of skin cancer.

Proline

Proline improves skin texture by aiding in the production of collagen and reducing the loss of collagen through the aging process. It is needed to repair tissue after a major sunburn or severe burn. It also helps in the healing of cartilage and the strengthening of joints, tendons, and the heart muscle. It works with vitamin C to promote healthy connective tissue.

Proline is obtained primarily from meat sources, dairy products, and eggs.

Serine

Serine is needed for the proper metabolism of fats and fatty acids, the growth of muscle, and the maintenance of a healthy immune system. It is a component of brain proteins and the protective myelin sheaths that cover nerve fibers. A supplement of D-serine improved memory, learning, and problem-solving in a group of elderly people. It is important in RNA and DNA function, cell membrane formation, and creatine synthesis. It also aids in the production of immunoglobulins and antibodies. However, serine levels in the body that are too high may have adverse effects on the immune system.

Serine can be made from glycine in the body, but this process requires the presence of sufficient amounts of vitamins B_3 and B_6 and folic acid. Food sources of serine include meat and soy foods, as well as many foods that often cause allergic reactions, such as dairy products, wheat gluten, and peanuts. It is included as a natural moisturizing agent in many cosmetics and skin-care preparations.

Taurine

High concentrations of taurine are found in the heart muscle, white blood cells, skeletal muscle, and central nervous system. It is a building block of all the other amino acids as well as a key component of bile, which is needed for the digestion of fats, the absorption of fat-soluble vitamins, and the control of serum cholesterol levels. Taurine can be useful for people with atherosclerosis, edema, heart disorders, hypertension, or hypoglycemia. It is vital for the proper utilization of sodium, potassium, calcium, and magnesium, and it has been shown to play a particular role in sparing the loss of potassium from the heart muscle. This helps to prevent the development of potentially dangerous cardiac arrhythmias.

Taurine has a protective effect on the brain, particularly if the brain is dehydrated. It is used to treat anxiety, epilepsy, hyperactivity, poor brain function, and seizures.

Taurine is found in concentrations up to four times greater in the brains of children than in those of adults. It may be that a deficiency of taurine in the developing brain is involved in seizures. Zinc deficiency also is commonly found in people with epilepsy, and this may play a part in the deficiency of taurine. Taurine is also associated with zinc in maintaining eye function; a deficiency of both may impair vision. Taurine supplementation may benefit children with Down syndrome and muscular dystrophy. This amino acid is also used in some clinics for breast cancer treatment.

Excessive losses of taurine through the urine can be caused by many metabolic disorders. Cardiac arrhythmias, disorders of platelet formation, intestinal problems, an overgrowth of candida, physical or emotional stress, a zinc deficiency, and excessive consumption of alcohol are all associated with high urinary losses of taurine. Excessive alcohol consumption also causes the body to lose its ability to utilize taurine properly. Taurine supplementation may reduce symptoms of alcohol withdrawal. People with cirrhosis caused by alcohol often experience severe leg cramping, especially while sleeping. Patients with chronic liver disease who took 4 grams of taurine daily for four weeks had a reduction in the frequency, duration, and intensity of leg cramps. Whether taurine works to lessen leg cramps in people who do not have significant liver disease is unknown. Diabetes increases the body's requirements for taurine; conversely, supplementation with taurine and cystine may decrease the need for insulin.

Taurine is found in eggs, fish, meat, and milk, but not in vegetable proteins. It can be synthesized from cysteine in the liver and from methionine elsewhere in the body, as long as sufficient quantities of vitamin B_6 are present. For vegetarians, synthesis by the body is crucial. For individuals with genetic or metabolic disorders that prevent the synthesis of taurine, taurine supplementation is required.

Threonine

Threonine is an essential amino acid that helps to maintain the proper protein balance in the body. It is important for the formation of collagen, elastin, and tooth enamel, and aids liver and lipotropic function when combined with aspartic acid and methionine. A precursor of the amino acids glycine and serine, threonine is present in the heart, central nervous system, and skeletal muscle, and helps to prevent fatty buildup in the liver. It enhances the immune system by aiding in the production of antibodies and may be helpful in treating some types of depression.

Because the threonine content of grains is low, vegetarians are more likely than others to have deficiencies.

Tryptophan

Tryptophan is an essential amino acid necessary for the production of vitamin B_3 (niacin). It is used by the brain to produce serotonin, a necessary neurotransmitter that transfers nerve impulses from one cell to another and is responsible for normal sleep. Consequently, tryptophan helps to combat depression and insomnia and to stabilize moods. But it is most commonly used to treat sleep problems. Serotonin also is related to mood. A group of depressed young adults took tryptophan, vitamin B_6 (pyridoxine), and a form of niacin (nicotinamide) for seven days. Mood improved according to two standard measures of depression, and no side effects were noted. This combination may hold promise for quickly improving depressed mood.

Tryptophan helps to control hyperactivity in children, alleviates stress, is good for the heart, aids in weight control by reducing appetite, and enhances the release of growth hormone. It is good for migraine headaches and may reduce some of the effects of nicotine. Sufficient amounts of vitamins B_6 and C, folate, and magnesium are necessary for the formation of tryptophan, which in turn is required for the formation of serotonin. A study reported in the *Archives of General Psychiatry* found that women with a history of bulimia nervosa, an eating disorder, experienced relapses after they took an amino acid mixture lacking tryptophan. Researchers believe that insufficient tryptophan altered brain serotonin levels and, consequently, the transmission of nerve impulses. A lack of tryptophan and magnesium may contribute to coronary artery spasms.

The best dietary sources of tryptophan include brown rice, cottage cheese, meat, peanuts, and soy protein. In November 1989, the U.S. Centers for Disease Control (CDC) reported evidence linking L-tryptophan supplements to a blood disorder called eosinophilia-myalgia syndrome (EMS). Several hundred cases of this illness—which is characterized by an elevated white blood cell count and can also cause such symptoms as fatigue, muscular pain, respiratory ailments, edema, and rash—were reported. After the CDC established an association between the blood disorder and products containing L-tryptophan in New Mexico, the U.S. Food and Drug Administration (FDA) first warned consumers to stop taking L-tryptophan supplements, then recalled all products in which L-tryptophan was the sole or a major component. According to the FDA, at least thirty-eight deaths could be attributed to the tryptophan supplements.

Subsequent research showed that it was contaminants in the supplements, *not* the tryptophan, that was probably responsible for the problem. In 2005, tryptophan supplements were sold again in the United States after the FDA carefully reviewed the new source of tryptophan and deemed it acceptable.

Tyrosine

Tyrosine is important to overall metabolism. It is a precursor of adrenaline and the neurotransmitters norepinephrine and dopamine, which regulate mood and stimulate metabolism and the nervous system. Tyrosine acts as a mood elevator; a lack of adequate amounts of tyrosine leads to a deficiency of norepinephrine in the brain, which in turn can result in depression. It also acts as a mild antioxidant, suppresses the appetite, and helps to reduce body fat. It aids in the production of melanin (the pigment responsible for skin and hair color) and in the functions of the adrenal, thyroid, and pituitary glands. It is also involved in the metabolism of the amino acid phenylalanine.

Tyrosine attaches to iodine atoms to form active thyroid hormones. Not surprisingly, low plasma levels of tyrosine have been associated with hypothyroidism. Symptoms of tyrosine deficiency can also include low blood pressure, low body temperature (such as cold hands and feet), and restless legs syndrome.

Supplemental L-tyrosine has been used for stress reduction, and research suggests it may be helpful against chronic fatigue and narcolepsy. It has been used to help individuals suffering from anxiety, depression, low sex drive, allergies, and headaches, as well as persons undergoing withdrawal from drugs. It may also help people with Parkinson's disease.

Natural sources of tyrosine include almonds, avocados, bananas, dairy products, lima beans, pumpkin seeds, and sesame seeds. Tyrosine can also be produced from phenylalanine in the body. Supplements of L-tyrosine should be taken at bedtime or with a high-carbohydrate meal so that it does not have to compete for absorption with other amino acids.

Persons taking monoamine oxidase (MAO) inhibitors, commonly prescribed for depression, must strictly limit their intake of foods containing tyrosine and should *not* take any supplements containing L-tyrosine, as it may lead to a sudden and dangerous rise in blood pressure. Anyone who takes prescription medication for depression should discuss necessary dietary restrictions with his or her physician.

Valine

Valine, an essential amino acid, has a stimulant effect. It is needed for muscle metabolism, tissue repair, and the maintenance of a proper nitrogen balance in the body. Valine is found in high concentrations in muscle tissue. It is one of the branched-chain amino acids, which means that it can be used as an energy source by muscle tissue. When valine was taken along with arginine and serine, the combination of amino acids led to less fatigue during intense exercise. Serum ketone bodies went up, indicating that more energy was being burned from fat. It may be helpful in treating liver and gallbladder disease, and it is good for correcting the type of severe amino acid deficiencies that can be caused by drug addiction. An excessively high level of valine may lead to such symptoms as a crawling sensation in the skin and even hallucinations.

Dietary sources of valine include dairy products, grains, meat, mushrooms, peanuts, and soy protein. Supplemental L-valine should always be taken in balance with the other branched-chain amino acids, L-isoleucine and L-leucine (*see* ISOLEUCINE earlier in this section).

Antioxidants

INTRODUCTION

Antioxidants are natural compounds that help protect the body from harmful free radicals. These are atoms or groups of atoms that can cause damage to cells, impairing the immune system and leading to infections and various degenerative diseases such as heart disease and cancer. Antioxidants therefore play a beneficial role in the prevention of disease. Free radical damage is thought by scientists to be the basis for the aging process as well. (*See* FREE RADICALS on page 186.)

There are a number of known free radicals that occur in the body, the most common of which are oxygen-derived free radicals, such as superoxide radicals and hydroxyl radicals, hypochlorite radicals, hydrogen peroxide, various lipid peroxides, and nitric oxide. They may be formed by exposure to radiation, including exposure to the sun's rays; exposure to toxic chemicals such as those found in cigarette smoke, polluted air, and industrial and household chemicals; and various metabolic processes, such as the process of breaking down stored fat molecules for use as an energy source.

Free radicals are normally kept in check by the action of *free radical scavengers* that occur naturally in the body. These scavengers neutralize the free radicals. Certain enzymes serve this vital function. Four important enzymes that neutralize free radicals are superoxide dismutase (SOD), methionine reductase, catalase, and glutathione peroxidase.

The body makes these as a matter of course. There are also a number of phytochemicals and nutrients that act as antioxidants, including vitamin A, beta-carotene and other carotenoids, flavonoids, vitamins C and E, and the mineral selenium. Researchers have found that eggplant contains high levels of chlorogenic acid, which has proven to be a highly effective antioxidant. Another antioxidant is the hormone melatonin, which is a powerful free radical neutralizer. Certain herbs have antioxidant properties as well.

Although many antioxidants can be obtained from food sources such as sprouted grains and fresh fruits and vegetables, it is difficult to get enough of them from these sources to hold back the free radicals constantly being generated in our polluted environment. We can minimize free radical damage by taking supplements of key nutrients. A high intake of antioxidant nutrients appears to be especially protective against cancer.

Antioxidants work synergistically in giving protection against free radical damage, so it is better to take smaller doses of several different antioxidants than a large amount of only one. For example, while beta-carotene by itself is an excellent antioxidant, a mix of natural carotenoids provides more health benefits than beta-carotene alone. There are many good combination formulas available that make it easy to take multiple antioxidants every day. Similarly, taking antioxidants together—for example, beta-carotene with vitamin E and vitamin C—appears to be more effective than taking any one alone.

Some of the major antioxidants are described in the sections that follow.

THE ANTIOXIDANTS

Alpha-Lipoic Acid

Alpha-lipoic acid (ALA) is a powerful antioxidant—both on its own and as a "recycler" of vitamin E and vitamin C. It can restore the antioxidant properties of these vitamins after they have neutralized free radicals. ALA also stimulates the body's production of glutathione and aids in the absorption of coenzyme Q_{10}, both important antioxidants. Because ALA is soluble in both water and fat, it can move into all parts of cells to deactivate free radicals.

Supplemental ALA has been used for almost three decades in Europe to treat peripheral nerve degeneration and to help control blood sugar levels in people with diabetes. Some people with diabetes also develop a painful neuropathy. Alpha-lipoic acid (600 milligrams) was useful at reducing pain, improving quality of life, and reducing the debilitating side effects of the condition after only forty days. It also helps to detoxify the liver of metal pollutants, block cataract formation, protect nerve tissues against oxidative stress, and reduce blood cholesterol levels. It can be used with carnitine to provide an antiaging effect. ALA is known also as a metabolic antioxidant, because without it, cells cannot use sugar to produce energy. The body does not produce large amounts of ALA, but because it is found naturally in only a few foods, including spinach, broccoli, potatoes, brewer's yeast, and organ meats, supplementation may be necessary.

Bilberry

The herb bilberry (*Vaccinium myrtillus*), a European relative of the American blueberry, contains natural antioxidants that keep capillary walls strong and flexible. They also help to maintain the flexibility of the walls of red blood cells and allow them to pass through the capillaries more freely. Everyone knows that vitamins C and E are good sources of antioxidants, but bilberry, which contains anthocyanidins, also acts as an antioxidant. In individuals who had recently suffered a heart attack (myocardial infarction), the herb bilberry was shown to improve stamina. This was felt to be due to the herb's antioxidant properties. This review also demonstrated less oxidative stress as measured by the lower oxidation of LDL cholesterol. Bilberry could prove to be a helpful supplement for those recovering from a recent heart attack. It also helps to lower blood pressure, inhibit clot formation, and enhance blood supply to the nervous system. Studies indicate that anthocyanidins can provide up to fifty times the antioxidant protection of vitamin E and ten times the protection of vitamin C. In addition, this herb protects the eyes and may enhance vision; supports and strengthens collagen structures; inhibits the growth of bacteria; acts as an anti-inflammatory; and has antiaging and anticarcinogenic effects. One study that looked at the effects of bilberry on night vision found that vision was not improved with the amounts that are typically sold. Tests have shown that the compound glucoquinine, found in bilberry leaves, helps to lower blood sugar levels.

Burdock

The herb burdock (*Arctium lappa*) was tested by researchers at the Chia Nan University of Pharmacy and Science in Taiwan for its antioxidant properties. They found that burdock is a powerful antioxidant, capable of scavenging hydrogen peroxide and superoxide radicals. It also showed a marked scavenging effect against hydroxyl radicals. The study showed also that burdock and vitamin E quench more free radicals when used in combination. Burdock also might protect against cancer by helping to control cell mutation.

Carotenoids

See VITAMIN A AND THE CAROTENOIDS later in this section.

Coenzyme Q$_{10}$

Coenzyme Q$_{10}$ is an antioxidant that is structurally similar to vitamin E. It plays a crucial role in the generation of cellular energy, is a significant immunologic stimulant, increases circulation, has antiaging effects, and is beneficial for the cardiovascular system. Also known as *ubiquinone* (from *quinone,* a type of coenzyme, and *ubiquitous,* because it exists everywhere in the body), coenzyme Q$_{10}$ is found in highest concentrations in the heart, followed by the liver, kidney, spleen, and pancreas. Within the mitochondria, the cells' energy-production centers, coenzyme Q_{10} helps to metabolize fats and carbohydrates. It also helps to maintain the flexibility of cell membranes.

Various research reports suggest that coenzyme Q_{10} also may be beneficial in treating cancer, AIDS, muscular dystrophy, allergies, gastric ulcers, myopathy, Parkinson's disease, and deafness. More recently, coenzyme Q_{10} has been shown to improve the lives of people with chronic heart disease. Those who took 100 milligrams three times daily of coenzyme Q_{10} were better able to perform regular activities and engage in exercise. In addition, the chances of dying of heart disease or anything else was cut in half.

Natural sources of coenzyme Q_{10} include meats, peanuts, sardines, and spinach. (*See* NATURAL FOOD SUPPLEMENTS starting on page 208 for more on coenzyme Q_{10}.)

Curcumin (Turmeric)

Found in the spice turmeric, the phytochemical curcumin has antioxidant properties that prevent the formation of and neutralize existing free radicals. It stops precancerous changes within DNA and interferes with enzymes necessary for cancer progression. Curcumin stops the oxidation of cholesterol, thus protecting against the formation of plaque in the arteries. In a study of chronic smokers, those who took curcumin excreted a substantially lower level of mutagens (substances that induce cells to mutate) in their urine, a reflection of how well the body is dealing with these cancer-causing substances. Curcumin has been shown to be of benefit to some patients with advanced pancreatic cancer. It may also calm an overactive immune system in patients with ulcerative colitis, reducing inflammation, redness, and soreness. In one study, curcumin helped keep patients with ulcerative colitis from experiencing intestinal flare-ups. But it does not seem to be effective for other inflammatory conditions such as psoriasis. Curcumin also blocks toxic compounds from reaching or reacting with body tissues and may prevent cataracts. Impressive findings were noted for people with prediabetes. In a well-designed research study, taking curcumin from an extract of 250 milligrams of curcuminoids per capsule, six times daily, reduced the likelihood of developing type 2 diabetes. No one who got the curcumin developed diabetes over the nine-month period, while 16 percent of those who were not given curcumin did develop diabetes. The curcumin seems to improve the ability of the pancreas to make insulin.

Curcumin should not be taken by anyone who has biliary tract obstruction or is taking anticoagulants, as curcumin stimulates bile secretion and acts as a blood thinner.

Flavonoids

Flavonoids are especially potent antioxidants and metal chelators. They are the largest category of plant compounds called polyphenols. They are chemical compounds that plants produce to protect themselves from parasites, bacteria, and cell injury. More than 4,000 chemically unique flavonoids are known; they occur in fruits, vegetables, spices, seeds, nuts, flowers, and bark. Wine (particularly red wine), apples, blueberries, bilberries, onions, soy products, and tea are some of the best food sources of flavonoids. Certain flavonoids in fruits and vegetables have much greater antioxidant activity than vitamins C and E or beta-carotene. In fact, flavonoids protect the antioxidant vitamins from oxidative damage. Regularly having a high flavonoid intake is associated with a blood-pressure-lowering effect similar to what is seen from eating a low-salt diet or following the Mediterranean diet.

Numerous medicinal herbs contain therapeutic amounts of flavonoids; they often are a major component of an herb's medicinal activity, which include helping prevent heart disease and cancer and reducing the incidence of neurodegenerative diseases.

Natural sources of the flavonoids include almonds, apples, broccoli, citrus fruits, tea, tomatoes, onions, soybeans, and red wine. In the United States, the greatest intake of flavonoids comes from citrus fruits, tea, and wine.

Garlic

This versatile healing herb also has antioxidant properties. The sulfhydryl (sulfur and hydrogen) compounds in garlic are potent chelators of toxic heavy metals, binding with them so that they can be excreted. These same compounds are effective protectants against oxidation and free radicals.

Garlic aids in the detoxification of peroxides such as hydrogen peroxide and helps to prevent fats from being oxidized and deposited in tissues and arteries. Garlic also contains antioxidant nutrients such as vitamins A and C and selenium.

Studies on aged garlic extract (AGE) have shown that the aging process substantially boosts garlic's antioxidant potential. AGE protects against DNA damage, keeps blood vessels healthy, and guards against radiation and sunlight damage. According to researcher and nutritionist Robert I-San Lin, PhD, aged garlic extract can prevent liver damage caused by carbon tetrachloride, a common indoor pollutant and free radical generator. Overall, aged garlic supplements provide a greater concentration of garlic's beneficial compounds. It is particularly helpful in reducing oxidation associated with aging. If you're worried about "garlic breath" putting a strain on your social life, choose an odorless and tasteless form such as Kyolic aged garlic extract from Wakunaga of America (https://kyolic.com/). Aged garlic extract reduces blood cholesterol levels, thus lowering the risk of heart attack; provides protection from heart disease by preventing clots that can lead to heart attacks and strokes; and helps lower high blood pressure. Timed-release garlic has been shown to reduce blood cholesterol levels, and to lower fasting blood sugar levels in patients with type 2 diabetes. An aged garlic extract was shown to boost immune function. During cold and flu season, healthy people were recruited to take a garlic extract for ninety days. At the end of the study, those who took garlic and those in the

FREE RADICALS

A free radical is an atom or group of atoms that contains at least one unpaired electron. Electrons are negatively charged particles that usually occur in pairs, forming a chemically stable arrangement. If an electron is unpaired, another atom or molecule can easily bond with it, causing a chemical reaction. Because they join so readily with other compounds, free radicals can effect dramatic changes in the body, and they can cause a lot of oxidative damage. Each free radical may exist for only a tiny fraction of a second, but the damage it leaves behind can be irreversible, particularly damage to heart muscle cells, nerve cells, and certain immune system sensor cells.

Free radicals are normally present in the body in small numbers. Oxygen-charged particles are created in the body as we breathe. Diets rich in antioxidants can more than neutralize these particles. Dietary supplements rich in antioxidants act in the same way. Biochemical processes naturally lead to the formation of free radicals, and under normal circumstances the body can keep them in check. Indeed, not all free radicals are bad. Free radicals produced by the immune system destroy viruses and bacteria. Other free radicals are involved in producing vital hormones and activating enzymes that are needed for life. We need free radicals to produce energy and various substances that the body requires. If there is excessive free radical formation, however, damage to cells and tissues can occur. The formation of a large number of free radicals stimulates the formation of more free radicals, leading to even more damage.

Many different factors can lead to an excess of free radicals. Exposure to radiation, whether from the sun or small amounts from medical X-rays, activates the formation of free radicals, as does exposure to environmental pollutants such as tobacco smoke and automobile exhaust. Diet also can contribute to the formation of free radicals. When the body obtains nutrients through the diet, it utilizes oxygen and these nutrients to create energy. In this oxidation process, oxygen molecules containing unpaired electrons are released. These oxygen free radicals can cause damage to the body if produced in extremely large amounts. Being overweight or consuming a diet that is high in fat can increase free radical activity because oxidation occurs more readily in fat molecules than it does in carbohydrate or protein molecules. Cooking fats at high temperatures, particularly frying foods in oil, can produce large numbers of free radicals.

The presence of a dangerous number of free radicals can alter the way in which the cells code genetic material.

Changes in protein structure can occur as a result of errors in protein synthesis. The body's immune system may then see this altered protein as a foreign substance and try to destroy it. The formation of mutated proteins can eventually damage the immune system and lead to leukemia and other types of cancer, as well as to many other diseases.

In addition to damaging genetic material, free radicals can destroy the protective cell membranes. Calcium levels in the body may be upset as well. Over time, the body produces more free radicals than it does scavengers. The resulting imbalance contributes to the aging process.

Substances known as antioxidants neutralize free radicals by binding to their free electrons. Antioxidants available in supplement form include the enzymes superoxide dismutase and glutathione peroxidase; vitamin A, beta-carotene, and vitamins C and E; the minerals selenium and zinc; and the hormone melatonin. By destroying free radicals, antioxidants help to detoxify and protect the body.

placebo group had the same number of colds or the flu, but those taking garlic had reduced cold and flu severity, with a reduction in the number of symptoms, the number of days functioning suboptimally, and the number of work/school days missed.

Ginkgo Biloba

Ginkgo biloba is an herb with powerful antioxidant effects in the brain, retina, and cardiovascular system. It is well known for its ability to enhance circulation, and a study reported in the *Journal of the American Medical Association* (*JAMA*) showed that it has a measurable effect on dementia in people with Alzheimer's disease and people recovering from strokes. Other studies indicate that it can improve both long- and short-term memory and enhance concentration.

Ginkgo biloba has also been used to treat hearing problems, impotence, and macular degeneration. According to their teachers and parents, children and adolescents with ADHD who took 80 to 120 milligrams per day of ginkgo biloba were better behaved. The children were taking a medication for their ADHD, so the ginkgo biloba was considered an adjuvant therapy.

Anyone who takes prescription anticoagulant (blood-thinning) medication or who uses over-the-counter painkillers regularly should consult a health care provider before using ginkgo biloba, as the combination may result in internal bleeding.

Glutathione

Glutathione is a protein that is produced in the liver from the amino acids cysteine, glutamic acid, and glycine. It is a powerful antioxidant that inhibits the formation of and protects against cellular damage from free radicals. It helps to defend the body against damage from cigarette smoking, exposure to radiation, cancer chemotherapy, and toxins such as alcohol. As a detoxifier of heavy metals and drugs, it aids in the treatment of blood and liver disorders.

Glutathione protects cells in several ways. It neutralizes oxygen molecules before they can harm cells. Together with selenium, it forms the enzyme glutathione peroxidase, which neutralizes hydrogen peroxide. It is also a component of another antioxidant enzyme, glutathione-S-transferase, which is a broad-spectrum liver-detoxifying enzyme.

Glutathione protects not only individual cells but also the tissues of the arteries, brain, heart, immune cells, kidneys, lenses of the eyes, liver, lungs, and skin against oxidant damage. It plays a role in preventing cancer, especially liver cancer, and may actually target carcinogens, make them water-soluble, and then help escort them from the body. It may also have an antiaging effect. The rate at which we age is directly correlated with reduced concentrations of glutathione in cellular fluids; as we grow older, glutathione levels drop, resulting in a decreased ability to deactivate free radicals.

Glutathione can be taken in supplement form. The production of glutathione by the body can be boosted by taking supplemental dehydroepiandrosterone (DHEA), a hormone; N-acetylcysteine or L-cysteine; and L-methionine. Studies suggest that this may be a better way of raising glutathione levels than taking glutathione itself, but check with your health care professional if you have any hormonal problems.

Grape Seed Extract
See OLIGOMERIC PROANTHOCYANIDINS later in this section.

Green Tea
Tea is the most commonly consumed beverage around the world after water. Green tea contains compounds known as polyphenols, including phytochemicals that have antioxidant, antibacterial, antiviral, and health-enhancing properties. Tests on epigallocatechin gallate (EGCG), a particular type of polyphenol in green tea, have shown that it is able to penetrate the body's cells and shield DNA from hydrogen peroxide, a potent free radical. Epidemiological studies have shown that green tea protects against cancer, lowers cholesterol levels, and reduces the clotting tendency of the blood. Because green tea boosts immune function and acts as an antiviral and anti-inflammatory agent, it may help prevent cancer. In one study, it was shown to prevent symptoms associated with colds and flu, and even reduced the number of these illnesses. It also shows promise as a weight-loss aid that can promote the burning of fat and help to regulate blood sugar and insulin levels. Instead of drinking green tea, a supplement containing known quantities of it can produce weight loss—especially as fat—and lower blood pressure and "bad" (LDL) cholesterol. A green tea extract containing 858.6 milligrams of EGCG produced significant weight loss and reduction in waist circumference in overweight and obese women. The women also experienced reductions in total cholesterol and LDL cholesterol.

Green tea is simply the dried leaves of the tea plant. All green teas are from the species *Camellia sinensis*, but depending on the locale where they are grown and on the processing, they can be quite different. Chinese teas are predominant and comprise about 90 percent of what is sold. There are numerous regional Chinese teas, the best-known being *lung ching* (dragon well).

Other teas from Japan are equally good. Japanese green teas are of two basic types, *sencha* or *gyokuro*. Sencha is grown in the full sun, while gyokuro is shaded a few weeks before it is harvested. While there are many brands, the basic difference is that gyokuro makes a sweeter, darker green tea than sencha, which is somewhat grassy in flavor. It also costs over twice as much. Gyokuro is the source of the special handmade powdered tea used in the traditional tea ceremony.

Green tea is not fermented and has more polyphenols than black tea. Black tea undergoes natural fermentation, which converts tannins, astringent phytochemicals, into more complex compounds. This fermentation process destroys some of black tea's polyphenols, and it was once thought that it was thus rendered less effective as an antioxidant. Tests have shown, however, that both green and black teas contain about the same amount of antioxidant polyphenols, but that there are different combinations of antioxidants in black teas and green teas depending on the method of processing. Black tea lowers blood sugar and raises insulin levels after a meal. The polyphenolic content of black tea is thought to stimulate the pancreas to release insulin.

Green tea does contain caffeine (15 to 25 milligrams per ¾ cup), but it is less than in similar amounts of coffee (80 to 115 milligrams per ¾ cup) or caffeinated carbonated beverages (38 to 46 milligrams per can). Those who have heart problems or sensitivity to caffeine or are pregnant may want to limit their intake of caffeine. Green tea contains vitamin K, which can make anticoagulant medication less effective. Consult your health provider if you are using them.

Methionine

A unique amino acid, methionine neutralizes hydroxyl radicals, one of the most dangerous types of free radicals. Most often a by-product of reactions between heavy metals and less toxic free radicals, hydroxyl radicals can be formed also during strenuous exercise or exposure to high levels of radiation and can damage any type of body tissue.

N-Acetylcysteine (NAC)

The sulfur-containing amino acid cysteine is needed to produce the free radical fighter glutathione and to help maintain it at adequate levels in the cells. N-acetylcysteine (NAC) is a more stable form of cysteine that can be taken in supplement form.

NAC is used by the liver and the lymphocytes to detoxify chemicals and other poisons. It is a powerful detoxifier of alcohol, tobacco smoke, and environmental pollutants, all of which are immune suppressors. Taking supplemental NAC can boost the levels of protective enzymes in the body, thus slowing some of the cellular damage that is characteristic of aging. NAC supplementation may also decrease both the frequency and duration of infectious diseases. It has been used in the management of AIDS and chronic bronchitis. Infertile men benefited from taking 600 milligrams of NAC. After six weeks, the men experienced increases in sperm count and mobility and in testosterone levels. Markers of oxidation decreased in the body, which may have been the reason for these positive findings.

People with diabetes should not take supplemental NAC without first consulting a health care provider, as it can interfere with the effectiveness of insulin.

Nicotinamide Adenine Dinucleotide (NADH)

Also known as coenzyme 1, nicotinamide adenine dinucleotide with high-energy hydrogen, or NADH, is the "spark" that ignites energy production in the body's cells.

NADH's high antioxidant capacity derives from its ability to reduce levels of substances. NADH plays a central role in DNA repair and maintenance, and in the cellular immune defense system. Studies report that NADH also can inhibit the autoxidation of the neurotransmitter dopamine, which causes the release of toxic chemicals that may damage sensitive parts of the brain.

Oligomeric Proanthocyanidins (OPCs)

Oligomeric proanthocyanidins (OPCs) are naturally occurring substances present in a variety of food and botanical sources. They are unique phytochemicals known as flavonoids that have powerful antioxidant capabilities. OPCs are highly water soluble, so the body is able to absorb them rapidly. Clinical tests suggest that OPCs may be as much as fifty times more potent than vitamin E and twenty times more potent than vitamin C in terms of bioavailable antioxidant activity. What's more, OPCs work with the antioxidant glutathione to recycle and restore oxidized vitamin C, thus increasing the vitamin's effectiveness. Because they are able to cross the blood-brain barrier, OPCs can protect the brain and spinal nerves against free radical damage. In addition to their antioxidant activity, OPCs protect the liver from damage caused by toxic doses of acetaminophen, a nonprescription pain reliever; they strengthen and repair connective tissue, including that of the cardiovascular system; and they support the immune system and slow aging. They also moderate allergic and inflammatory responses by reducing histamine production. OPC supplementation was shown to improve the gum disease gingivitis. Following a 21-day placebo-controlled trial, those receiving OPC supplementation demonstrated fewer areas of gum bleeding and significantly improved gingivitis rating scores.

OPCs are found throughout plant life; however, the two main sources are pine bark extract (Pycnogenol), produced from a French coastal pine tree, and grape seed extract, made from the seeds of the wine grape (*Vitis vinifera*). Pycnogenol was the first source of OPCs discovered, and the process for extracting it was patented in the 1950s. Pycnogenol is a trademarked name for pine bark extract, not a generic term for OPCs from other sources.

Pycnogenol

See OLIGOMERIC PROANTHOCYANIDINS above.

Selenium

Selenium is an essential trace mineral that functions as an antioxidant in partnership with vitamin E to protect tissues and cell membranes. Among other things, it increases antioxidant enzyme levels in cells. Selenium is also an integral component of the antioxidant enzyme glutathione peroxidase (each molecule of this enzyme contains four atoms of selenium). Glutathione peroxidase targets harmful hydrogen peroxide in the body and converts it into water. It is a particularly important guardian of blood cells and of the heart, liver, and lungs.

Numerous plants contain selenium, including garlic, asparagus, and grains, but the levels depend on soil content, which varies from one geographic region to another.

Use caution when taking supplemental selenium. A maximum safe dose is up to 400 micrograms daily. A Danish study showed that those taking 300 micrograms or more of selenium for ten years had a 60 percent increased chance of dying compared to those with lower intakes of selenium. Amounts higher than 1,000 micrograms (1 milligram) daily may be toxic.

The best natural sources of selenium include Brazil nuts (over 500 micrograms per ounce!), brown rice, seafood, eggs, tuna, and buckwheat.

Silymarin

Extracted from the seeds of the herb milk thistle, silymarin has been used for centuries to treat liver disease. The active ingredients in milk thistle are several types of flavonoids (powerful antioxidants) known collectively as silymarin.

Silymarin guards the liver from oxidative damage. It also protects the liver from toxins, drugs, and the effects of alcohol, and promotes the growth of new liver cells. In addition, silymarin increases levels of glutathione, superoxide dismutase, and catalase, potent antioxidant enzymes that protect the liver. It also has been shown to reduce insulin resistance, which may help patients with diabetes. In one study, patients with diabetes who received silymarin experienced better control of blood glucose and better blood tests related to liver function. A newer study confirmed these findings in people with type 2 diabetes. Those taking 140 milligrams three times daily experienced significant lowering of fasting blood sugar and total cholesterol after 45 days of treatment. Also, HDL cholesterol, the one protective against heart disease, increased.

Superoxide Dismutase

Superoxide dismutase (SOD) is an enzyme. SOD revitalizes cells and reduces the rate of cell destruction. It neutralizes the most common, and possibly the most dangerous, free radicals—superoxide radicals. Superoxide radicals instigate the breakdown of synovial fluid, the lubricant for the body's joints. This leads to friction and, ultimately, inflammation.

SOD works synergistically with the enzyme catalase, which is abundant throughout the body. Catalase removes hydrogen peroxide by-products created by SOD reactions.

SOD also aids in the body's utilization of zinc, copper, and manganese. Its levels tend to decline with age, while free radical production increases. Its potential as an antiaging treatment is currently being explored.

Chemically speaking, there are two forms of this enzyme. The copper/zinc form (known as Cu/Zn SOD) exerts its antioxidant properties in the cytoplasm of cells. This is the watery fluid that surrounds all the other cellular components. Metabolic activity that takes place in the cytoplasm results in the production of free radicals, and Cu/Zn neutralizes them. The manganese form (Mn SOD) is active in the mitochondria, structures within cells where energy is produced. The production of cellular energy also leads to the creation of free radicals.

SOD occurs naturally in barley grass, broccoli, Brussels sprouts, cabbage, wheatgrass, and most green plants. It is also available in supplement form. SOD supplements in pill form must be enteric coated—that is, coated with a protective substance that allows the pill to pass intact through the stomach acid into the small intestines to be absorbed. Cell Guard from Biotec Food Corporation and KAL S.O.D. 3000 from Nutraceutical Corporation are good sources of SOD.

Vitamin A and the Carotenoids

A class of phytochemicals, carotenoids are fat-soluble pigments found in yellow, red, green, and orange vegetables and fruits. They are a potent family of antioxidants that include alpha-carotene, beta-carotene, lycopene, lutein, and zeaxanthin. Of the more than five hundred carotenoids found in nature, about fifty can be converted into vitamin A in the body.

Carotenoids quench singlet oxygen, which is not, chemically speaking, a free radical, but is nevertheless highly reactive and can damage body molecules. Carotenoids also act as anticancer agents, decrease the risk of cataracts and age-related macular degeneration, and inhibit heart disease.

Studies have shown that carotenoids found in tomato juice (lycopene), carrots (alpha- and beta-carotene), and spinach (lutein) may help to protect against cancer by reducing oxidative and other damage to DNA. Together, the antioxidants alpha-lipoic acid, coenzyme Q_{10}, vitamin C, and vitamin E help conserve carotenoids in tissues. Another carotenoid, astaxanthin, when taken as a supplement, was shown to be well-absorbed and tended to reduce damage to fat particles floating in the blood. This means that astaxanthin may be a beneficial supplement to reduce the risk of heart disease. Over two years, lutein (10 milligrams) and zeaxanthin (4 milligrams) daily were instrumental in preserving vision and slowing the progression of age-related macular degeneration.

The body converts beta-carotene into vitamin A as needed. Any leftover beta-carotene then acts as an antioxidant, breaking free radical chain reactions and preventing the oxidation of cholesterol. It reduces the oxidation of DNA and disables reactive oxygen species molecules generated by exposure to sunlight and air pollution, preventing damage to eyes, lungs, and skin.

One laboratory study found that taking very high doses of supplemental beta-carotene alone (50,000 international units or more daily) may interfere with the normal control of cell division. It is best to take a carotenoid complex containing a variety of carotenoids.

Natural sources of vitamin A include liver, whole milk, whole eggs, cheddar cheese, and beta-carotene foods. Natural sources of the carotenoids in general include sweet potatoes, carrots, spinach, corn, sweet peppers, spirulina, and kale.

Vitamin C

Vitamin C is a very powerful antioxidant that also recharges other antioxidants, such as vitamin E, to keep them potent. Its water solubility makes it an efficient free radical scavenger in body fluids. Some studies have shown that vitamin C is the first line of antioxidant defense in plasma against many different kinds of free radicals. The cells of the brain and spinal cord, which frequently incur free radical damage, can be protected by significant amounts of vitamin C. This vitamin also guards against atherosclerosis by preventing damage to artery walls. Vitamin C acts as a more potent free radical scavenger in the presence of the phytochemical hesperidin.

Natural sources of vitamin C include citrus fruits, papaya, Brussels sprouts, broccoli, and strawberries.

Vitamin E

Vitamin E is a powerful antioxidant that prevents the oxidation of lipids (fats). Fat oxidation has been implicated in the process that leads to atherosclerosis. Vitamin E is fat soluble, and since cell membranes are composed of lipids, it effectively prevents the cells' protective coatings from becoming rancid as a result of the assault of free radicals.

Vitamin E also improves oxygen utilization, enhances immune response, plays a role in the prevention of cataracts caused by free radical damage, and may reduce the risk of coronary artery disease.

The natural form of vitamin E (d-alpha-tocopherol) is superior to the synthetic version (dl-alpha-tocopherol).

New evidence suggests that zinc is needed to maintain normal blood concentrations of vitamin E. Selenium enhances vitamin E uptake.

For information regarding dosage and safety of vitamin E supplements, consult the VITAMINS section earlier in this book. Natural sources of vitamin E include nuts, soybeans, spinach, sunflower seeds, asparagus, and sweet potatoes.

Zinc

Zinc's main antioxidant function is in the prevention of fat oxidation. In addition, it is a constituent of the antioxidant enzyme superoxide dismutase (SOD). Zinc is also needed for proper maintenance of vitamin E levels in the blood and aids in the absorption of vitamin A.

Enzymes

INTRODUCTION

The late Dr. Edward Howell, a physician and pioneer in enzyme research, called enzymes the "sparks of life." These energized protein molecules play a necessary role in virtually all of the biochemical activities that go on in the body.

They are essential for digesting food, for stimulating the brain, for providing cellular energy, and for repairing all tissues, organs, and cells. Life as we know it could not exist without the action of enzymes, even in the presence of sufficient amounts of vitamins, minerals, water, and other nutrients.

In their primary role, enzymes are catalysts—substances that accelerate and precipitate the hundreds of thousands of biochemical reactions in the body that control life's processes. If it were not for the catalytic action of enzymes, most of these reactions would take place far too slowly to sustain life. Enzymes are not consumed in the reactions they facilitate.

Each enzyme has a specific function in the body that no other enzyme can fulfill. The chemical shape of each enzyme is specialized so that it can initiate a reaction only in a certain substance, or in a group of closely related substances, and not in others. The substance on which an enzyme acts is called the *substrate*. Because there must be a different enzyme for every substrate, the body must produce a great number of different enzymes.

THE FUNCTIONS OF ENZYMES

Enzymes assist in practically all bodily functions. Digestive enzymes break down food particles for energy. This chemical reaction is called *hydrolysis*, and it involves using water to break the chemical bonds to turn food into energy. The stored energy is later converted by other enzymes for use by the body as required. Iron is concentrated in the blood by the action of enzymes; other enzymes in the blood help the blood to coagulate in order to stop bleeding. Uricolytic enzymes catalyze the conversion of uric acid into urea. Respiratory enzymes aid in eliminating carbon dioxide from the lungs. Enzymes assist the kidneys, liver, lungs, colon, and skin in removing wastes and toxins from the body. Enzymes also utilize the nutrients ingested by the body to construct new muscle tissue, nerve cells, bone, skin, and glandular tissue. One enzyme can take dietary phosphorus and convert it into bone. Enzymes prompt the oxidation of glucose, which creates energy for the cells. Enzymes also protect the blood from dangerous waste materials by converting these substances to forms that are easily eliminated by the body. Indeed, the functions of enzymes are so many and so diverse that it would be impossible to name them all.

Enzymes are often divided into two groups: digestive enzymes and metabolic enzymes. Digestive enzymes are secreted along the gastrointestinal tract and break down foods, enabling the nutrients to be absorbed into the bloodstream for use in various bodily functions. If you don't make enough digestive enzymes, you will experience any or all of the following symptoms: bloating, gas, indigestion, diarrhea, and pain. Of the macronutrients—carbohydrates, proteins, and fats—people have the most trouble digesting fats, followed by proteins and carbohydrates. Those who are lactose intolerant lack the enzymes needed to break down milk sugar. When choosing an enzyme supplement, make sure that it addresses your specific digestion needs. There are three main categories of digestive enzymes: amylase, protease, and lipase.

- *Amylase,* found in saliva and in the pancreatic and intestinal juices, breaks down carbohydrates. It begins to act as soon as you start chewing. (This is why it is important to chew your food well.) Different types of amylase break down specific types of sugars. For example, lactase breaks down lactose (milk sugar), maltase breaks down maltose (malt sugar), and sucrase breaks down sucrose (cane and beet sugar).

- *Protease,* found in the stomach juices and also in the pancreatic and intestinal juices, helps to digest protein.

- *Lipase,* found in the stomach and pancreatic juices, and also present in fats in foods, aids in fat digestion.

Another component of the digestive process is hydrochloric acid. While not technically an enzyme itself, it interacts with digestive enzymes as they perform their functions.

Metabolic enzymes are enzymes that catalyze the various chemical reactions within the cells, such as energy production and detoxification. Metabolic enzymes govern the activities of all the body's organs, tissues, and cells. They are the workers that build the body from proteins, carbohydrates, and fats. Metabolic enzymes are found doing their specific work in the blood, organs, and tissues. Each body tissue has its own specific set of metabolic enzymes.

Two particularly important metabolic enzymes are superoxide dismutase (SOD) and its partner, catalase. SOD is an antioxidant that protects the cells by attacking a common free radical, superoxide. (*See* SUPEROXIDE DISMUTASE *under* ANTIOXIDANTS earlier in the book.) Catalase breaks down hydrogen peroxide, a metabolic waste product, and liberates oxygen for the body to use.

The body uses most of its enzyme-producing potential to produce about two dozen enzymes. These control the breakdown and utilization of proteins, fats, and carbohydrates to create the hundreds of metabolic enzymes necessary to maintain the rest of the tissues and organs in their functions.

FOOD ENZYMES

While the body manufactures a supply of enzymes, it also can and should obtain enzymes from food. In fact, the body's ability to manufacture enzymes is being seriously taxed by our diet of processed and highly cooked food. Unfortunately, enzymes are extremely sensitive to heat. Low to moderate heat (118°F or above) destroys most enzymes in food. To obtain enzymes from the diet, some people find benefit from eating raw foods. Eating raw foods or taking enzyme supplements helps prevent depletion of the body's own enzymes and thus reduces the stress on the body. Since enzymes are made from protein, it is essential to consume adequate amounts of protein in the diet.

Who should take enzyme supplements? Anyone who has a malabsorption problem or a yeast infection (candidiasis), or is over age sixty and whose digestive process seems to be stalling out, resulting in unpleasant symptoms. Ingredients should include pancreatin, lipase, amylase, and protease. This combination ensures digestion and absorption of amino acids, fat-soluble nutrients, and carbohydrates. Bromelain, derived from pineapple stems, along with papain, derived from the papaya fruit, also are welcome. Specific problems can be addressed by the addition of specific enzymes. For instance, people who have trouble with dairy sugars should consider lactase; people who can't digest legumes might try legumase. Hydrochloric acid supplements also might be necessary in the form of betaine hydrochloride taken as capsules at the start of each meal.

Enzymes can be found naturally in many different foods, from both plant and animal sources. Avocados, papayas, pineapples, bananas, and mangoes are all high in enzymes. Sprouts are the richest source. Unripe papaya and pineapple are excellent sources of enzymes. The enzymes extracted from papaya and pineapple—papain and bromelain, respectively—are proteolytic enzymes, which break down proteins. Many fat-containing foods also supply lipase, which breaks down fats. In fact, fat in food exposed only to pancreatic lipase (the lipase produced by the body) in the intestines is not as well digested as fat that is first worked on in the stomach by food lipase. Pancreatic lipase digests fat in a highly alkaline environment (the intestines), whereas lipase found in food fats works in a more acidic environment (the stomach). The optimal extraction of nutrients from fats depends on the work of different fat-digesting enzymes in successive stages.

Hydrochloric acid (HCl) comes in several different forms, including lysine HCl and betaine HCl. Betaine HCl is derived from sugar beets. When new, HCl capsules and tablets are almost white in color, but sometimes they can turn a deep purple color when they age. Supplemental HCl is not sold in powder or liquid form because contact with the teeth can damage tooth enamel. HCl has a sulfur-like odor.

Superoxide dismutase occurs naturally in a variety of food sources, including alfalfa, barley grass, broccoli, Brussels sprouts, cabbage, wheatgrass, and most dark green plants.

As powerful as they are, enzymes cannot act alone. They require adequate amounts of other substances, known as coenzymes, to be fully active. Among the most important coenzymes are the B-complex vitamins, vitamin C, vitamin E, and zinc.

COMMERCIALLY AVAILABLE ENZYMES

The majority of commercially available enzymes are digestive enzymes extracted from various sources. Enzymes are not manufactured synthetically. Most commercial enzyme products are made from animal enzymes, such as pancreatin and pepsin, which help in the digestion of food once it has reached the lower stomach and the intestinal tract. Some companies make their supplements from enzymes extracted from aspergillus, a type of fungus. Be sure to read labels. Those from animals are usually more concentrated than those grown from this fungus.

These enzymes begin their predigestive work in the upper stomach. All of these products are used primarily to aid the digestion of foods and absorption of nutrients, especially protein. If proteins are not completely digested, undigested protein particles may make their way into the bloodstream through the intestinal wall with other nutrients. This phenomenon is known as *leaky gut syndrome*, and it can result in allergic reactions that may be more or less severe, depending upon the strength of the immune system. This is one reason why the proper digestion of proteins is so important.

Any enzyme that acts on protein and prepares it for absorption is called a proteolytic enzyme. Proteolytic enzymes available in supplement form include pepsin, trypsin, rennin, pancreatin, chymotrypsin, bromelain, and papain. In addition to aiding digestion, proteolytic enzymes have been shown to be beneficial as anti-inflammatory agents. Pancreatin, derived from secretions of animal pancreas, is a focus of cancer research, because people with cancer are often deficient in this enzyme. Pancreatin is used in the treatment of digestive problems, viral infections, and sports injuries, as well as pancreatic insufficiency, food allergies, cystic fibrosis, autoimmune disorders, and other chronic illnesses.

Also available in supplement form are the antioxidant enzymes superoxide dismutase (SOD) and catalase.

The following table lists some common enzymes and their substrates (the substance acted upon).

ENZYME	SUBSTRATE
Amylase	Carbohydrates
Bromelain	Proteins
Cellulase	Fiber
Chymopapain	Proteins
Diastase	Carbohydrates
Glucoamylase	Carbohydrates
Hemicellulase	Carbohydrates
Hyaluronidase	Proteins, adhesions, fibrin

ENZYME	SUBSTRATE
Invertase	Carbohydrates
Lactase	Lactose (milk sugar)
Lipase	Fats
Maltase	Carbohydrates
Pancreatin	Proteins, fats, carbohydrates
Papain	Proteins, fats, carbohydrates
Pectinase	Carbohydrates
Pepsin	Proteins
Phytase	Carbohydrates
Plasmin	Proteins
Protease	Proteins
Rennin	Proteins
Trypsin	Proteins

If you decide to supplement, keep in mind that the way you respond to an enzyme may vary depending on the manufacturer. The good thing about digestive enzymes is that they work right away, so if you find you are not digesting a certain food—even after you have taken the enzyme—try another brand. Enzyme supplements may not be for everyone. During pregnancy, it is a rule to be careful with supplements in general. Nursing mothers also should be careful about supplements, to avoid affecting their milk. People who have hemophilia or who take anticoagulants (blood thinners) should consult their health care providers before taking large amounts of enzymes. Anyone contemplating surgery where there is a high risk of bleeding should ask his or her physician for advice before taking any supplement.

WHAT'S ON THE SHELVES

Enzymes are available over the counter in tablet, capsule, powder, and liquid forms. They may be sold in combination with each other or as separate items. Some enzyme products also contain garlic to aid digestion.

For maximum benefit, any digestive enzyme supplement you choose should contain all of the major enzyme groups—amylase, protease, and lipase. Digestive enzymes should be taken with meals. You can make your own digestive enzymes by drying papaya seeds, grinding them in a pepper mill, and sprinkling them on your food. These have a peppery taste.

If you take supplemental superoxide dismutase (SOD), make sure to choose a product that is enteric coated—that is, coated with a protective substance that allows the SOD to pass intact through the stomach acid to be absorbed in the small intestine. Do not crush or chew these pills. All forms of enzymes should be kept in a reasonably cool place to ensure potency because they are susceptible to moisture.

Research has shown that as we grow older, the body's ability to produce enzymes decreases. At the same time, malabsorption of nutrients, tissue breakdown, and chronic health conditions increase. Taking supplemental enzymes can help to ensure that you continue to get the full nutritional value from your foods. We believe that enzyme supplementation is vital for elderly persons. In addition, most patients with cystic fibrosis require enzyme supplements. This disease affects the pancreas and renders it unable to make adequate amounts of all digestive enzymes. Be sure to check with your health care provider to determine what product is right for you.

The following are a few recommended enzyme complex products:

- AbsorbAid from Nature's Sources is made from plant enzymes and includes lipase, amylase, and protease from bromelain, as well as cellulase and lactase. It has been shown to significantly improve the absorption of nutrients, especially essential fatty acids and zinc.

- Acid-Ease from Enzymatic Therapy is a digestive aid from natural plant sources that includes amylase, lipase, and cellulase, as well as the soothing herbs marshmallow root and slippery elm.

- All Complete Enzymes from TriMedica, Inc., is a blend of plant enzymes that provide a full range of essential enzymes, plus coenzymes for added effectiveness. It is designed to adapt to various body temperatures and pH levels without losing potency. Ingredients include amylase, lipase, bromelain, papain, protease, cellulase, acidophilus, bifidus, and trace minerals.

- Bio-Gestin from Biotec Foods (a division of AgriGenic Food Corporation) is freeze-dried mature green papaya containing papain and chymopapain. The naturally sweet taste of the papaya makes these especially good capsules to open and sprinkle over food before eating.

- Digestive Aid #34 Food Enzymes from Carlson Laboratories contains pancreatin and ox bile, with enough capability in each tablet to digest 34 grams of protein, 120 grams of carbohydrate, and 21 grams of fat. Ox bile is a beneficial supplement for people with gallbladder disorders.

- Daily Essential Enzymes from Source Naturals is a full-spectrum digestive enzyme supplement containing protease (acid stable), lipase, amylase, cellulase, and lactase. The powder in the capsules has very little taste of its own, and the contents may be added to food that is not hot (over 110°F) by sprinkling over food. (This is a good option for vegetarians who want to avoid gelatin capsules.) This supplement is designed to work in both the acidic environment of the stomach and the more alkaline environment of the intestines.

- Mega-Zyme from Enzymatic Therapy is an extra-strength pancreatic and digestive enzyme tablet. Each tablet contains protease, amylase, lipase, trypsin, papain, bromelain, and lysozyme.

- Vegetarian Enzyme Complex from Futurebiotics contains protease, amylase, cellulase, lipase, papain, and bromelain.

Other sources for quality enzyme supplements available only through health care professionals include:

- Milco-zyme, a two-part enzyme supplement with glutamic acid HCl, betaine HCl, papain, pepsin, and an enteric-coated side of the same tablet with pancreatin, lipase, amylase, and bromelain.

- Carozyme, which contains betaine HCl, trypsin, chymotrypsin, bromelain, pancreatin, mannitol, thymus extract, lipase, amylase, and papain.

- Proteolytic Enzymes, made with enteric-coated trypsin and chymotrypsin.

- Karbozyme (not to be confused with the sound-alike product above), which contains pancreatin, sodium bicarbonate, and potassium bicarbonate.

- MM-Zyme, which contains pancreatic lipase, bromelain, amylase, raw pancreas extract, papain, trypsin, chymotrypsin, and selenium.

Finally, while not technically an enzyme product, Bioperine 10 from Nature's Plus also enhances the digestion and absorption of nutrients. It contains an extract of black pepper (*Piper nigrum*), and when taken with food or with vitamin, mineral, or herbal supplements, it may help food to digest and accelerates the distribution of nutrients throughout the body. However, not all vitamin, mineral, and herbal supplements have been tested in clinical studies.

Natural Food Supplements

INTRODUCTION

Natural food supplements include a wide variety of products. Almost all health food stores carry them, and a number of drugstores, supermarkets, and mass market/club stores stock them on their shelves as well. In general, natural food supplements are composed of, derived from, or by-products of foods that provide health benefits. In some cases, health benefit claims made by manufacturers are based upon a supplement's use in traditional healing; in other cases, they are based on modern scientific research. Today, label claims are regulated by the Food and Drug Administration and the Federal Trade Commission to be true, not misleading, and based on science.

Food supplements can be high in certain nutrients, contain active ingredients that aid digestive or metabolic processes, or provide a combination of nutrients and active ingredients. It is important to point out that some unscrupulous manufacturers make false promises. It is therefore vital to be an informed consumer.

Many natural food supplements have been known to work for years; these products are medically endorsed only when they are "discovered" by researchers deemed acceptable by these groups.

Such recent discoveries include garlic, aloe vera, fiber, and fish oils—substances that have been used for centuries in many parts of the world. In a review by the head of the American Botanical Council, Mark Blumenthal, several herbs have not only been used a long time but have also stood up to rigorous scientific testing. He makes an argument for the strong science behind St. John's wort to help with depression, garlic to help people with heart disease, ginseng to improve sexual function in males, and echinacea to boost immunity.

WHAT'S ON THE SHELVES

Food supplements come in many shapes and forms—tablets, capsules, powders, liquids, jellies, creams, biscuits, wafers, granules, and more. Product packaging depends entirely on the nature of the food supplement's composition.

The potency of these products varies. Because they are made up of perishable foods, food derivatives, or food by-products, their potency may be affected by the length of time they sit on a shelf or by the temperature at which they are kept. If you don't understand how a product is to be used, ask questions or read the available literature on the particular supplement. All products sold today need to have a "sell by" date on the label. If there isn't one, contact the manufacturer and tell them the code on your box.

If you have never used a natural food supplement, you may be uncomfortable about buying and using one for the first time. This is normal. Keep in mind that once you become familiar with its use and benefits, you won't give the idea of using it a second thought.

Acidophilus
See Lactobacillus acidophilus in this section.

Adenosine Triphosphate (ATP)

Adenosine triphosphate (ATP) is a compound that serves as the immediate source of energy for the body's cells, notably muscle cells. It increases energy and stamina, builds muscular density, increases muscular strength, buffers lactic acid buildup (the reason for sore, achy muscles after physical activity), delays fatigue, and preserves muscle fibers. ATP is produced naturally in the body from adenine, a nitrogen-containing compound; ribose, a type of sugar; and phosphate units, each containing one phosphorus atom and four oxygen atoms.

Alfalfa

One of the most mineral-rich foods known, alfalfa has roots that grow as much as 130 feet into the earth. Alfalfa is available in liquid extract form and is good to use while fasting because of its chlorophyll and nutrient content. It contains digestive-aiding enzymes, amino acids, and carbohydrates. It also contains calcium, magnesium, phosphorus, potassium, plus virtually all known vitamins. The minerals are in a balanced form, which promotes absorption. These minerals are alkaline but have a neutralizing effect on the intestinal tract.

If you need a mineral supplement, alfalfa is a good choice. It has helped many arthritis sufferers. Alfalfa, wheatgrass, barley, and spirulina, all of which contain chlorophyll, have been found to aid in the healing of intestinal ulcers, gastritis, liver disorders, eczema, hemorrhoids, asthma, high blood pressure, anemia, constipation, body and breath odor, bleeding gums, infections, burns, athlete's foot, and cancer.

Aloe Vera

This plant is known for its healing effect and is used in many cosmetic and hair care products. There are over two hundred different species of aloe that grow in dry regions around the world.

Aloe vera is commonly known as a skin healer, moisturizer, and softener. It is dramatically effective on burns of all types, and is also good for cuts, insect stings, bruises, acne and blemishes, poison ivy, welts, skin ulcers, and eczema.

Taken internally, 98 or 99 percent pure aloe vera juice is known to aid in the healing of stomach disorders, ulcers, constipation, hemorrhoids, rectal itching, colitis, and all colon problems. People with gastroesophageal reflux disease (GERD) benefited from taking aloe vera in a syrup. The eight main symptoms of GERD (heartburn, food regurgitation, flatulence, belching, dysphagia, nausea, vomiting, and acid regurgitation) improved after four weeks. Thus, aloe vera may be helpful for managing symptoms of GERD.

Aloe vera can also be helpful against infections, varicose veins, skin cancer, and arthritis, and is used in the management of AIDS.

We have had excellent results using colon cleansers containing psyllium husks in combination with aloe vera juice. We have found this combination to be good for food allergy and colon disorder sufferers. Psyllium keeps the folds and pockets in the colon free of toxic material that gathers there. The aloe vera not only has a healing effect, but if constipation or diarrhea is present, it will return the stools to normal.

It takes a few weeks to cleanse the colon, but regular periodic use will keep the colon clean. As with any substance, it is possible to develop intolerance to aloe vera juice and/or psyllium husks, so this treatment should not be used on an ongoing basis.

Barley Grass
Barley grass contains small amounts of calcium, iron, all the essential amino acids, chlorophyll, flavonoids, vitamin B_{12}, vitamin C, and many minerals, plus enzymes. This food heals stomach, duodenal, and colon disorders as well as pancreatitis, and is an effective anti-inflammatory.

Bee By-Products
See Bee Pollen, Bee Propolis, Honey, and Royal Jelly, all in this section.

Bee Pollen

Bee pollen is a powderlike material that is produced by the anthers of flowering plants and gathered by bees. It is composed of 10 to 15 percent protein and also contains B-complex vitamins, vitamin C, essential fatty acids, enzymes, carotene, calcium, copper, iron, magnesium, potassium, manganese, sodium, plant sterols, and simple sugars.

Like other bee products, bee pollen has an antimicrobial effect. In addition, it is useful for combating fatigue, depression, cancer, and colon disorders. It is also helpful for people with allergies because it strengthens the immune system.

It is best to obtain bee pollen from a local source, as this increases its antiallergenic properties. Fresh bee pollen should not cling together or form clumps, and it should be sold in a tightly sealed container. Some people (an estimated 0.05 percent of the population) may be allergic to bee pollen. It is best to try taking a small amount at first and watch for a developing rash, wheezing, discomfort, or any other signs of a reaction. If such symptoms occur, discontinue taking bee pollen.

Bee Propolis

Bee propolis is a resinous substance collected from various plants by bees. Bees use propolis, together with beeswax, in the construction of hives. As a supplement, it is an excellent aid against bacterial infections. Bee propolis is believed to stimulate phagocytosis, the process by which some white blood cells destroy bacteria.

Propolis is beneficial as a salve for abrasions and bruises because of its antibacterial effect. Good results have been reported on the use of propolis against inflammation of the mucous membranes of the mouth and throat, dry cough and throat, halitosis, tonsillitis, ulcers, and acne, and for the stimulation of the immune system. A newer study showed that bee propolis may help people with type 2 diabetes. Sixty people with type 2 diabetes took 900 milligrams of bee propolis daily for twelve weeks. This was enough time to see a benefit in lowering fasting blood sugar and hemoglobin A1c. Also, the bee propolis group had total cholesterol levels close to where they started, while others in a placebo group experienced an increase in total cholesterol. Type 2 diabetes management involves a number of things like diet and exercise, but bee propolis may be another beneficial natural product.

Be sure that any bee products you use smell and taste fresh. All bee products should be in tightly sealed containers. It is best to purchase these products from a manufacturer who specializes in bee products. If you are using bee products for allergies, it is best to obtain products that are produced within a ten-mile radius of your home. This way, you get a minute dose of pollen to desensitize you to the local pollen in the area.

Beta-1,3-Glucan

Beta-1,3-glucan is a polysaccharide (a complex type of carbohydrate molecule) with immune-stimulating properties. Specifically, it stimulates the activity of macrophages (immune cells that destroy cellular debris), microorganisms, and abnormal cells by surrounding and digesting them.

Beta-1,3-D-glucan is a supplemental form of beta-1,3-glucan made from the cell walls of baker's yeast. Despite its origin, it does not contain any yeast proteins. It is useful for treating many bacterial, viral, and fungal diseases. It can also kill tumor cells and increase bone marrow production. Yeast beta-glucan (900 milligrams a day) taken during cold and flu season seemed to reduce the severity of an upper respiratory infection during the first week after an infection developed, but not during the entire time the infection was present. In addition, compared to a group who didn't get the beta-glucan, those who did felt happier and less stressed.

Because of its ability to protect the immune system, beta-1,3-D-glucan may protect against the effects of aging. Studies done as early as the 1970s have found that it can reduce the size of cancerous tumors in rats. Further investigation has shown beta-1,3-D-glucan to be a potent agent for healing sores and ulcers in women who have undergone mastectomies.

Bifidobacterium bifidum

Bifidobacterium bifidum aids in the synthesis of the B vitamins by creating healthy intestinal flora. *B. bifidum* is the predominant healthy organism in the intestinal flora and establishes a healthy environment for the manufacture of the B-complex vitamins and vitamin K.

When you take antibiotics, the "friendly" bacteria in your digestive tract are destroyed along with the harmful bacteria. Supplementing your diet with *B. bifidum* helps you maintain healthy intestinal flora and helps strengthen the intestinal wall. Unhealthy flora can result in the liberation of abnormally high levels of ammonia as protein-containing foods are digested. This irritates the intestinal membranes. In addition, the ammonia is absorbed into the bloodstream and must be detoxified by the liver, or it will cause nausea, a decrease in appetite, vomiting, and other toxic reactions. By promoting the proper digestion of foods, the friendly bacteria also aid in preventing digestive disorders such as constipation and gas, as well as food allergies. If digestion is poor, the activity of intestinal bacteria on undigested food may lead to excessive production of the body chemical histamine, which triggers allergic symptoms.

Yeast infections of the vaginal tract respond very favorably to douching with *B. bifidum* preparations. These microorganisms destroy the pathogenic organisms. When used as an enema, *B. bifidum* also helps establish a healthy intestinal environment. It improves bowel function by aiding peristalsis and results in the production of a softer, smoother stool. Harmful bacteria are kept in check, and toxic wastes that have accumulated in the intestines are destroyed and/or eliminated from the body. For people with irritable bowel syndrome, taking one strain of bifidobacteria (MIMBb75) produced positive results. The participants had less pain/discomfort, distension/bloating, urgency, and digestive disorders; and had an improved quality of life. This specific strain, MIMBb75, offers promise for people with irritable bowel syndrome, according to the authors of this article.

B. bifidum may be useful in the treatment of cirrhosis of the liver and chronic hepatitis; by improving digestion, it reduces the strain on the liver. Many people who do not respond to L. acidophilus react positively to B. bifidum. Many experts consider B. bifidum to be preferable to L. acidophilus for children and for adults with liver disorders. This product needs to be taken every day or the body will go back to its usual state of bacteria growth.

Bifidus
See Bifidobacterium bifidum above.

Bovine Cartilage
Cleaned, dried, and powdered bovine cartilage is a supplement that helps to accelerate wound healing and reduce inflammation. Like shark cartilage, it has been shown to be helpful for psoriasis, all types of arthritis, and ulcerative colitis.

Brewer's Yeast
See Yeast in this section.

Cellulose
See under Fiber in this section.

Cerasomal-cis-9-cetylmyristoleate
This is a modified version of a medium-chain fatty acid, cetylmyristoleate, which is found in nuts, vegetables, and animal tissue. It appears to be a very promising development in arthritis research. Studies in laboratory rats have shown it to have anti-inflammatory effects, and early clinical studies in people suggest it may be beneficial for many with osteoarthritis, rheumatoid arthritis, and psoriatic arthritis, as well as psoriasis. It

is believed to work by normalizing the functioning of the immune system and reducing the production of pro-inflammatory prostaglandins.

Chlorella

Chlorella is a tiny single-celled water-grown alga containing a nucleus and an enormous amount of readily available chlorophyll. It also contains protein (approximately 58 percent), carbohydrates, all of the B vitamins, vitamins C and E, amino acids, and rare trace minerals. In fact, it is virtually a complete food. It contains more vitamin B_{12} than liver, plus a considerable amount of beta-carotene. It has a strong cell wall, however, which makes it difficult to gain access to its nutrients. Consequently, it requires factory processing to be effective. For women with painful menstrual periods, chlorella may be of some help. Use of 1,500 milligrams daily helped reduce common side effects like pain, nausea, and lack of energy. These benefits were attributed to the anti-inflammatory and antioxidative effects of chlorella.

Chlorella is one of the few edible species of water-grown algae. The chlorophyll in chlorella can help speed the cleansing of the bloodstream. Chlorella is very high in RNA and DNA, and has been found to protect against the effects of ultraviolet radiation. Studies show that chlorella is an excellent source of protein, especially for people who cannot or who choose not to eat meat. It is available from Sun Chlorella USA. (*See* sunchlorella .com for further information.)

Chlorophyll

See under Chlorella and "Green Drinks" in this section.

Chondroitin Sulfate

Chondroitin sulfate is an important element in the creation of cartilage. Cartilage is the tough yet flexible connective tissue found in the joints, where it acts as a cushion, and in other parts of the body, such as the tip of the nose and the outer ear.

Chemically, chondroitins belong to a group of substances classified as *glycosaminoglycans* (also referred to as *mucopolysaccharides*), which are complex types of carbohydrate molecules. Glycosaminoglycans in turn attach to proteins such as collagen and elastin, forming even more complex substances designated *proteoglycans,* which are a vital component of cartilage tissue. Chondroitin sulfate attracts water to the proteoglycans and holds it there, which is important for maintaining healthy joint cartilage. It can also protect existing cartilage from premature degeneration by blocking certain enzymes that destroy cartilage and prevent nutrients from being transported to the cartilage for repair. In one study of patients with osteoarthritis of the knee who used chondroitin, the disease progressed more slowly and they had less pain compared to a group that was not treated. It was more effective in patients with mild knee pain than in those with severe pain.

Taking supplemental chondroitin sulfate, usually derived from powdered shark cartilage or cow trachea cartilage, has been shown to be helpful in the treatment of osteoarthritis. Many times it is used in conjunction with glucosamine for even more effective therapy. The supplements are usually taken together in pill form. Neither chondroitin sulfate nor glucosamine has shown any toxic effects, but there are potential side effects for certain people. The Arthritis Foundation recommends exercising caution in taking these supplements for treatment of osteoarthritis. Let your physician know you are taking these supplements and discuss any allergies or potential reactions. Use caution in taking chondroitin sulfate if you are taking anticoagulants (blood thinners) or daily aspirin, as it is chemically similar to the blood thinner heparin. Pregnant women should not take these supplements, as there has not been sufficient study regarding their safety and potential side effects during pregnancy.

Twinlab manufactures a few good products containing chondroitin sulfate. Glucosamine Plus from Only Natural is a good source of glucosamine.

Citrin

Citrin is a trademarked name for a standardized herbal extract from the fruit of the *Garcinia cambogia* plant (Indian berry). It inhibits the synthesis of fatty acids in the liver, promotes the burning of body fat as fuel, and suppresses the appetite. Its main usefulness is in treating obesity; it may also aid in preventing or slowing atherosclerosis and heart disease. It does not affect the nervous system or have any known side effects. Citrin is found in a number of products sold by various manufacturers. Some studies suggest that GarCitrin, a similar extract made from *Garcinia cambogia*, may be more effective for weight loss than Citrin.

Coenzyme A

Coenzyme A, a substance manufactured by body cells from pantothenic acid (vitamin B_5), is at the center of the whole metabolic process. It performs a vital role in the process by which the cells generate energy from glucose. Indeed, it helps produce around 90 percent of the energy the body needs to function. Coenzyme A also begins the metabolism of fatty acids. A lack of sufficient coenzyme A can result in stiff, sore muscles and a decrease in energy. Taken as a supplement, coenzyme A increases energy, supports the manufacture of substances critical for the brain and adrenal glands, helps with the manufacture of connective tissue, and supports the immune system. Studies suggest that coenzyme A may be as, if not more, beneficial than coenzyme Q_{10}.

Coenzyme Q_{10}

Coenzyme Q_{10} is present in the mitochondria of all the cells in the body. It is vital because it carries into the cells the energy-laden protons and electrons that are used to produce adenosine triphosphate (ATP), the immediate source of cellular energy. (*See* Adenosine Triphosphate [ATP] earlier in this section.) This is a constant process because the body can store only a small quantity of ATP at any one time. It is believed that as many as 75 percent of people over fifty may be deficient in coenzyme Q_{10}. A lack of sufficient coenzyme Q_{10} can lead to cardiovascular disease. Without enough of it, the heart cannot circulate the blood effectively. Coenzyme Q_{10} has varied applications, including migraine prevention, improving energy levels, lowering blood pressure, and the management of chronic cardiac failure. It has *not* been shown to help with glucose management, prevent oxidation of bad cholesterol, enhance blood flow from the heart, or inhibit periodontal disease. In Japan, coenzyme Q_{10} has been approved for use in treating congestive heart failure. (*See* ANTIOXIDANTS earlier in this chapter for a discussion of coenzyme Q_{10} as an antioxidant.)

Colostrum

Colostrum is a thin, yellowish fluid secreted by the mammary glands of mammalian mothers in the first days after giving birth, before the production of true milk begins. It contains high levels of protein and growth factors, as well as immune factors that help to protect the newborn against infection. Taken as a supplement, colostrum can boost the immune system by enhancing the ability of the thymus gland to create T cells and also can help the body to burn fat and build lean muscle. It may also accelerate the healing of injuries, increase vitality and stamina, and have an antiaging effect. In a study done in older adults of the effects of eight weeks of supplementation with bovine colostrum compared with whey protein, bovine colostrum (60 grams) was better at increasing leg muscle strength and keeping bones strong by allowing calcium to remain inside them. Both whey protein and bovine colostrum improved upper body strength, muscle thickness and mass, and cognition.

Supplemental colostrum usually contains bovine (cow) colostrum. Good sources include Colostrum Plus from Symbiotics and Colostrum Prime Life from Jarrow Formulas.

Corn Germ

Using a process that isolates the embryo of the corn plant, which contains the most usable nutrients, corn germ is made. Corn germ has a longer shelf life than wheat germ and is higher in some nutrients, especially zinc. Corn germ contains ten times the amount of zinc found in wheat germ.

You can use corn germ to bread chicken or fish. It is also good when added to cereals and used as a topping.

Creatine

Creatine (creatine monohydrate) is a compound produced by metabolic processes in the body. When muscles are in use, the compound adenosine triphosphate (ATP) is broken down into two other compounds—adenosine diphosphate (ADP) and inorganic phosphate. This process produces the body's cellular energy, which, among other things, powers the muscles. Each such burst of energy is very fleeting.

However, with the addition of creatine, ADP can be transformed back to ATP, the source of cellular energy. Taken as a supplement, creatine can increase both endurance and strength, making possible extended workout time. Longer workouts in turn can result in a real increase in lean muscle mass, and do not simply puff up the muscle with water.

Creatine is particularly popular with athletes. The use of creatine for muscle-depleting illnesses and the natural wasting of muscles that comes with age is also being studied. In one study, elderly men and women had improved upper body grip strength and lower body muscle endurance after using creatine. They were less fatigued in general and experienced no side effects from the supplement.

Creatine should be used in combination with a balanced, nutritionally complete diet. Vegetarians do not get enough dietary creatine—since it comes exclusively from animal-based foods—and may need supplementation, especially if they exercise. Vegetarians who received 20 grams daily of creatine experienced improved memory, maybe because they weren't getting enough from their diet. No change was observed in a group of meat eaters in the same study. Those who eat animal-based foods consume about 2 grams a day. You should not take it with fruit juices, as this combination results in the production of creatinine, which is difficult for the kidneys to process. Never exceed the recommended dose. Smaller doses (about 2.5 grams) rather than 5 or more grams seemed to be just as effective in growing new muscles during a workout.

Dehydroepiandrosterone (DHEA)

Dehydroepiandrosterone (DHEA) is a hormone that is produced primarily by the adrenal glands and is found naturally in the human body. It is an important base from which other key substances, including the hormones testosterone, progesterone, and corticosterone, can be derived, either directly or indirectly. The amount of DHEA produced by the body declines with age, particularly after age forty. Research indicates that taking DHEA supplements may help to prevent cancer, arterial disease, multiple sclerosis, and Alzheimer's disease; may be beneficial in the treatment of lupus and osteoporosis; may enhance the activity of the immune system; and may help to improve memory.

Caution should be exercised when taking this supplement. Some physicians believe that taking high doses of DHEA suppresses the body's natural ability to synthesize this hormone. Further, laboratory studies have shown that high doses can lead to liver damage. DHEA is on the banned substance list of the World Anti-Doping Agency, because it is thought to increase testosterone levels. After four weeks, men and women who took 100 milligrams daily of DHEA experienced increases in testosterone, but women had a greater increase than men. Other hormone levels changed, indicating that DHEA at this amount has an effect in the body and that some of these changes can be used to see if an athlete is doping. If you take supplemental DHEA, it is important also to take supplements of the antioxidant vitamins C and E and the antioxidant mineral selenium to prevent oxidative damage to the liver. Possible side effects of taking DHEA include excess growth of facial hair in women. This can often be avoided by starting with a dose of 10 milligrams daily. 7-Keto DHEA is a derivative of DHEA that is not converted into estrogen or testosterone, which is good for women concerned about breast cancer and for men concerned about prostate cancer. 7-Keto DHEA is a good and safer alternative to DHEA and has the same benefits.

Desiccated Liver

Desiccated liver is concentrated dried liver that is put into powdered or tablet form. This form of liver contains vitamins A, D, and C; the B-complex vitamins; and the minerals calcium, copper, phosphorus, and iron. Desiccated liver is good for people with anemia and aids in building healthy red blood cells. It is known to increase energy, aid in liver disorders, and help relieve stress in the body. Use only a product made from liver derived from cattle raised organically.

Dimethylglycine (DMG)

Dimethylglycine (DMG) is a derivative of glycine, the simplest of the amino acids. It acts as a building block for many important substances, including the amino acid methionine, choline, a number of important hormones and neurotransmitters, and DNA.

Low levels of DMG are present in meats, seeds, and grains. It is a safe, nontoxic food substance that does not build up in the body. No deficiency symptoms are associated with a lack of DMG in the diet, but taking supplemental DMG can have a wide range of beneficial effects, including helping the body maintain high energy levels and boosting mental acuity. DMG has been found to enhance the immune system and to reduce elevated blood cholesterol and triglyceride levels. It improves oxygen utilization by the body, helps to normalize blood pressure and blood glucose levels, and improves the functioning of many important organs. It may also be useful for controlling epileptic seizures. Some people have used DMG as a substitute for pangamic acid, a supplement that is no longer available in the United States but that is widely used in Russia to treat heart disease, liver disease, alcohol and drug addiction, and other problems. DMG is thought to increase pangamic acid levels in the body.

Dimethylsulfoxide (DMSO)

Dimethylsulfoxide (DMSO) is a by-product of wood processing for papermaking. It is a somewhat oily liquid that looks like mineral oil and has a slightly garlicky odor. Because it is an excellent solvent, it is widely used as a degreaser, paint thinner, and antifreeze. However, it also has remarkable therapeutic properties, especially for the healing of injuries. Applying DMSO on sprained ankles, pulled muscles, dislocated joints, and even at the site of simple fractures can virtually eliminate the pain. It also promotes immune system activity.

DMSO is absorbed through the skin and enters the bloodstream by osmosis through capillary walls. It is then distributed through the circulatory system and ultimately is excreted through the urine. Because of the properties of DMSO, it will take any contaminants on the skin or in the product directly into the bloodstream. For this reason, only pure DMSO from a health food source can be used. The use of hardware-store DMSO could cause serious health problems. DMSO has been used successfully in the treatment of brain and spinal cord damage, arthritis, Down syndrome, sciatica and other back problems, keloids, acne, burns, musculoskeletal problems, sports injuries, cancer, sinusitis, headaches, skin ulcers, herpes, and cataracts. The use of DMSO may result in a garlicky body odor. This is temporary and is not a cause for concern.

Essential Fatty Acids (EFAs)

Fatty acids are the basic building blocks of which fats and oils are composed. Contrary to popular myth, the body does need some of the right kind of fat. The fatty acids that are necessary for health and that cannot be made by the body are called *essential fatty acids* (EFAs). EFAs must be supplied through the diet.

EFAs have desirable effects on many disorders. They improve the skin and hair, reduce blood pressure, aid in the prevention of arthritis, lower cholesterol and triglyceride levels, and reduce the risk of blood clot formation. They are beneficial for candidiasis, cardiovascular disease, eczema, and psoriasis. Found in high concentrations in the brain, EFAs aid in the transmission of nerve impulses, and are needed for the normal development and functioning of the brain. A deficiency of EFAs can lead to an impaired ability to learn and recall information. Infant formulas now contain ARA and DHA, essential fats for infants, which may promote better learning.

Every living cell in the body needs EFAs. They are essential for rebuilding and producing new cells. They are also used by the body for the production of prostaglandins, hormonelike substances that act as chemical messengers and regulators of various body processes.

There are two basic categories of EFAs, designated *omega-3* and *omega-6,* based on their chemical structures. Omega-3 EFAs, including alpha-linolenic and eicosapentaenoic acid (EPA), are found in fresh deepwater fish, fish oil, and certain vegetable oils, among them canola oil, flaxseed oil, and walnut oil. Omega-6 EFAs, which include linoleic and gamma-linolenic acids, are found primarily in raw nuts, seeds, and legumes, and in unsaturated vegetable oils, such as borage oil, grape seed oil, primrose oil, sesame oil, and soybean oil. One study reported in the British medical journal *Lancet* has shown that omega-3 fatty acids, which create a more stable arterial plaque, are better for your heart than the omega-6 variety. We recommend that you try to increase your consumption of omega-3s at the expense of the omega-6s. In order to supply EFAs, these oils must be consumed in pure liquid or supplement form and must not be subjected to heat, either in processing or cooking. Heat destroys EFAs. Worse, it results in the creation of dangerous free radicals. (*See* ANTIOXIDANTS earlier in this book.) If oils are hydrogenated (processed to make the oil more solid, as is commonly done in the production of margarine), the linoleic acid is converted into trans-fatty acids, which are not beneficial to the body.

The daily requirement for EFAs is satisfied by an amount equivalent to 10 to 20 percent of total fat intake. The most essential of the EFAs is linoleic acid.

A number of sources of EFAs are recommended in this book, among them fish oils, flaxseeds and flaxseed oil, and primrose oil. If you are taking any of these oils, you need to cut back on linoleic-rich oils such as corn, sunflower, and cottonseed oil to avoid getting too much of the omega-6 fats.

Emu Oil

Emu oil is an excellent source of linoleic acid, linolenic acid, and oleic acid. Linolenic acid has anti-inflammatory properties. It can be used topically for the relief of rashes, hemorrhoids, poison ivy, insect bites, arthritis, joint aches, and muscle strains, and it has been known to stop the pain of burns. It can also be used as a facial moisturizer to reduce wrinkles and lines. Thunder Ridge Emu is a good source for emu oil.

Fish Oil

Fish oil is a good source of omega-3 EFAs. Salmon, herring, tuna (limit to 1 serving per week), and sardines are good sources of fish oil because they have a higher fat content and provide more omega-3 factors than other fishes.

For instance, 4 ounces of salmon contains 1,000 to 4,600 milligrams of omega-3 fatty acids, while 4 ounces of cod (a low-fat fish) contains only about 300 milligrams. Menhaden, another type of fish, supplies most of the oil used in dietary supplements because it is rich in omega-3s.

Carlson Laboratories markets a good Norwegian salmon oil that we recommend. Cod-liver oil from Norway is the most commonly used fish oil and is milder tasting than other varieties. The late author Don Dale Alexander claimed it was excellent for arthritis. He has marketed an oil containing 13,800 international units of vitamin A and 1,380 international units of vitamin D per tablespoon. However, we do not recommend that you rely on cod-liver oil as a source of the EFAs. You would have to overdose on vitamins A and D to obtain the amount of fatty acids you need.

People with diabetes have been cautioned not to take fish oil supplements because fish oil may slightly raise blood cholesterol levels. However, the benefit of such oils in reducing triglyceride levels outweighs this risk. People with diabetes should check with their health care provider, but they should consume fish anyway for its EFAs.

Flaxseeds and Flaxseed Oil

Flaxseeds are rich in omega-3 EFAs, magnesium, potassium, and fiber. The omega-3s in plant-based foods are not in a bioactive form, which means the body has to process them before it can use them. In contrast, omega-3s from fish are ready for the body to use. Most experts agree that the body uses only 10 percent or less of omega-3s from plant-based foods. Both seeds and oils are also a good source of the B vitamins, protein, and zinc. They are low in saturated fats and calories and contain no cholesterol. The nutty taste of ground flaxseeds is pleasant, and they can be mixed with water or any fruit or vegetable juice. They can also be added to salads, soups, yogurt, cereals, baked goods, or fresh juices. You can grind these tiny seeds in a coffee grinder.

If you prefer not to eat the seeds, you can use flaxseed oil as an alternative. Like the seeds from which it is extracted, organic cold-pressed flaxseed oil is rich in EFAs. Several studies have shown that it can reduce the pain, inflammation, and swelling of arthritis. It has been found to lower blood cholesterol and triglyceride levels, and to help reduce the hardening effects of cholesterol on cell membranes.

Grape Seed Oil

Of the many natural sources of EFAs, grape seed oil is among the highest in linoleic acid and among the lowest in saturated fats. Grape seed oil is rich in omega-6 oils, which are essential, but usually we get more than enough omega-6s in our diet, so use it sparingly. It contains no cholesterol and no sodium. It has a light, nutty taste that brings out the flavor in many foods. Unlike most other oils, it can be heated to temperatures as high as 485°F without producing dangerous and possibly carcinogenic free radicals. These features make it good for use in cooking. Buy only grape seed oil that is cold-pressed and contains no preservatives. A grape seed extract was helpful at reducing blood pressure in people with pre-hypertension. The participants in the study were randomized to receive tablets containing 200 milligrams, 400 milligrams, or a placebo, but those who were nonsmokers and took the larger amount got the most blood-pressure-lowering effect.

Primrose Oil

Primrose oil (also known as evening primrose oil) contains 9 to 10 percent gamma-linolenic acid (GLA). It is an anti-inflammatory fatty acid and may help reduce the likelihood of developing cancer, diabetes, heart disease, and Alzheimer's disease. It relieves pain and inflammation; enhances the release of sex hormones, including estrogen and testosterone; aids in lowering cholesterol levels; and is beneficial for cirrhosis of the liver.

Many women have found that primrose oil supplements relieve unpleasant menopausal symptoms such as hot flashes. Women in menopause reaped benefit from taking 500 milligrams of evening primrose oil daily for six weeks. Those who took the oil had hot flashes that were less frequent and severe and didn't last as long as those in the placebo group. In addition, the women taking the oil were more involved socially and had better sex lives. Because it promotes the production of estrogen, women suffering from breast cancer that is diagnosed as estrogen-receptor positive (estrogen-related) should avoid or limit their intake of primrose oil. Black currant seed oil is a good substitute.

Evening Primrose Oil

See Primrose Oil above.

Fiber

Found in many foods, fiber helps to lower blood cholesterol levels and stabilize blood sugar levels. It helps prevent colon cancer, constipation, hemorrhoids, obesity, and many other disorders. Fiber is also good for removing certain toxic metals from the body. Because the refining process has removed much of the natural fiber from our foods, the typical American diet is lacking in fiber.

There are seven basic classifications of fiber: bran, cellulose, gum, hemicellulose, lignin, mucilage, and pectin. Each form has its own function. It is best to rotate among several different supplemental fiber sources. Start with small amounts and gradually increase your intake until your stools are the proper consistency. Also, be aware that while today's average diet is lacking in fiber, consuming excessive amounts may decrease the absorption of zinc, iron, and calcium. Always take supplemental fiber separately from other medications or supplements. Otherwise, it can lessen their strength and effectiveness.

In addition to using a fiber supplement, you should make sure to get fiber through your diet. Make sure your diet contains these high-fiber foods:

- Whole-grain cereals and flours.

- Brown rice.

- Agar-agar (made from the algae genus *Gelidium*; also called *dai choy goh*).

- All kinds of bran.

- Fresh fruit.

- Dried prunes.

- Nuts.

- Seeds (especially flaxseeds).

- Beans.

- Lentils.

- Peas.

- Fresh raw vegetables.

Eat several of these foods daily. When eating organic produce, leave the skin on apples and potatoes. Coat chicken in corn bran or oats for baking. Add extra bran to cereals and breads. Unsalted, unbuttered popcorn is also excellent for added fiber.

Bran, Gums, and Mucilages

Both gums and mucilages help to regulate blood glucose levels, aid in lowering cholesterol, and help in the removal of toxins. They are found in oatmeal, oat bran, sesame seeds, and dried beans. Gums and mucilages are soluble fibers that foster the growth of healthy bacteria, which in turn discourage the growth of harmful ones. If you are taking any probiotics—for example, bifidobacteria—it is best to take it with one of these fibers.

One of the following should be part of your daily dietary plan:

- *Fennel seed.* Fennel is an herb that is helpful for digestive purposes. The seeds of this plant help to rid the intestinal tract of mucus and aid in relieving flatulence.

- *Glucomannan.* Derived from the tuber of the amorphophallus plant, it picks up and removes fat from the colon wall. This substance is good for diabetes, as it has been recognized for normalizing blood sugar and is good for people with hypoglycemia. Glucomannan expands to sixty times its own weight, thereby helping to curb the appetite. Taking 2 to 3 capsules with a large glass of water thirty minutes before meals is helpful for reducing allergic reactions and some symptoms associated with high and low blood sugar disorders. Always be sure to drink a large glass of water when taking glucomannan in capsule or pill form, as capsules can lodge in the throat and expand there, causing breathing problems. Glucomannan is tasteless and odorless and can be added to foods to help normalize blood sugar.

- *Guar gum.* Extracted from the seeds of the guar plant, guar gum is good for the treatment of diabetes and for curbing the appetite. It also has the ability to reduce the levels of cholesterol, triglycerides, and low-density lipoproteins in the blood, and binds with toxic substances and carries them out of the body. Guar gum tablets must be chewed thoroughly or sucked gradually, not swallowed whole, and should be taken with lots of water, because guar gum has a tendency to ball up in the throat when mixed with saliva. It should not be used by individuals who have difficulty swallowing or who have had gastrointestinal surgery. Some persons with colon disorders may have trouble using guar gum.

- *Oat bran and rice bran.* Bran is the broken coat of the seed of cereal grain that has been separated from the flour or meal by sifting or bolting. It helps to lower cholesterol.

- *Psyllium seed.* Psyllium is a grain grown in India that is utilized for its fiber content. A good intestinal cleanser and stool softener, it is one of the most popular fibers used. It thickens very quickly when mixed with liquid and must be consumed immediately. Some doctors recommend Metamucil, which contains psyllium hydrophilic mucilloid as a laxative and fiber supplement. However, we prefer less processing and all-natural products.

Cellulose

Cellulose is an indigestible carbohydrate (or insoluble fiber) found in the outer layer of vegetables and fruits. It is good for hemorrhoids, varicose veins, colitis, and constipation, and for the removal of cancer-causing substances from the colon wall.

It is found in apples, beets, Brazil nuts, broccoli, carrots, celery, green beans, lima beans, pears, peas, and whole grains.

Hemicellulose

Hemicellulose is an indigestible complex carbohydrate that absorbs water. It is good for promoting weight loss, relieving constipation, preventing colon cancer, and controlling carcinogens in the intestinal tract. Hemicellulose is found in apples, bananas, beans, beets, cabbage, corn, green leafy vegetables, pears, peppers, and whole-grain cereals.

Lignin

This form of fiber is good for lowering cholesterol levels. It helps to prevent the formation of gallstones by binding with bile acids and removing cholesterol before stones can form. It is beneficial for persons with diabetes or colon cancer. Those who eat a lot of dietary lignins have been shown to have better cognitive function than those who eat a low-lignin diet.

Lignins are found in all plants but especially in alfalfa, berries, Brazil nuts, broccoli, carrots, green beans, peaches, peas, potatoes, seed oils, strawberries, tomatoes, and whole grains.

Pectin

Because it slows the absorption of food after meals, pectin is good for people with diabetes. It also removes unwanted metals and toxins, reduces the side effects of radiation therapy, helps lower cholesterol, and reduces the risk of heart disease and gallstones. Pectin is found in apples, bananas, beets, cabbage, carrots, citrus fruits, dried peas, and okra.

Combination Fiber Supplements

There are many products available that combine two or more different types of fiber, or that combine fiber with other ingredients. Be sure you buy one that has both soluble and insoluble fiber. Two products of this kind that we recommend are:

- ABC Multi-Fiber Blend from Aerobic Life Industries. This formula contains psyllium and oat bran and provides approximately 3 grams of soluble fiber and 4 grams of insoluble fiber per serving.

- Super Cleanse from Nature's Secret. This formula combines gums with cellulose, hemicellulose, pectin, and lignin, plus herbs that support and cleanse the blood and internal organs.

Fish Oil

See under Essential Fatty Acids in this section.

5-Hydroxy L-Tryptophan (5-HTP)

5-HTP is a substance that is created naturally in the body from the amino acid tryptophan, and that in turn is used by the body to produce serotonin, an important neurotransmitter. Supplemental 5-HTP is derived from the seeds of the griffonia plant (*Griffonia simplicifolia*), which is native to West Africa. It can be used to aid in weight loss, insomnia, and depression. People with different levels of severity of depression benefited within two weeks from taking 5-HTP, and the response was comparable to a drug used to treat depression.

5-HTP should be used together with a high-carbohydrate food or liquid such as orange juice, and as part of a comprehensive nutritional program. It may not benefit everyone who takes it. If you regularly take large doses of 5-HTP (more than 300 milligrams daily), you should undergo blood testing for eosinophil (a type of white blood cell) levels every three months. HTP.Calm from Natural Balance is a good source of 5-HTP. You should avoid this supplement if you are taking antidepressants.

Flaxseeds and Flaxseed Oil

See under Essential Fatty Acids in this section.

Garlic

Garlic is one of the most valuable foods on this planet. It has been used since biblical times and is mentioned in the literature of the ancient Hebrews, Greeks, Babylonians, Romans, and Egyptians. The builders of the pyramids supposedly ate garlic daily for endurance and strength.

Garlic lowers blood pressure through the actions of one of its components, methyl-allyl-trisulfide, which dilates blood vessels. It thins the blood by inhibiting platelet aggregation, which reduces the risk of blood clots and aids in preventing heart attacks.

It also lowers serum cholesterol levels and aids in digestion. Garlic is useful for many diseases and illnesses, including cancer. It is a potent immune system stimulant and a natural antibiotic. It should be consumed daily. It can be eaten fresh, taken in supplement form, or used to prepare garlic oil. According to one study, garlic had special benefit during cold and flu season. A group of people who took 2.56 grams of aged garlic daily had less severe symptoms associated with developing a cold or the flu and were sick fewer days, compared to others who did not get the garlic. Those taking the garlic also had improved immune systems.

Garlic contains an amino acid derivative, alliin. When garlic is consumed, the enzyme alliinase, which converts alliin to allicin, is released. Allicin has an antibiotic effect; it exerts an antibacterial effect estimated to be equivalent to 1 percent of that of penicillin. Because of its antibiotic properties, garlic was used to treat wounds and infections and to prevent gangrene during World War I.

Garlic is also effective against fungal infections, including athlete's foot, systemic candidiasis, and yeast vaginitis. There is some evidence that it may also destroy certain viruses, such as those associated with fever blisters, genital herpes, a form of the common cold, smallpox, and a type of influenza.

Garlic oil is good for the heart and colon, and is effective in the treatment of arthritis, candidiasis, and circulation problems. To make garlic oil, add peeled whole garlic cloves to a quart of olive or canola oil. Experiment to find the number of cloves that gives the degree of flavor you like. Be sure to wash your hands thoroughly and rinse the garlic after peeling and before placing it in the oil. The peel may contain mold and bacteria that can contaminate the oil.

Keep garlic oil refrigerated. This mixture will keep for up to a month before you need to replace it with fresh oil. Garlic oil can be used for sautéing, in salad dressings, and in a variety of other ways. If you find the odor too strong after you eat garlic, chew some sprigs of parsley or mint, or caraway or fennel seeds.

An alternative to fresh garlic is Kyolic from Wakunaga of America (https://kyolic.com/). Kyolic is an odorless, "sociable" garlic product, and is available in tablet, capsule, and oil extract forms.

Ginkgo Biloba

The ornamental tree *Ginkgo biloba* originated in China thousands of years ago, and now grows in temperate climates throughout the world. The extract of its fan-shaped leaves is one of the world's most popular herbal products. It has been reported in scientific journals to enhance blood circulation and to increase the supply of oxygen to the heart, brain, and all bodily parts. This makes it useful for improving memory and relieving muscle pains. It also acts as an antioxidant, has antiaging effects, reduces blood pressure, inhibits blood clotting, and is helpful for tinnitus, vertigo, hearing loss, impotence, and Raynaud's disease.

Ginkgo biloba is widely known as the "smart herb" of our time. It has even been said to slow the early progression of Alzheimer's disease in some individuals. In one study of the very old (over eighty-five years of age), ginkgo biloba was shown to slow the progression of dementia and memory decline. There also was no increased risk of bleeding, as had been reported in earlier studies. One large study in nearly 3,000 people over the age of seventy found that ginkgo biloba did not reduce the likelihood of developing Alzheimer's disease. In this Alzheimer's study, there were no increased risks from using the herb and no differences in the development of other disease like heart disease and stroke between those who took ginkgo biloba and those who got a placebo.

Ginseng

Ginseng is used throughout the Far East as a general tonic to combat weakness and give extra energy. There are a number of different varieties of ginseng:

- *Eleutherococcus senticosus* (Siberian ginseng)

- *Panax quinquefolius* (American ginseng)

- *Panax ginseng* (Chinese or Korean ginseng)

- *Panax japonicum* (Japanese ginseng)

Panax ginseng is the most widely used species. Early Native Americans were familiar with ginseng and used it for stomach and bronchial disorders, asthma, and neck pain. Russian scientists claim that the ginseng root stimulates both physical and mental activity, improves endocrine gland function, and has a positive effect on the sex glands. It has been shown to help men regain sexual function. Ginseng is beneficial for fatigue because it spares glycogen (the form of glucose stored in the liver and muscle cells) by increasing the use of fatty acids as an energy source. It is used to enhance athletic performance, to rejuvenate, to increase longevity, and to detoxify and normalize the entire system. Many studies have shown ginseng to be effective at improving energy levels, endurance, and alertness. Cancer patients who used ginseng reported a better quality of life, especially related to mood and socialization. Postmenopausal women who used 500 milligrams of ginseng daily experienced improved quality of life, fewer menopause-related symptoms, and better sexual function.

In lower doses, ginseng seems to raise blood pressure, while higher amounts appear to reduce blood pressure. Research suggests that high doses of ginseng may be helpful for inflammatory diseases such as rheumatoid arthritis, without the side effects of steroids, and may also protect against the harmful effects of radiation. Ginseng is beneficial for people with diabetes because it decreases the level of the hormone cortisol in the blood (cortisol interferes with the function of insulin). Normal individuals who were tested with one of several specially prepared ginseng formulas experienced less blood sugar response after a meal, but the level was not low enough to be harmful. Other parts of the ginseng plant used in this study had no effect on blood sugar levels. A portion of the ginseng rootlet referred to as Rg1 seemed to be the most important regulator of blood sugar response to foods. Nevertheless, people with hypoglycemia should avoid using large amounts of ginseng.

The root is sold in many forms: as a whole root or root pieces, which are either untreated or blanched; as a powder or powdered extract; as a liquid extract or concentrate; in granules for instant tea; as a tincture; in an oil base; and in tablets and capsules. These products should not contain sugar or added color and should be pure ginseng. Many supplement manufacturers add ginseng to combination products, but these often contain such low amounts that they may not be effective.

We advise following the Russian approach to using ginseng: Take it for fifteen to twenty days, followed by a rest period of two weeks. Avoid long-term usage of high doses. Ginseng should not be used by people with high blood pressure, or during pregnancy or lactation.

Glucomannan

See under Fiber in this section.

Glucosamine

This is one of a number of substances classified as an *amino sugar*. Unlike other forms of sugar in the body, amino sugars are components of carbohydrates that are incorporated into the structure of body tissues, rather than being used as a source of energy. Glucosamine is thus involved in the formation of the nails, tendons, skin, eyes, bones, ligaments, and heart valves. It also plays a role in the mucous secretions of the digestive, respiratory, and urinary tracts.

Glucosamine is made in the body from the simple carbohydrate glucose and the amino acid glutamine. It is found in high concentrations in joint structures. It is also available as a supplement, in the form of glucosamine sulfate, which helps to combat both the causes and symptoms of osteoarthritis. Glucosamine has been studied in nearly 200 clinical trials. Although not all the participants in these studies responded to the supplements, most did. For patients with osteoarthritis of the knee, glucosamine was more effective than taking nothing and reduced the likelihood of needing a knee replacement. Glucosamine was also shown to help with acute injuries such as one would get from exercise. Athletes with recent knee injuries healed faster in terms of knee flexion and extension when using glucosamine compared to a group who took nothing.

It can also slightly reduce the destruction of cartilage and depression caused by taking nonsteroidal anti-inflammatory drugs (NSAIDs), which are commonly prescribed for people with arthritis. Glucosamine may be taken in conjunction with chondroitin sulfate for an even greater effect on osteoarthritis (*see* Chondroitin Sulfate in this section).

In addition to having benefits for people with osteoarthritis, supplemental glucosamine can be helpful for asthma, bursitis, candidiasis, food allergies, osteoporosis, respiratory allergies, tendinitis, vaginitis, and various skin problems. The product GS-500 from Enzymatic Therapy is a good source of glucosamine. GlucosaMend from Source Naturals is another recommended product. A related compound is N-acetylglucosamine (NAG), available as N-A-G from Source Naturals.

Grape Seed Oil

See under Essential Fatty Acids in this section.

"Green Drinks"

"Green drinks" are natural food formulas made from plants that are good detoxifiers and blood cleansers, as well as sources of chlorophyll, minerals, enzymes, and other important nutrients. Greens help neutralize acid buildup in the blood. Eating a Western diet, which is high in meat, dairy, and grains, produces an excess of hydrogen ions in the blood, making it acidic. An adequate intake of fruits and vegetables can counteract this effect, but few of us consume enough of these foods. The green drinks leave an alkaline residue upon digestion, just like fruits and vegetables. This neutralizes the acid from the other foods. Generally, green drinks are sold in powdered form to be mixed just before use. Many different companies market green drink formulas. We recommend buying organic green drinks. In addition, those that provide the greatest number of different plants offer a broader range of antioxidant protection. The following are some recommended products:

- BarleyLife from AIM International. This product contains a combination of barley juice and kelp.

- Earth Source Greens & More from Solgar. This formula combines four organically grown grasses (alfalfa, barley, kamut, and wheat), Hawaiian blue-green spirulina, and Chinese chlorella with three potent immune-stimulating mushrooms (maitake, reishi, and shiitake), plus powdered broccoli, carrots, and red beets, which supply phytonutrients. Its fruit flavor comes from fresh fruit powders.

- Green Magma from Green Foods Corporation. Green Magma is a pure, natural juice of young barley leaves that are organically grown in Japan and are pesticide-free. Brown rice is added to supply vitamins B_1 (thiamine) and B_3 (niacin) and linoleic acid. Green Magma contains thousands of enzymes, which play an important role in the metabolism of the body (*see* ENZYMES earlier in this book), plus a high concentration of superoxide dismutase (SOD). The powdered product may be added to juice or quality water.

- Kyo-Green from Wakunaga of America. This is a combination of barley, wheatgrass, kelp, and the green algae chlorella. The barley and wheatgrass are organically grown. It is a highly concentrated natural source of chlorophyll, amino acids, vitamins and minerals, carotene, and enzymes. Chlorella is a rich natural source of vitamin A, and kelp supplies iodine and other valuable minerals. (*See* Chlorella and Kelp in this section.)

- ProGreens from NutriCology (Allergy Research Group). ProGreens includes organic alfalfa, barley, oat, and wheatgrass juice powders; natural fiber; wheat sprouts; blue-green algae; sea algae; fructooligosaccharides (FOS); lecithin; standardized bioflavonoid extracts; along with royal jelly and bee pollen; beet and spinach extracts; acerola juice powder; natural vitamin E; and the herbs astragalus, echinacea, licorice, Siberian ginseng, and suma.

Green Papaya

Green (unripe) papaya is an excellent source of vitamins, minerals, and enzymes. Ounce for ounce, it contains more vitamin A than carrots and more vitamin C than oranges, as well as abundant B vitamins and vitamin E. The complex of enzymes it contains helps to digest proteins, carbohydrates, and fats.

Green papaya can be eaten fresh or taken in supplement form. Papain is the most abundant, most active enzyme in both the fresh fruit and the powdered supplement form. Papain possesses very powerful digestive action.

Guar Gum

See under Fiber in this section.

Hemicellulose

See under Fiber in this section.

Honey

Bees produce honey by mixing nectar, which is a sweet substance secreted by flowers, with bee enzymes. Honey is a highly concentrated source of many essential nutrients, including large amounts of carbohydrates (sugars), some minerals, B-complex vitamins, and vitamins C, D, and E.

Honey is used to promote energy and healing. It has been shown to be an effective treatment for relieving symptoms of coughing from an upper respiratory tract infection in people two to eighteen years of age. The FDA and leading medical groups have called the effectiveness of most cold and flu preparations into question. Honey offers a natural and effective alternative. It is a natural antiseptic and makes a good salve for burns and wounds. Honey is also used for sweetening foods and beverages. It varies somewhat in color and taste depending on the origin of the flower and nectar, but in general it is approximately twice as sweet as sugar, so not as much is needed for sweetening purposes.

People who have diabetes or hypoglycemia should be careful when consuming honey and its by-products. These substances affect blood sugar levels in the same way that refined sugars do. Tupelo honey contains more fructose than other types of honey and it is absorbed at a slower rate, so some people with hypoglycemia can use this type sparingly without ill effects.

Buy only unfiltered, unheated, unprocessed honey, and *never* give honey to an infant under one year of age. In its natural form, honey can contain spores of the bacteria that cause botulism. This poses no problem for adults and older children, but in infants and those with compromised immune systems, the spores can colonize the digestive tract and produce the deadly botulin toxin there. Honey is safe for babies after age one.

Inosine

Inosine occurs naturally in the human body. It is involved in the rebuilding of adenosine triphosphate (ATP) and stimulates the production of a compound designated 2,3-diphosphoglycerate (2,3-DPG), which is needed in the transportation of oxygen to muscle cells for the production of energy. Weight and endurance trainers have found supplemental inosine to be beneficial; it is believed to increase muscle development and blood circulation. It also enhances immune function.

If you have kidney problems or gout, you should not take inosine because it can increase the production of uric acid. For best results, use the dosage recommended by the manufacturer for your body size, and take it 45 to 60 minutes prior to exercising.

Inositol Hexaphosphate (IP$_6$)

Inositol hexaphosphate (IP$_6$, also known as phytic acid) is a compound consisting of the B vitamin inositol plus six phosphate groups. Found naturally in many foods, including wheat, rice, and legumes, it is a powerful antioxidant that has many positive effects on the body. Laboratory studies suggest it may fight cancer, prevent and treat heart disease, prevent kidney stones and liver disease, and also reduce cholesterol levels and prevent the inappropriate formation of blood clots, a major cause of heart attacks. IP$_6$ inhibits the activity of free radicals in the body, which slows the type of abnormal cell division associated with cancer and tumor growth. It works best very early in the development of malignant tumors, before the malignancy can even be recognized by the immune system. The cells are then normalized and begin to grow in the usual manner again.

IP$_6$ contains a substance designated beta-1,3-D-glucan, which helps to maintain a strong immune system in people undergoing chemotherapy and radiation. IP$_6$ protects the heart by preventing the formation of blood clots in blood vessels and reducing the levels of cholesterol and triglycerides (fats) in the bloodstream. It protects the liver by preventing fatty deposits from accumulating there. Studies have shown that a diet high in IP$_6$ is associated with a lower incidence of cancer of the breast, colon, and prostate.

Significant amounts of IP$_6$ are found in foods such as beans, brown rice, whole-kernel corn, sesame seeds, wheat bran, cornbread, grape juice, raisins, and mulberries. It can also be taken in supplement form. Some studies have shown that IP$_6$ may interfere with the body's absorption of minerals, so supplements should not be taken within one hour of meals. IP$_6$ from Jarrow

Formulas and Cell Forté IP-6 and Inositol from Enzymatic Therapy are recommended sources of IP_6.

Kelp

Kelp is a type of seaweed that can be eaten raw, but it is usually dried, granulated, or ground into powder. It is also available in a liquid form that can be added to drinking water. Granulated or powdered kelp can be used as a condiment and for flavoring, as a salt substitute. If you find the taste unappealing, you can purchase it in tablet form.

Kelp is a rich source of vitamins, especially the B vitamins, as well as of many valuable minerals and trace elements. It is reported to be very beneficial to brain tissue, the membranes surrounding the brain, the sensory nerves, and the spinal cord, as well as the nails and blood vessels. It has been used in the treatment of thyroid problems because of its iodine content and is useful for other conditions as varied as hair loss, obesity, and ulcers. It protects against the effects of radiation and softens stools. Kelp is recommended as a daily dietary supplement, especially for people with mineral deficiencies.

Kombucha Tea

The kombucha, or Manchurian, "mushroom" has reputedly been used in Asian countries and in Russia for centuries. The kombucha itself is not eaten. Rather, a tea is made by fermenting it for about a week in a mixture of water, sugar, and green or black tea, with apple cider vinegar or a bit of previously made tea added. Kept in this mixture, the kombucha reproduces, and the daughter mushrooms can then be used to produce more tea.

Although commonly referred to as a mushroom, kombucha is actually a combination of a number of different elements, including lichen, bacteria, and yeast. Kombucha tea contains a variety of different nutrients and other health-promoting substances. It is a natural energy booster and detoxifier that may also help slow or reverse the aging process.

Because of the way in which it has traditionally been propagated (one at a time, by individual users), kombucha may be difficult to find. Many people who have them received a daughter mushroom as a gift from a friend, although there are some herbal companies that sell both the mushrooms and the bottled tea commercially.

Lactobacillus acidophilus

Lactobacillus acidophilus is a type of "friendly" bacteria that assists in the digestion of proteins, a process in which lactic acid, hydrogen peroxide, enzymes, B vitamins, and antibiotic substances that inhibit pathogenic organisms are produced. Acidophilus has antifungal properties, helps to reduce blood cholesterol levels, aids digestion, and enhances the absorption of nutrients.

The flora in the healthy colon should consist of at least 85 percent lactobacilli and 15 percent coliform bacteria. However, the typical colon bacteria count today is the reverse. This can result in gas, bloating, intestinal and systemic toxicity, constipation, and malabsorption of nutrients, and is conducive to an overgrowth of candida. Taking an acidophilus supplement helps to combat all of these problems by returning the intestinal flora to a healthier balance. In addition, acidophilus may help to detoxify harmful substances. Between 5 and 30 percent of those who take antibiotics develop antibiotic-associated diarrhea, and *Lactobacillus acidophilus* may prevent it.

There are many good acidophilus supplements available. Acidophilus products come in tablet, capsule, and powdered forms. We recommend using the powdered form. Natren markets quality products that contain very high numbers of organisms. Other good nondairy acidophilus supplements include Primadophilus from Nature's Way, Probiotic All-Flora from New Chapter, and Mega Probiotic from DaVinci Labs.

Acidophilus can die at high temperatures. Whatever product you choose, keep it in a cool, dry place—refrigerate but do not freeze it. Take acidophilus on an empty stomach in the morning and one hour before each meal. If you are taking antibiotics, do not take the antibiotics and acidophilus simultaneously.

Lactoferrin

Lactoferrin is a protein that occurs naturally in human bile, tears, mucus, saliva, and milk. Because it binds with free iron in the body, it plays an important role in regulating iron levels (and, in turn, growth) and aids in preventing and fighting infection by depriving disease-causing organisms of the iron they need to grow and multiply. It also plays a role in the functioning of lymphocytes, a type of white blood cell important for immunity. Taken in supplement form, it may boost immune function and help in combating both infectious and inflammatory conditions. It may also benefit intestinal health.

Lecithin

Lecithin is a type of lipid that is needed by every living cell in the human body. Cell membranes, which regulate the passage of nutrients into and out of the cells, are largely composed of lecithin. The protective sheaths surrounding the brain are composed of lecithin, and the muscles and nerve cells also contain this essential fatty substance.

Lecithin consists mostly of the B vitamin choline, and also contains linoleic acid and inositol. Although lecithin is a lipid, it is partly soluble in water and thus acts as an emulsifying agent. This is why many processed foods contain lecithin.

This nutrient helps to prevent arteriosclerosis, protects against cardiovascular disease, improves brain function, and aids in the absorption of thiamine by the liver and vitamin A by the intestine. It is also known to promote energy and is needed to help repair damage to the liver caused by alcoholism. Lecithin enables fats, such as cholesterol and other lipids, to be dispersed in water and removed from the body. The vital organs and arteries are thus protected from fatty buildup.

Lecithin would be a wise addition to anyone's diet. It is especially valuable for older adults. Women aged forty to sixty benefited from a high dose of lecithin (1,200 milligrams) more than a lower dose (600 milligrams). Women who had initially complained of fatigue had more vigor and experienced lowering of blood pressure. Any adult who is taking niacin for high serum cholesterol and triglycerides should also include lecithin in his or her program. Two tablespoons of lecithin granules can be sprinkled on cereals and soups or added to juices or breads. Lecithin also comes in capsule form. Taking one 1,200-milligram capsule before each meal helps in the digestion of fats and the absorption of fat-soluble vitamins. A mixture of lecithin and soy stanols has been shown to be an effective cholesterol-lowering supplement. It can reduce the amount of cholesterol absorbed from the diet, thereby reducing both total cholesterol and LDL ("bad" cholesterol).

Most lecithin is derived from soybeans, but egg lecithin has become popular. This type of lecithin is extracted from the yolks of fresh eggs. Egg lecithin may hold promise for those suffering from AIDS, herpes, chronic fatigue syndrome, and immune disorders associated with aging. Studies have shown that it works better for people with these disorders than soy lecithin does. Other sources of lecithin include brewer's yeast, grains, legumes, fish, and wheat germ.

Lignin
See under Fiber in this section.

Maitake
Maitake (*Grifola frondosa*) is a mushroom that has a long history of use in traditional Chinese and Japanese herbology and cooking. It grows wild in Japan, as well as in some wooded areas in eastern North America. Because maitake is difficult to cultivate, however, only relatively recently have the mushrooms become widely available.

Maitake is considered an adaptogen, which means that it helps the body adapt to stress and normalizes bodily functions. Its healing properties are thought to be related to its high content of a polysaccharide called beta-1,6-glucan, which is considered very powerful. In laboratory studies, this substance has been shown to prevent carcinogenesis, inhibit the growth of cancerous tumors, kill HIV, and enhance the activity of key immune cells known as T-helper cells or CD4 cells. Maitake may also be useful for diabetes, chronic fatigue syndrome, chronic hepatitis, obesity, and high blood pressure. A Japanese study found that maitake may promote ovulation in women with polycystic ovary disease. Some women took the standard drug (clomiphene citrate), and others received an extract of maitake. The percentage of women who ovulated was not statistically different between the two groups (93 percent for the drug group and 77 percent in the maitake group).

Maitake can be eaten in food or taken as a supplement. Buy organically grown dried mushrooms (when using them in cooking, soak them in water or broth for half an hour first), or purchase maitake in capsule, extract, or tea form. Some of the capsule supplements contain a small amount of vitamin C, which enhances the effectiveness of the active ingredient in maitake by aiding in its absorption.

Melatonin

The hormone melatonin is naturally produced by the pineal gland, a cone-shaped structure in the brain. The body's pattern of melatonin production is similar to that of the other "antiaging" hormones, human growth hormone (HGH) and dehydroepiandrosterone (DHEA). Throughout early life, melatonin is produced in abundance. It was thought for some time that the production of melatonin begins to drop at puberty and then continues to decline steadily as we age. This may not be true, according to research done at the Harvard Medical School. Researchers say that older people who were on aspirin therapy might have skewed the results because taking aspirin reduces melatonin levels in the body.

Research has demonstrated that melatonin may have several profound long-term effects on the body. As one of the most powerful antioxidants ever discovered—with a greater range of effectiveness than vitamin C, vitamin E, or beta-carotene—melatonin helps prevent harmful oxidation reactions from occurring. In this way, melatonin may prevent the changes that lead to hypertension and heart attack and may reduce the risk of certain kinds of cancer. Melatonin also has been found to stimulate the immune system; have a major role in the production of estrogen, testosterone, and possibly other hormones, helping to prevent cancers involving the reproductive system; and slow the growth of existing malignancies. Studies suggest that if melatonin is taken in the mornings, tumor growth may be stimulated, but if it is taken in the evenings, tumor growth tends to be slowed. In addition, as melatonin is secreted cyclically, in response to the fall of darkness at the end of each day, the hormone helps our bodies keep in sync with the rhythms of day and night. Thus, melatonin helps regulate sleep.

Research on melatonin continues, and with it, knowledge is increasing about the functions of melatonin in the body and the effects of melatonin supplementation. Melatonin is the internal sleep facilitator in humans. Both human research studies and anecdotal evidence indicate that melatonin supplements can be an effective and side-effect-free sleep aid both for adults suffering from insomnia and for children with autism, epilepsy, Down syndrome, cerebral palsy, and other problems that can cause sleep disorders. There is evidence that supplemental melatonin can induce sleep by reducing restlessness before sleep, and correct sleep patterns during sleep so you feel rested upon awakening. Sleeping disorders increase with age, and melatonin has been shown to help. Subjects over fifty-five years of age who used 2 milligrams of time-released melatonin had better quality of sleep and felt more alert in the morning. It has been shown to be effective in those who suffer from minor sleep disorders when used on a regular basis, and episodically for jet lag or shift workers. In addition, in a rare condition resulting in nocturnal hypertension, patients using melatonin experienced a reduction in blood pressure while they slept. For patients with mild cognitive impairment, melatonin allowed for better performance on several tests that assess cognitive function. Mental acuity was thought to improve because the patients slept better and felt refreshed in the morning.

Animal and other laboratory research indicates that melatonin supplementation may help prevent age-related disorders and perhaps extend life. Melatonin can be taken to ease PMS symptoms; stimulate the immune system; prevent memory loss, arteriosclerosis, and stroke; and treat cancer and Alzheimer's disease. People who suffer from migraines (two to eight per month) tried melatonin as a potential treatment. The study found that 3 milligrams of melatonin is better than taking nothing for migraine prevention, more tolerable than amitriptyline (a common drug used to treat migraines), and just as effective as 25 milligrams of amitriptyline.

Although no toxic levels of melatonin have been found, it is a powerful hormone, and some researchers feel that certain people probably should not use this supplement until further information is available. Included in this category are pregnant and nursing women; people with severe allergies or autoimmune diseases; people with immune system cancers, such as lymphoma and leukemia; and healthy children, who already produce sufficient amounts of the hormone. Because high doses of melatonin have been found to act as a contraceptive, women who wish to become pregnant also might want to avoid taking this supplement.

Melatonin should be taken two hours or less before bedtime. This schedule is designed to release the added hormone at the same time that natural production peaks. A sustained-release form is best if you frequently awaken after several

MAINTAINING YOUR MELATONIN LEVEL NATURALLY

As darkness falls at the end of each day, melatonin production rises. In the morning, when daylight hits the retina, neural impulses cause production of the hormone to slow. Clearly, light and darkness are the primary factors that set the rhythms of melatonin production. However, they are not the only factors involved. In fact, it has been found that a variety of regular daily routines can strengthen the rhythm of melatonin production. Here are a few simple ways in which you can help your body maintain high levels of this important hormone:

- Eat regular meals. The rhythm of melatonin production is strengthened by regular daily routines. Keep your mealtimes as regular as possible to keep your body in sync with the rhythms of the day.

- Keep your diet light at night. When melatonin production begins after nightfall, the digestive process is slowed. Thus, any heavy foods eaten close to bedtime may lead to digestive problems, which can make it difficult to sleep. To get the sleep you need, eat small, light meals in the late evening.

- Avoid stimulants. Stimulants such as coffee, tea, and caffeine-containing medications and soft drinks can interfere with melatonin production by interfering with your sleep. As much as possible, eliminate these stimulants from your diet and lifestyle. Or at the very least, allow at least four to five hours between the time you consume them and bedtime.

- Avoid exercising late at night. Vigorous activity delays melatonin secretion. If you exercise in the morning, you will reinforce healthful sleeping habits that lead to regular melatonin production. For best results, do your morning exercise outdoors, in the morning light.

hours' sleep; a sublingual form is best if you are very ill or suffer from malabsorption. When you awaken after melatonin-assisted sleep, you should feel refreshed—not tired or groggy. If you do experience grogginess, you should reduce the dosage. (To learn how you can maintain or increase your melatonin levels through daily routines, *see* Maintaining Your Melatonin Level Naturally on page 249.)

Methylsulfonylmethane (MSM)

Methylsulfonylmethane (MSM, also known as dimethylsulfone) is a naturally occurring organic sulfur compound found in plant and animal tissues that is essential for optimum health. It is a derivative of dimethylsulfoxide (DMSO) that has remarkable therapeutic properties, especially for the healing of injuries. It can also help to detoxify the body on a cellular level. MSM helps to nourish the hair, skin, and nails; relieve pain and inflammation; reduce allergy problems; and promote gastrointestinal health. It has also been found to aid immune function, and there have been reports of benefits to patients with heartburn, arthritis, lung problems, migraines, and muscle pain. MSM is present naturally in foods such as fresh fish, meat, plants, fruit, and milk. However, it can be eliminated by even moderate processing, including drying or heating.

Most North Americans today eat considerable amounts of processed food, and MSM is normally either not present at all or present only in very small amounts in the typical diet. Most people therefore would probably benefit from supplementation.

Research suggests that we require a constant supply of MSM for optimum good health, as sulfur is one of the essential minerals. Commonly recommended dosage levels are about 2,000 milligrams (2 grams) per day taken in divided doses, with the morning and evening meals, but it is best to start out at 1,000 milligrams (1 gram) per day to avoid a too-rapid rate of detoxification. Higher doses (3,000 milligrams twice a day) were shown to be safe and effective at helping patients with osteoarthritis perform daily activities and feel better in general. The positive effects in this study occurred in eighty-four days. However, benefits could become evident in as few as two to twenty-one days and can be enhanced by vitamin C supplementation. In addition, when MSM was combined with sternum collagen II, pain and soreness decreased in a group of patients with osteoarthritis. MSM is found in a variety of products from the following companies: Aerobic Life Industries, Allergy Research Group, Bluebonnet Nutrition, Jarrow, and Natrol.

Mucilage
See under Fiber in this section.

Nicotinamide Adenine Dinucleotide (NADH)
NADH is a form of vitamin B_3 (niacin) that is essential for the production of various neurotransmitters and cellular energy. NADH, which is also known as coenzyme 1, also acts as an antioxidant (*see under* ANTIOXIDANTS starting on page 179).

As we age, natural levels of NADH decline, which can lead to reduced levels of both energy and significant brain chemicals. Taking supplemental NADH can result in improvements in the biochemistry of energy production, especially in the brain and nervous systems. NADH shows promise as a therapy for Parkinson's disease because it results in an increase in brain levels of the neurotransmitter dopamine, which is deficient in people with this disorder.

People with Alzheimer's disease may be helped by this supplement as well. Some people suffering from chronic fatigue syndrome (CFS) have shown significant improvement with NADH therapy.

Oat Bran
See under Fiber in this section.

Octacosanol

Octacosanol is a naturally derived wheat germ oil concentrate. Although it would be possible to extract octacosanol from whole wheat, 10 pounds of wheat would be needed to obtain just 1,000 micrograms of octacosanol. Wheat germ has long been known for its many benefits. Today, extracts of wheat germ weighing only 2 milligrams offer remarkable benefits as well.

Octacosanol has been clinically proven to increase oxygen utilization during exercise and improve glycogen stores in muscle tissue. As a result, it increases physical endurance, improves reaction time, reduces high-altitude stress, and aids in tissue oxygenation. This substance can greatly benefit those who experience muscle pain after exercise or have a lowered endurance level. It is good for muscular dystrophies and other neuromuscular disorders as well. It also reduces blood cholesterol levels.

Olive Leaf Extract

Olive leaf extract is an herbal supplement that has been shown to be effective against virtually all the viruses and bacteria on which it has been tested. Laboratory studies suggest that olive leaf extract interferes with viral infection becoming established and/or spreading, either by rendering viruses incapable of infecting cells or by preventing them from reproducing. It has been shown to help protect against infection by such viruses as human immunodeficiency virus (HIV), herpesviruses, and influenza viruses. It is useful for such disorders as pneumonia, sore throat, sinusitis, and skin diseases such as chronic infections and rashes, as well as for fungal and bacterial infections. Olivir 15 from DaVinci Laboratories is a good source of olive leaf extract that has been tested in clinical trials.

Pectin

See under Fiber in this section.

Perilla

Perilla (*Perilla frutescens*) is an Asian plant that is a member of the mint family. It has been prescribed by Asian herbalists for the relief of cough and lung ailments and for certain types of food poisoning, as well as to prevent the flu and restore energy balance. It may aid in increasing learning ability and is also used as a culinary herb. Investigators in Thailand tested perilla oil in people with mild to moderate dementia. The perilla oil was not effective at improving cognition but did lower total cholesterol and LDL cholesterol.

Perilla comes in several forms, including seed oil. This is an unsaturated oil that contains linolenic, linoleic, and oleic acids. Perilla oil is available in capsule form. Studies suggest that it may be an effective and safe source of essential omega-3 fatty acids.

Phosphatidylcholine (PC)

Phosphatidylcholine (PC) is a component of lecithin. (*See* Lecithin in this section.) Taken as a supplement, it helps to break down fats and can be helpful in preventing atherosclerosis (hardening of the arteries due to fatty plaques in the blood vessels), heart disease, gallstones, and liver problems. It has also shown substantial benefits for people with neurological disorders, memory loss, and depression.

PC is known to be safe and effective; however, people with bipolar mood disorder should not take large amounts.

Phosphatidylserine (PS)

Phosphatidylserine (PS) is a substance classified as a phospholipid (a phosphorus-containing lipid) that is needed by every cell in the body and is especially abundant in nerve cells. PS is the most important of the phospholipids and is crucial for the maintenance of healthy cell membranes. Although the brain normally produces enough PS, production dwindles as we age, which can result in deficiency. The Food and Drug Administration has granted PS a Qualified Health Claim. Products that contain PS can claim either of these statements:

- Phosphatidylserine (PS) may reduce the risk of cognitive dysfunction in the elderly. *Very limited and preliminary scientific research suggests that PS may reduce the risk of cognitive dysfunction in the elderly. FDA concludes that there is very little scientific evidence supporting this claim.*

- Phosphatidylserine (PS) may reduce the risk of dementia in the elderly. *Very limited and preliminary scientific research suggests that PS may reduce the risk of dementia in the elderly. FDA concludes that there is little scientific evidence supporting this claim.*

Supplemental PS, which is compounded from soybean oil in products sold in the United States, has been said to reduce symptoms of depression and Alzheimer's disease, and to enhance memory and learning abilities. Some of the earlier studies on this product focused on PS from cow brains, which is no longer sold in the United States. That was a different product chemically from the soy-based product sold today and results may not be the same. Some people have experienced nausea as a result of taking PS; however, taking it with food can help to avoid this. No danger has been reported with long-term use of the soy-based supplement. Its safety for pregnant women has not been determined.

Primrose Oil
See under Essential Fatty Acids in this section.

Probiotics
Probiotics are beneficial bacteria normally present in the digestive tract. They are vital for proper digestion and also perform a number of other useful functions, such as preventing the overgrowth of yeast and other pathogens and synthesizing vitamin K. The probiotics most often used as supplements are acidophilus and bifidobacteria. (*See Lactobacillus acidophilus* and/or *Bifidobacterium bifidum* in this section.)

Cultured, or fermented, foods also contain various types and amounts of beneficial bacteria. These foods include buttermilk, cheese, kefir, miso, sauerkraut, tempeh, umeboshi, and yogurt.

Progesterone Cream

Progesterone is a hormone that is produced primarily by the ovaries and also by the adrenal glands. It works in partnership with estrogen to regulate menstrual cycles and is important for the maintenance of pregnancy. In addition to its role in the female reproductive system, it has a number of other important effects: it stimulates the activity of bone-building cells called osteoblasts; exerts an antidepressant and calming effect in the brain; helps to regulate blood sugar levels; and plays a role in maintaining the myelin sheaths that protect nerve cells. It can be used by the body to produce other hormones, including DHEA, estrogen, testosterone, and cortisol, as needed. A deficiency of progesterone, on the other hand, can exacerbate symptoms of premenstrual syndrome (PMS) and menopausal discomfort and may increase the risk of osteoporosis. Progesterone deficiency becomes increasingly common in women as they approach menopause and can start as early as age thirty-five. Symptoms can include night sweats, hot flashes, depression, and premenstrual discomfort.

Supplemental progesterone is available in cream form. The hormone is absorbed through the skin after the cream is applied, and it passes directly into the bloodstream for transport to sites where progesterone is needed. As these are biologically active substances, consult your health care professional before using them.

Propolis
See Bee Propolis in this section.

Psyllium Seed
See under Fiber in this section.

Red Yeast Rice
Red yeast rice is a food product created by fermenting rice with

a strain of red yeast (*Monascus purpureus* Went yeast). It is also sometimes referred to as Monascus rice or, in Chinese, *Hung-chu* or *Hong-Qu*. It has long been used in China and Japan as a food and as a remedy for digestive ailments and poor circulation. More recently, red yeast rice extract, taken in supplement form, has been found both to reduce overall blood cholesterol levels and to improve the ratio of HDL ("good" cholesterol) to LDL ("bad" cholesterol). A study conducted by the University of California, Los Angeles, School of Medicine found that people who took red yeast rice and maintained a low-fat diet reduced their overall cholesterol levels by an average of 40 points over a period of twelve weeks. The extract contains a number of cholesterol-lowering compounds known as *statins*. One of these is lovastatin, a substance also sold as a prescription drug under the brand name Mevacor. Lovastatin acts to lower cholesterol by inhibiting the action of an enzyme designated HMG-CoA reductase, which in turn limits the rate at which the body produces cholesterol. Studies have shown statins to lower cholesterol levels and reduce the risk of heart attack. Unlike prescription products, red yeast rice extract has shown no serious adverse side effects in clinical trials. Smaller amounts of lovastatin from a plant as opposed to drugs are required to be effective. This is because it is thought that the natural compounds in the plant work synergistically with the active ingredient. Merck, which sells Mevacor, asked the FDA to ban red yeast rice extract. The FDA considered Merck's request but decided to allow companies to continue to sell it. However, the FDA did mandate that there cannot be any mention of lowering cholesterol levels or reducing heart disease risk. Check with your health care professional before using red yeast rice.

Reishi

See Shiitake and Reishi in this section.

Rice Bran

See under Fiber in this section.

Royal Jelly

Royal jelly is a thick, milky substance that is secreted from the pharyngeal glands of a special group of young nurse bees between their sixth and twelfth days of life. When honey and pollen are combined and refined within the young nurse bee, royal jelly is naturally created. This substance contains all of the B-complex vitamins, including a high concentration of pantothenic acid (vitamin B_5) and vitamin B_6 (pyridoxine), and is the only natural source of pure acetylcholine. Royal jelly also contains minerals, enzymes, hormones, eighteen amino acids, antibacterial and antibiotic components, and vitamins A, C, D, and E. It is useful for bronchial asthma, liver disease, pancreatitis, insomnia, stomach ulcers, kidney disease, bone fractures, and skin disorders, and it strengthens the immune system. Women who were experiencing symptoms associated with menopause benefited from taking 1,000 milligrams daily over eight weeks. This product must be combined with honey to preserve its potency. Royal jelly spoils easily. Keep it refrigerated and make sure it is tightly sealed when purchased.

S-Adenosylmethionine (SAMe)

S-adenosylmethionine (SAMe) is a derivative of the amino acid methionine that is formed in the body when methionine combines with adenosine triphosphate (ATP), the major source of cellular energy. Taken as a supplement, SAMe has a variety of positive effects:

- It is an effective antidepressant.

- It is beneficial for disorders of the joints and connective tissue, including arthritis and fibromyalgia.

- It promotes the health of the liver.

- It may lower levels of homocysteine, an amino acid that is associated with cardiovascular disease.

- It may help to slow the aging process.

SAMe works closely with folic acid, choline, and vitamins B_6 and B_{12}. It is one of a class of substances called *methyl donors*. As the name implies, methyl donors are compounds that "donate" units called methyl groups, which contain hydrogen and carbon atoms, to other substances. This process is called *methylation,* and it is one way in which the body protects itself from damage on the cellular level.

Among other things, methyl donors help to protect against such serious disorders as cancer, heart disease, neurological disorders, and many age-related problems, and facilitate the manufacture of DNA and brain neurotransmitters. SAMe increases catechol-O-methyltransferase (COMT) enzyme activity, which has been shown to somewhat lessen aggressive symptoms in schizophrenia. In addition, brain waves of elderly patients with depression responded favorably with SAMe at different doses. The effect was observed at one hour and lasted up to six. Use of SAMe alone without other medications was not effective in making most individuals with depression feel better. However, those with mild depression fared well with 800 milligrams of SAMe daily, indicating that for those without severe depression, SAMe may be an effective and safe treatment option. In patients with AIDS, depressive symptoms were improved with SAMe, and the change was noted after one week of treatment. SAMe has also been shown to be effective when coupled with drugs classified as selective serotonin reuptake inhibitors (SSRIs). If you are taking medications for depression, check with your health care provider before using SAMe.

Taking supplemental SAMe may also increase natural levels of glutathione, an antioxidant; phosphatidylcholine, which aids in the metabolism of fats; and the hormone melatonin. A small number of people have experienced minor nausea, gastrointestinal disturbances, and headaches as a result of taking high doses, but otherwise no notable side effects have been reported. Although SAMe is considered very safe, anyone with bipolar mood disorder should consult a physician before taking this supplement. Do not give to a child under twelve. SAMe should always be taken on an empty stomach. Be sure what you purchase is actually SAMe, because there have been some knockoffs. It is rather costly.

Sea Cucumber

Sea cucumbers, also known as *bêche de mer* and *trepang,* are not actually cucumbers, but are marine animals related to starfish and sea urchins. They have been used in China for thousands of years as a treatment for arthritis. Modern research has confirmed they are beneficial for musculoskeletal inflammatory diseases, especially rheumatoid arthritis, osteoarthritis, and ankylosing spondylitis, a rheumatic disease that affects the spine.

Researchers believe that sea cucumbers improve the balance of prostaglandins, which regulate the inflammatory process. They also contain substances known as chondroitins, which are often lacking in people with arthritis and connective tissue disorders (*see* Chondroitin Sulfate in this section). In addition, sea cucumbers provide vitamins A, B_1 (thiamine), B_2 (riboflavin), B_3 (niacin), and C, as well as the minerals calcium, iron, magnesium, and zinc.

Sea Mussel

The green-lipped mussel (*Perna canaliculus*) is a species of edible shellfish. These mussels contain numerous amino acids, the building blocks of body proteins, in addition to enzymes and essential trace elements. The minerals they contain are present in a balance similar to that in blood plasma, and these minerals are naturally chelated by the amino acids, making for better assimilation into the body.

Sea mussel aids in the functioning of the cardiovascular system, the lymphatic system, the endocrine system, the eyes, connective tissues, and mucous membranes. They help to reduce inflammation and relieve the pain and stiffness of arthritis. They also promote the healing of wounds and burns.

Shark Cartilage

The tough, elastic material that makes up the skeleton of the shark is dried and pulverized (finely powdered) to make this food supplement. Shark cartilage contains a number of active components, the most important of which is a type of protein that acts as an angiogenesis inhibitor—that is, it supposedly acts to suppress the development of new blood vessels. This would make it valuable in fighting a number of disorders. Many cancerous tumors, for instance, are able to grow only because they induce the body to develop new networks of blood vessels to supply them with nutrients.

Shark cartilage is said to suppress this process, so that tumors are deprived of their source of nourishment and often begin to shrink. Many patients with advanced stages of cancer of the breast, colon, prostate, and other organs have sought shark cartilage as a means to avoid disease progression. To date, however, studies show that shark cartilage has no impact on disease progression, and many patients had adverse side effects from using the product.

There are certain eye disorders, such as diabetic retinopathy and macular degeneration, that are characterized by the growth of new blood vessels within the eye; because they grow in inappropriate places, the presence of these blood vessels can lead to blindness. Such diseases also may respond well to shark cartilage. Other conditions for which shark cartilage is useful include arthritis, psoriasis, and regional enteritis (inflammation of the lining of the bowels). In addition to angiogenesis-inhibiting protein, shark cartilage contains calcium (approximately 16 percent) and phosphorus (approximately 8 percent), which are absorbed as nutrients, and mucopolysaccharides that act to stimulate the immune system.

Shark cartilage is available in powder and capsule forms. Exercise caution when buying shark cartilage, as the purity and correct processing of the product are vital to its effectiveness. Not all shark cartilage products contain only 100 percent pure shark cartilage, so read labels carefully.

Pure shark cartilage is white in color. If you are taking large quantities of shark cartilage, it may be wise to increase your supplementation of certain minerals, especially magnesium and potassium, to maintain a proper mineral balance in the body. Shark cartilage should *not* be taken by pregnant women or children, or by persons who have recently undergone surgery or suffered a heart attack.

Shiitake and Reishi

Shiitake and reishi are Japanese mushrooms with a delicate texture, strong stems, and well-defined undersides. They are attractive and have impressive health-promoting properties.

Shiitake (*Lentinus edodes*) contain a polysaccharide, lentinan, that strengthens the immune system by increasing T cell function. Shiitake mushrooms contain eighteen amino acids, seven of which are essential amino acids. They are rich in B vitamins, especially vitamins B_1 (thiamine), B_2 (riboflavin), and B_3 (niacin). When sun-dried, they contain high amounts of vitamin D. These mushrooms are considered delicacies and are entirely edible.

Reishi (*Ganoderma lucidum*) have been popular for at least two thousand years in the Far East. They were rated number one on ancient Chinese lists of superior medicines and were believed to give eternal youth and longevity.

Today, both shiitake and reishi mushrooms are used to treat a variety of disorders and to promote vitality. They are used to prevent high blood pressure and heart disease, to control and lower cholesterol, to build resistance to disease, and to treat fatigue and viral infections. They are also known to have antitumor properties valuable in treating cancer.

The mushrooms are available fresh or dried for use in foods (soak dried mushrooms in warm water or broth for 30 minutes before using), as well as in supplements in capsule, pill, and extract form.

Spirulina

Spirulina is a microalgae that thrives in hot, sunny climates and in alkaline waters around the world, and produces twenty times as much protein as soybeans growing on an equal-sized area of land. It contains concentrations of nutrients unlike any other single grain, herb, or plant. Among its valuable components are gamma-linolenic acid (GLA), linoleic and arachidonic acids, vitamin B_{12} (needed, especially by vegetarians, for healthy red blood cells), iron, a high level of protein (60 to 70 percent), essential amino acids, and the nucleic acids RNA and DNA, along with chlorophyll, and phycocyanin, a blue pigment that is found only in blue-green algae and that has increased the survival rate of mice with liver cancer in laboratory experiments. Spirulina has been clinically tested and has shown a variety of effects. Those with the common cold experienced less sneezing and congestion. Others showed lowered cholesterol levels and blood pressure. The use of spirulina helped promote weight loss in a group of obese individuals with high blood pressure. Use of 2 grams daily of *Spirulina maxima* produced weight loss, reductions in waist circumferences, and improvements in LDL cholesterol and insulin sensitivity. The authors suggested that this may offer a new tool to help hypertensive people lose weight. Finally, those who used spirulina as part of their regular diet had reduced post-exercise muscle soreness that may have allowed them to have longer workout sessions.

Spirulina is a naturally digestible food that aids in protecting the immune system, in cholesterol reduction, and in mineral absorption. Because it supplies nutrients needed to help cleanse and heal, while also curbing the appetite, it is beneficial for people who are fasting. A person with hypoglycemia may benefit from using this food supplement between meals because its high protein content helps stabilize blood sugar levels.

Torula Yeast

See Yeast in this section.

Wheat Germ

Wheat germ is the embryo of the wheat berry. It is a good source of vitamin E; most of the B vitamins; the minerals calcium, magnesium, and phosphorus; and several trace elements.

One problem with wheat germ is that it spoils easily. If you purchase wheat germ separately from the flour, make sure the product is fresh. It should be either vacuum-packed or refrigerated, with a packing date or a label stating the date by which the product should be used. Toasted wheat germ has a longer shelf life, but the raw product is better because it is unprocessed. Wheat germ oil capsules are also available.

Wheatgrass

Wheatgrass is a rich nutritional food that was popularized by the late Dr. Ann Wigmore, an educator and founder of the Hippocrates Health Institute in Boston. Wheatgrass contains a great variety of vitamins, minerals, and trace elements. According to Dr. Wigmore, 1 pound of fresh wheatgrass is equal in nutritional value to nearly 25 pounds of the choicest vegetables.

Dr. Wigmore reported that wheatgrass therapy, along with "living foods," helped to eliminate cancerous growths and helped many other disorders, including mental health problems. The molecular structure of chlorophyll resembles that of hemoglobin, the oxygen-carrying protein of red blood cells, and this may be the reason for the effectiveness of wheatgrass. The key difference between the two is that the metallic atom in the middle of each molecule of human hemoglobin is iron, while the metallic atom at the center of a molecule of chlorophyll is magnesium. In experiments on anemic animals, blood counts returned to normal after four to five days of receiving chlorophyll.

Whey Protein

Whey is a normal by-product of cheesemaking; it is the liquid that is left when the solids in milk come together and are pressed into solid form. Filtering and purifying produce whey protein. Then the water is removed to produce a powder that, while high in quality protein, is free of fat and lactose (milk sugar).

This supplement helps to build lean body mass by increasing the body's production of muscle protein. A 30-gram serving of whey protein contains nearly all of the essential amino acids necessary each day. For this reason, it is popular among athletes and bodybuilders, and may also help to protect against muscle wasting in people with such diseases as AIDS and cancer. In addition to its effect on muscles, it appears to inhibit the proliferation of cancer cells, protect against free radical damage, and enhance immune function. Compared to soy protein, whey seems more effective at promoting weight loss. Some recommended whey protein supplements include Enhanced Life Extension Whey Protein from Life Extension, Molkosan from A. Vogel/Bioforce USA, and Whey to Go from Solgar.

Yeast

Yeast are single-celled organisms that can multiply at extremely rapid rates, doubling in number in two hours. Yeast is rich in many basic nutrients, such as the B vitamins (except for vitamin B_{12}), sixteen amino acids, and at least fourteen different minerals. The protein content of yeast is responsible for 52 percent of its weight. Yeast is also high in phosphorus.

There are various media on which yeast may be grown. Brewer's yeast, also known as nutritional yeast, is grown on hops, a bitter herb that is also used as an ingredient in beer. Torula yeast is grown on blackstrap molasses or wood pulp. A liquid yeast product from Switzerland called Bio-Strath, distributed by A. Vogel/Bioforce USA, is derived from herbs, honey, and malt. It is a natural product that we highly recommend.

Live baker's yeast should be avoided. Live yeast cells actually deplete the body of B vitamins and other nutrients. In nutritional yeast, these live cells are destroyed, leaving the beneficial nutrients behind.

Yeast may be consumed in juice or water and is a good energy booster between meals. It can also be added to the diet to aid in treating certain disorders. It helps in sugar metabolism and is good for eczema, heart disorders, gout, nervousness, and fatigue. By enhancing the immune system, yeast is useful for people undergoing radiation therapy or chemotherapy for cancer. Yeast also seems to increase mental and physical efficiency.

Specialty Supplements

In addition to the substances discussed above, there are many natural food supplements designed for specific circumstances.

There are too many of these products for us to discuss all of them here, but some that we feel are to be highly recommended are the following:

- Allergy Relief formulas from bioAllers. These are eight homeopathic formulas designed to relieve allergies by combining homeopathic remedies with specific allergens to help strengthen resistance to those allergens. Formulas include Animal Hair/Dander; Grain/Dairy; Grass Pollen; Mold/Yeast/Dust; Pollen/Hayfever; Sinus & Allergy Nasal Spray; and Tree Pollen.

- Betatene. This is a dietary supplement of mixed carotenoids, including alpha- and beta-carotene, lutein, lycopene, zeaxanthin, and cryptoxanthin. It is intended to help maintain a healthy and strong immune system.

- Bone Maximizer from Metabolic Response Modifiers. This is a combination supplement that contains microcrystalline hydroxyapatite concentrate (MCHC). MCHC is a source of bone proteins and highly absorbable calcium. Other ingredients include glucosamine, pregnenolone, vitamin D, magnesium, methylsulfonylmethane (MSM, a source of bioavailable sulfur), and other nutrients vital for bone health.

- Bone Support with Ostivone from Twinlab. This is a combination supplement designed to help maintain healthy bones. Ingredients include ipriflavone, calcium, vitamin D, magnesium, boron, and purified soy phytoestrogen extracts.

- Cardiaforce from A. Vogel/Bioforce USA. This hawthorn berry extract promotes healthy cardiovascular function, circulation, and heart muscle strength. It is a liquid supplement that is meant to be added to water and taken three times a day, before meals. It has no known interactions with other medications and should be taken over a period of several months, with periodic short interruptions.

- Cold, flu, and allergy season formulas from ZAND. This is a line of products designed to support health through the various allergy seasons of the year. Individual formulas include Insure Herbal, an echinacea and goldenseal formula; Decongest Herbal, a natural decongestant formula; Herbal-Mist throat spray; and Allergy Season Formula, which contains bromelain, nettle extract, quercetin, and vitamin B_5 (pantothenic acid). These formulas can be used individually or on a rotating basis.

- Noni from Earth's Bounty. Noni (*Morinda citrifolia*) is a small tree that grows in Hawaii and other tropical regions. The fruit of this plant has a long history of use for a wide variety of problems, including joint problems, pain, inflammation, digestive problems, and cardiovascular disorders. Its active compounds include phytochemicals, designated anthraquinones, enzymes, and alkaloids.

- Echinaforce from Bioforce USA. This is a liquid echinacea supplement that promotes natural disease resistance during the winter season and helps to maintain a healthy immune system.

- Fibroplex from Metagenics. This supplement contains vitamins B_1 (thiamine) and B_6 (pyridoxine), magnesium, manganese, and malic acid. It is designed to provide nutritional support for the nerves and muscles.

- Tummy Soothe from Nature's Way. Gastro-Soothe is a natural antacid that contains calcium carbonate and ginger to soothe the stomach.

- Jerusalem artichoke tablets. Jerusalem artichoke whole tuber flour (JAF) tablets are a good source of fructooligosaccharides (FOS), which support the growth of healthy intestinal flora.

- Kyolic Neuro-Logic from Wakunaga of America. This supplement contains aged garlic extract, ginkgo biloba extract, lecithin, acetyl-L-carnitine, and phosphatidylserine in a formula designed to improve memory and mental activity.

- Miracle 2000 from Century Systems is a combination supplement that contains twenty-seven vitamins and minerals, eighteen herbs, eight amino acids, and numerous ionic trace minerals.

- Nature's Answer line of herbal extracts designed for children. They are made using alcohol, like standard extracts, but the alcohol is then removed and replaced with glycerin, which is a preservative and a natural sweetener.

- Remifemin from Enzymatic Therapy. Remifemin is a standardized extract of black cohosh that has been used in Europe for over forty years for the treatment of menopausal symptoms. (*See* Black Cohosh *under* Herbs and Their Uses in HERBS later in this book.) This supplement does not affect hormone levels.

- VitaSerum from ABRA, Inc. This is a skin care product designed to protect against free radicals, stimulate cell renewal, and reduce the visible signs of aging. It contains vitamin C from acerola berries; herbal extracts of elder flower, green tea, grape seed, and horsetail; citrus and cranberry bioflavonoids; hyaluronic acid; zinc sulfate; and essential oils of lavender, rose geranium, and sweet lavender.

- Vita-Min-Herb for Men from the Synergy Company. This is a combination nutritional supplement that contains a balanced blend of all major vitamins and minerals, trace elements, and a variety of herbal extracts used to support men's health.

- Wellness line of products from Source Naturals. These supplements are designed to support optimal health and keep the immune system strong.

Herbs

INTRODUCTION

The medicinal benefits of herbs have been known for centuries. Records of Native American, Roman, Egyptian, Persian, and Hebrew medical practices show that herbs were used extensively to treat practically every known illness.

Many herbs contain powerful ingredients that, if used correctly, can help heal the body. The pharmaceutical industry was originally based upon the ability to isolate these ingredients and make them available in a purer form. Herbalists, however, contend that nature provides other ingredients in the same herbs to balance the more powerful ingredients.

These other components, though they may be less potent, may help to act as buffers, synergists, or counterbalances working in harmony with the more powerful ingredients. Therefore, when you use herbs in their complete form, your body's healing process utilizes a balance of ingredients provided by nature.

In the United States, herbal remedies were used widely until the early 1900s, when what was to become the modern pharmaceutical industry began isolating individual active compounds and producing drugs based on them. American medicine became almost exclusively committed to a medical system some practitioners call *allopathy,* which seeks to treat illness by producing a condition in the body that does not allow the disease to live or thrive. Over the years, most Americans have become conditioned to rely on synthetic, commercial drugs for relief.

Today, however, scientists are taking a second look at herbal remedies. Particularly in the past twenty years, a growing body of research (much of it done in Europe) has pointed to the therapeutic potential of numerous herbs. And big pharmaceutical companies are always on the lookout for plants to help with a variety of diseases. But a lot of work remains to be done; less than 1 percent of the estimated plant species on earth have been investigated for possible medicinal uses. In 1978, the German Commission E monographs were created, which describe the safety and effectiveness of herbs. This is still considered the most authoritative modern work on the subject.

Today's renewed interest in herbs reflects increasing concern about the side effects of powerful synthetic drugs, as well as the desire of many people to take charge of their own health, rather than merely submitting themselves to a sometimes-impersonal health care system. We are also rediscovering the healthful benefits of tasty herbs for cooking and aromatic herbs for enhancing and helping to balance mental, spiritual, and physical health.

Nature's pharmacy is an abundant one. Many herbs are rich in compounds that have a beneficial effect on certain tissues and organs and therefore can be used as medicines to treat, cure, or prevent disease. Herbal remedies can help nourish your immune system, stimulate the regeneration of damaged liver tissue, build the strength of the adrenal glands, counter the adverse side effects of chemotherapy, balance the endocrine system, stimulate milk production, and improve night vision, among other things.

Generally, medicinal herbs fall into two basic categories: *tonic* and *stimulating*.

Tonics help cells, tissues, and organs to maintain tone, or balance, throughout the body. Some tonics activate and invigorate bodily processes or parts. Other tonics supply important nutrients that cells, tissues, and organs need to function properly. Tonics ordinarily are taken regularly for three to nine months at a time to gently strengthen and improve overall health and/or certain organ functions.

Stimulating herbs have much stronger actions and are used to treat particular ailments. They should be taken in smaller doses than tonic herbs, and for shorter periods of time.

Just because an herb had a historical use doesn't necessarily mean it will work for your condition. There may be some trial and error with different herbs and herbal blends before you get satisfactory results. Today, some herbs have undergone processing to produce a standardized extract that targets specific conditions. Extracts are a good place to start if you have one of the targeted conditions because they have a known amount of the active compound, which is not the case with the herb itself.

PHYTOMEDICINALS: THE HEALING POWER OF HERBS

Ancient cultures had no idea why herbs worked—they simply knew that certain plants produced certain desired results.

Only in the last hundred years or so have chemists and pharmacists been isolating and purifying the beneficial chemical compounds in plants to produce reliable pharmaceutical drugs. About 25 percent of the prescription medicines sold today are (or were originally) derived from plants. For example:

- Morphine and codeine come from the opium poppy.

- Aspirin originated from willow bark.

- Digitalis, a heart muscle strengthener, is derived from the foxglove plant.

- Paclitaxel (Taxol), used in cancer chemotherapy, comes from the Pacific yew tree.

Phytomedicine, a recently coined term, refers to an herbal medicine that is a whole-plant preparation, rather than a single isolated chemical compound. (The prefix *phyto* comes from the Greek word *phyton,* meaning a plant.) The herbal preparation derived from a whole plant or plant part is considered the active entity, even though it may actually contain hundreds of individual active components. Phytomedicines are standardized, however—that is, they contain set percentages of specified active components—and their therapeutic values are backed by pharmacological and clinical studies and experience.

Phytomedicines are widely recognized in Europe, where they are categorized as plant-derived drugs. In Germany, for example, phytomedicines are considered "ethical drugs," and physicians prescribe them and pharmacists dispense them. In the United States, phytomedicines are sold as over-the-counter dietary supplements in health food stores and in some pharmacies. A few mainstream doctors, however, have begun prescribing herbal remedies along with standard drugs. Some health insurance companies cover the cost of herbal medicines when they are prescribed by health care professionals. The National Center for Complementary and Integrative Health (NCCIH), part of the National Institutes of Health, is funding research on herbal remedies (for more information, go to www.nccih.nih. gov). According to Dr. David M. Eisenberg at the Harvard Medical School, more than 18 percent of the U.S. population, or 38 million adults, use herbal supplements.

Although herbal supplements are not subject to the same standards as are prescription and over-the-counter drugs, they are regulated by the FDA. In fact, in July 2008 the FDA applied a set of regulations to supplements called Current Good Manufacturing Practices (CGMP). These rules ensure that all supplements are manufactured in a uniform way and that what appears on the label is what is in the product.

OTHER HERBAL HEALING SYSTEMS

The World Health Organization estimates that 80 percent of the earth's population today depends on plants to treat common ailments. Herbalism is an essential part of Ayurvedic (Indian), traditional Asian, Native American, and naturopathic medicines. Many homeopathic remedies are derived from plants as well. Homeopathic remedies are regulated by the FDA but are subject to slightly different rules than dietary supplements. The biggest difference is that unlike supplements, they can carry disease claims on the label. This means labels for homeopathic remedies used historically for cancer patients, for example, can say "helps prevent recurrence of cancer." Other supplements may not make such claims.

Oriental herbs are a recent addition to the American herb scene, with the influx of several popular Chinese herbs. The Chinese are today's foremost herbalists, drawing on thousands of years of experience in compounding and processing roots and herbs. In the Asian tradition, herbs are used to bring the whole body into balance and harmony. They are taken daily as a preventive measure, rather than as a treatment once illness has occurred. In the Orient, medicinal herbs often find their way into foods as seasoning and ingredients. Indeed, according to the late Chinese writer and scholar Lin Yutang, the Chinese view medicine and food as the same thing, believing that what is good for the body is medicine and at the same time is also food. Some of the Chinese herbs most readily found in U.S. herb and natural food stores include astragalus, Chinese ginseng, ginkgo biloba, gotu kola, licorice root, dong quai, ginger, and schizandra.

Every Native American nation has its own herbal medicine tradition based on the plants growing in the geographic area where it lives. Common among all Native American cultures is the spirituality attached to the gathering and use of herbs, and many peoples use the same herbs both medicinally and ceremonially. For the Navajos, for example, herbalism is a complex and specialized religion, in which the Navajo healer serves as both doctor and priest. Before plants are collected, prayers and offerings are made to the earth and the plant spirit. Herbs used in healing ceremonies are not thrown away but are reverently placed back into the earth. Much like the Asian approach, Native American herbalism aims to achieve balance within the total person. Medicinal and ceremonial herbs commonly used by Native American cultures include American ginseng, yarrow, black cohosh, boneset, echinacea, goldenseal, nettles, juniper, wild buckwheat, and dogwood.

As they have for centuries, indigenous rainforest tribes around the world rely on the forests for virtually all their medicines. They too have incorporated herbs into their religions and everyday lives. Researchers estimate that the world's rain forests contain literally thousands of potentially useful medicinal plants. Rain forests exist on every continent, though most research attention is currently directed at the rain forests of South America, particularly in the Amazon, and of the South Pacific Islands. Out of this rich storehouse of natural remedies, only a handful are now commonly found in health food stores, among them pau d'arco, boldo, cat's claw, kava, yerba maté, suma, yohimbe (not recommended), guarana, and passionflower. More and more rainforest remedies are becoming available.

USING MEDICINAL HERBS

Commercial herbal preparations are available in several different forms, including bulk herbs, medicinal herb blends, teas, oils, tinctures, fluid extracts, and tablets or capsules. Following are some of the ways in which herbal remedies can be used.

Essential Oils

Essential oils are highly concentrated extracts—typically obtained either by steam distillation or cold-pressing—from the flowers, leaves, roots, berries, stems, seeds, gums, needles, bark, or resins of numerous plants. They contain natural hormones, vitamins, antibiotics, and antiseptics. Essential oils typically come from anise, thyme, ginger, and chamomile. Some of these oils, and especially chamomile, appear to inhibit herpes simplex virus in a petri dish.

Known also as *volatile oils* because they evaporate easily in air, essential oils are soluble in vegetable oil, partially soluble in alcohol, and not soluble in water. Because they are so concentrated, they are likely to irritate mucous membranes and the stomach lining if taken internally. It is therefore best to use essential oils externally only, such as in poultices, inhalants, or bathwater, or on the skin (a few drops). The therapeutic properties of essential oils can help to remedy ailments ranging from insomnia to respiratory disorders to impotence to arthritis.

Extracts

An extract is a concentrate that results when crude herb is mixed with a suitable solvent, such as alcohol and/or water. Of the different herbal forms, extracts are generally the most effective because their active ingredients are more highly concentrated, and they can be standardized to a guaranteed potency. Extracts also have longer shelf lives than other herbal preparations. Fresh herbal extracts retain almost all of the original plant's benefits.

Alcohol-free extracts are available. When administered sublingually (drops are placed under the tongue), herbal extracts can be absorbed by the body quickly. This is an especially effective way for older adults and people with absorption problems to use herbs.

Plasters, Compresses, and Poultices

These are ways of applying herbal remedies directly to the skin. Plasters and compresses are cotton bandages soaked in infusions or decoctions and wrapped around the affected area or held on with pressure. Compresses are also warm. Poultices are made by moistening herbs, placing them on the skin, and holding them there with a bandage. Moistened and warmed herbal tea bags also help soothe and heal. Try using chamomile tea bags to relieve the itching and inflammation of insect bites and eczema.

Powders

Powders are dried herbs ground to a fine consistency. You can sprinkle them over food, stir them into a liquid such as juice or water for tonics, or add them to soup stocks. You also can take them in capsule or tablet form.

Salves, Ointments, and Creams

These preparations combine a medicinal herb with an oily base for external use. Creams are light and slightly oily, to blend with the skin's secretions and allow the active ingredients to penetrate the skin. The heavier and oilier salves and ointments apply protective remedies to the skin surface.

Syrups

Syrups are used to improve the taste of bitter herbal formulas and to administer soothing cough or throat medicines. Herbs often taken in syrup form include wild cherry, marshmallow root, and licorice.

Teas, Infusions, and Decoctions

People have been consuming herbal teas for as long as they have known how to heat water—since well before recorded history. Unlike green, black, and oolong teas, herbal teas can be made from virtually any plant, and from any part of the plant, including the roots, flowers, seeds, berries, or bark. There are some herbs, such as echinacea, ginkgo leaf, saw palmetto, and milk thistle, that are not effective at healing when taken in tea form because their active components are not water-soluble, and the concentration needed for medicinal potency is so high it can be obtained only from an extract, pill, or capsule.

Different herbal teas, which sometimes contain thousands of beneficial active compounds, have their own distinctive healing uses. The late botanical expert Varro Tyler, Ph.D., formerly professor emeritus of pharmacognosy (the study of natural drug properties) at Purdue University, taught that herbal teas are very good for relieving mild to moderate ailments such as upset stomach, sore throat, coughs, stuffy nose, and insomnia.

Many herbal teas are available in tea bag form. They can also be prepared from the raw herb. To make an herbal tea, gently crumble leaves and flowers and break roots and bark into pieces (cutting the herbs causes the essential oils to dissipate) and place them in a ceramic or glass container. Cover the herb parts with boiling water (do not bring the herbs themselves to a boil) and allow them to steep. Most herbs should be steeped for four to six minutes, although some herbal teas, such as chamomile, need to be steeped for fifteen to twenty minutes in a covered container in order to deliver their full therapeutic effect. Other herbs, such as ginseng root, can be boiled. Astragalus can be lightly simmered for several hours. In fact, in Asia, ginseng root, astragalus, dong quai, and other herbs are added to chicken broth to make a tonic soup that is both food and medicine.

Infusion is simply another term for tea. This is the easiest way to take herbal remedies. To make an infusion, you simply boil water and add leaves, stems, flowers, or powdered herbs—plant material whose active ingredients dissolve readily in hot water—then steep, strain, and drink the mixture as a tea.

A decoction is a tea made from thicker plant parts, such as bark, roots, seeds, or berries. These also contain lignin, a substance that is difficult to dissolve in water. Thus, decoctions require a more vigorous extraction method than infusions.

Tinctures

Plant components that are either insoluble or only partially soluble in water can be extracted with solvents such as alcohol or glycerol. The herb is soaked in the solvent for a period of time, then pressed to render the tincture. Tinctures can preserve extracted ingredients for twelve months or more.

Vinegars

Herbal vinegars can serve as both medicines and salad dressings. To make an herbal vinegar, add the herb or herbs of your choice to raw apple cider vinegar, balsamic vinegar, rice vinegar, or malt vinegar. Allow the herbs to steep for four days (agitate the container daily), strain, and then press through a straining cloth and bottle in a dark glass container.

Wines

Steeping herbs in wine is a novel and pleasant way to use them medicinally. Wine does not keep as long as the stronger alcohols, so refrigeration is a good idea.

TIPS AND PRECAUTIONS

However they are used, most herbs act gently and subtly. They do not produce the kind of dramatic, immediate results we expect from prescription drugs. Basically, herbs are balancers that work with the body to help it heal and regulate itself. They work better together than they do singly because the effect of one herb is usually supported and reinforced when combined with others.

While most herbs aren't likely to be harmful, keep in mind that "natural" isn't a synonym for "safe." Like synthetic drugs, herbal preparations may be toxic, cause allergic reactions, or affect your response to other medications.

Common sense, care, and forethought are needed when using herbs for either food or medicine. Here are some essential guidelines for herbal self-care:

- Use herbal self-care for minor ailments only, not for serious or life-threatening conditions.

- Use only recommended amounts for recommended periods of time.

- Use the correct herb. Buy your herbal remedies from a reputable company. If you collect or grow herbs on your own, be absolutely positive in your identification.

- Use the correct part of the plant. For instance, don't substitute roots for leaves. When buying fresh herbs, check to be sure which part of the herb is required for a remedy—the whole herb, flowers, fruit, leaves, stems, or roots.

- When using an herbal remedy for the first time, start with a small amount to test for possible allergic reactions.

- Don't take certain herbs if you are pregnant or planning to become pregnant.

- Don't take herbal remedies if you are nursing a baby.

- Don't give medicinal amounts of herbs to children without first consulting with your health care practitioner.

Buying Herbal Remedies

When choosing herbal remedies, select quality products from a reliable source. How do you know whether a manufacturer or supplier is reliable? Start by making a phone call to the manufacturer. Ask how long the company has been in business, if they are following the GMP guidelines from the FDA, and how they determine the identity and potency of the herbs they sell. Membership in trade groups such as the American Herbal Products Association (www.ahpa.org), while not a stamp of approval, does indicate the company's recognition of industry standards. The American Botanical Council provides regular updates on new science related to herbs (www.herbalgram.org). We recommend purchasing herbs sold by reputable companies that have been in the herb business for at least ten years.

If you wish to buy organically grown herbs, look for the "certified organic" label on the product. More than half of U.S. states have certification programs for organic farms and products. Federal standards are now implemented through a nationwide certification system under the USDA National Organic Program. More information on the regulations governing these producers can be found at https://www.ams.usda.gov/about-ams/programs-offices/national-organic-program.

Finally, look for herbal products that are standardized to contain a specific percentage of active ingredients extracted from the specific herb part known to be effective.

HERBS AND THEIR USES

The following table describes some of the most commonly used medicinal herbs, including which parts of each herb are used, its chemical and nutrient content, and its various uses.

HERB (SCIENTIFIC NAME)	PART(S) USED	PHYTOCHEMICAL AND NUTRIENT CONTENT
Acerola (*Malpighia glabra*)	Fruit.	Phytochemicals: Beta-carotene. Nutrients: Calcium, iron, magnesium, phosphorus, potassium, vitamins A, B_1, B_2, B_3, B_5, B_6, and C.
Alfalfa (*Medicago sativa*)	Flowers, leaves, petals, sprouted seeds.	Phytochemicals: Alpha-carotene, beta-carotene, beta-sitosterol, chlorophyll, coumarin, cryptoxanthin, daidzen, fumaric acid, genistein, limonene, lutein, saponin, stigmasterol, zeaxanthin. Nutrients: Calcium, copper, folate, iron, magnesium, manganese, phosphorus, potassium, silicon, zinc, vitamins A, B_1, B_2, B_3, B_5, B_6, C, D, E, and K.
Aloe (*Aloe vera*)	Pulp from insides of succulent leaves.	Phytochemicals: Acemannan, beta-carotene, beta-sitosterol, campesterol, cinnamic acid, coumarin, lignins, p-coumaric acid, saponins. Nutrients: Amino acids, calcium, folate, iron, magnesium, phosphorus, potassium, zinc, vitamins A, B_1, B_2, B_3, C, and E.

ACTIONS AND USES	COMMENTS
Has antioxidant, antifungal, and astringent properties. Helps to support the liver and hydrate the skin. Useful for diarrhea and fever.	A rainforest herb similar to the cherry. One of the richest natural sources of vitamin C; found in numerous multivitamin supplements.
Alkalizes and detoxifies the body. Acts as a diuretic, anti-inflammatory, and antifungal. Lowers cholesterol, balances blood sugar and hormones, and promotes pituitary gland function. Good for anemia, arthritis, ulcers, bleeding-related disorders, and disorders of the bones and joints, digestive system, and skin.	Must be used in fresh, raw form to provide all nutrients. Sprouts are especially effective. (Be sure to rinse them thoroughly before use to remove mold and bacteria.)
Acts as an astringent, emollient, antifungal, antibacterial, and antiviral. Applied topically, heals mouth sores and stimulates cell regeneration. Helps healing of burn wounds. Ingested, helps to lower cholesterol, reduces inflammation resulting from radiation therapy, increases blood vessel generation in lower extremities of people with poor circulation, soothes stomach irritation, aids healing, and acts as a laxative. May be good for patients with AIDS and for skin. It supports a healthy digestive system probably by increasing short-chain fatty acid production from the friendly bacteria in the colon.	Allergic reactions, though rare, may occur in susceptible persons. Before using, apply a small amount behind the ear or on the underarm. If stinging or rash occurs, do not use. *Caution:* Should not be taken internally during pregnancy.

HERB (SCIENTIFIC NAME)	PART(S) USED	PHYTOCHEMICAL AND NUTRIENT CONTENT
Anise (*Pimpinella anisum*)	Seeds, seed oil.	Phytochemicals: Alpha-pinene, apigenin, bergapten, caffeic acid, chlorogenic acid, eugenol, limonene, linalool, myristicin, rutin, scopoletin, squalene, stigmasterol, umbelliferone. Nutrients: Calcium, iron, magnesium, manganese, phosphorus, potassium, zinc, vitamins A, B_1, B_2, B_3, B_5, B_6, C, and E.
Annatto (*Bixa orellana*)	Leaves, roots, seeds.	Phytochemicals: Beta-carotene, bixin, cyanidin, ellagic acid, salicylic acid, saponin, tannins. Nutrients: Amino acids, calcium, iron, phosphorus, vitamins B_2, B_3, and C.
Ashwagandha (*Withania somnifera*)	Roots.	Phytochemicals: Alkaloids, beta-sitosterol, chlorogenic acid, scopoletin, withaferin. Nutrients: Amino acids, choline.
Astragalus (*Astragalus membranaceus*)	Roots.	Phytochemicals: Betaine, beta-sitosterol, formononetin, isoliquiritigenin. Nutrients: Calcium, choline, copper, essential fatty acids, iron, magnesium, manganese, potassium, zinc.
Barberry (*Berberis vulgaris*)	Bark, berries, roots.	Phytochemicals: Berbamine, berberine, beta-carotene, caffeic acid, kaempferol, lutein, quercetin, sinapic acid, zeaxanthin. Nutrients: Calcium, iron, magnesium, manganese, phosphorus, potassium, selenium, silicon, zinc, vitamins B_1, B_2, B_3, and C.

ACTIONS AND USES	COMMENTS
Aids digestion, clears mucus from air passages, combats infection, and promotes milk production in nursing mothers. Good for indigestion and for respiratory infections such as sinusitis. Also helpful for menopausal symptoms.	Used in many popular products as a fragrance and flavoring.
Has diuretic, antioxidant, antibacterial, anti-inflammatory, and expectorant properties. Helps to protect the liver and kidneys. May reduce blood sugar levels. Useful for indigestion, fever, coughs, burns, skin problems, and weight loss.	A rainforest herb used in skin care products as an emollient, and as an orange-yellow food coloring.
Rejuvenates and energizes the nervous system. Helps prevent stress-related disorders and stress-related depletion of vitamin C and cortisol. Increases physical endurance and improves sexual function. Has anti-inflammatory and antiaging effects. In laboratory studies, has modulated and stimulated immune function. Helps normalize thyroid hormones.	An Ayurvedic herb also known as Indian ginseng and winter cherry. An important herb in Ayurvedic medicine.
Acts as a tonic to protect the immune system. Aids adrenal gland function and digestion. Increases metabolism, produces spontaneous sweating, promotes healing, and provides energy to combat fatigue and prolonged stress. Increases stamina. Good for colds, flu, and immune-deficiency-related problems, including AIDS, cancer, and tumors. Effective for chronic lung weakness.	Also called huang qi. *Caution:* Do not use if fever is present.
Decreases heart rate, slows breathing, reduces bronchial constriction. Kills bacteria on the skin and stimulates intestinal movement. May reduce heart disease risk in people with type 2 diabetes.	*Caution:* Should not be used during pregnancy.

HERB (SCIENTIFIC NAME)	PART(S) USED	PHYTOCHEMICAL AND NUTRIENT CONTENT
Bayberry (*Myrica cerifera*)	Root bark.	Phytochemicals: Beta-carotene, gallic acid, myristic acid, phenol. Nutrients: Calcium, iron, magnesium, manganese, phosphorus, potassium, selenium, silicon, zinc, vitamins B_1, B_2, B_3, and C.
Bilberry (*Vaccinium myrtillus*)	Entire plant.	Phytochemicals: Anthocyanosides, beta-carotene, caffeic acid, caryophyllene, catechin, chlorogenic acid, ferulic acid, gallic acid, hyperoside, lutein, quercetin, quercitrin, ursolic acid, vanillic acid. Nutrients: Calcium, inositol, magnesium, manganese, phosphorus, potassium, selenium, silicon, sulfur, zinc, vitamins B_1, B_2, B_3, and C.
Birch (*Betula alba*)	Bark, leaves, sap.	Phytochemicals: Betulin, betulinic acid, hyperoside, luteolin and quercetin glycosides, methyl salicylate.
Black cohosh (*Cimicifuga racemosa*)	Rhizomes, roots.	Phytochemicals: Beta-carotene, cimicifugin, formononetin, gallic acid, phytosterols, salicylic acid, tannic acid, tannin. Nutrients: Calcium, chromium, iron, magnesium, manganese, phosphorus, potassium, selenium, silicon, zinc, vitamins B_1, B_2, B_3, and C.
Black walnut (*Juglans nigra*)	Husks, inner bark, leaves, nuts.	Phytochemicals: Beta-carotene, ellagic acid, juglone, myricetin, tannin. Nutrients: Calcium, iron, magnesium, manganese, phosphorus, potassium, selenium, silicon, zinc, vitamins B_1, B_2, B_3, and C.

ACTIONS AND USES	COMMENTS
Acts as a decongestant and astringent. Aids circulation, reduces fever. Helps stop bleeding. Good for circulatory disorders, fever, hypothyroidism, and ulcers. Also good for the eyes and the immune system.	The wax of the berries is used to make fragrant candles. *Caution:* Should not be used at high dosages or for prolonged periods. May temporarily irritate sensitive stomachs.
Acts as an antioxidant, diuretic, and urinary tract antiseptic. Keeps blood vessels flexible, allowing increased blood flow. Helps control insulin levels and strengthen connective tissue. Supports and strengthens collagen structures, inhibits the growth of bacteria, and has antiaging and anticarcinogenic effects. Useful for hypoglycemia, inflammation, stress, anxiety, night blindness, and cataracts. May help halt or prevent macular degeneration. Shown to be beneficial for people who recently had a heart attack. In a timed study, it allowed them to walk faster. In addition, oxidation of LDL cholesterol was reduced.	Also known as European blueberry. Related to the American blueberry. *Caution:* Interferes with iron absorption when taken internally. Should not be used by people with diabetes except under the supervision of a knowledgeable health professional.
Acts as a diuretic, anti-inflammatory, and pain reliever. Good for joint pain and urinary tract infections. Applied topically, good for boils and sores.	Betulinic acid in birch bark has been found to kill cancer cells.
Lowers blood pressure and cholesterol levels. Reduces mucus production. Helps cardiovascular and circulatory disorders. Relieves menopausal symptoms, menstrual cramps with back pain, morning sickness, and pain. Helpful for poisonous snakebites. Good for arthritis.	Also known as black snakeroot. *Caution:* Do not use during pregnancy or in the presence of chronic disease. There have been reports of liver problems associated with the use of this herb in certain individuals. Some products contain Asian Actaea and not black cohosh. Buy from a reputable company.
Aids digestion and acts as a laxative. Helps heal mouth and throat sores. Cleanses the body of some types of parasites. Good for bruising, fungal infection, herpes, poison ivy, and warts. May help lower blood pressure and cholesterol levels.	When boiled, the hulls produce a dye that is used to color wool.

HERB (SCIENTIFIC NAME)	PART(S) USED	PHYTOCHEMICAL AND NUTRIENT CONTENT
Blessed thistle (*Cnicus benedictus*)	Flowers, leaves, stems.	Phytochemicals: Beta-carotene, beta-sitosterol, cnicin, ferulic acid, kaempferol, luteolin, oleanolic acid, stigmasterol. Nutrients: Calcium, essential fatty acids, iron, magnesium, manganese, phosphorus, potassium, selenium, silicon, zinc, vitamins B_1, B_2, B_3, and C.
Blue cohosh (*Caulophyllum thalictroides*)	Roots.	Phytochemicals: Anagyrine, beta-carotene, caulophylline, caulophyllosaponin, caulosaponin, hederagenin, phytosterols, saponin. Nutrients: Calcium, iron, magnesium, manganese, phosphorus, potassium, selenium, zinc, vitamins B_1, B_2, B_3, and C.
Boldo (*Peumus boldus*)	Leaves.	Phytochemicals: Alpha-pinene, ascaridole, benzaldehyde, beta-pinene, boldin, boldine, camphor, coumarin, eugenol, farnesol, kaempferol, limonene, linalool, 1,8-cineole. Nutrients: Choline.
Boneset (*Eupatorium perfoliatum*)	Flower petals, leaves.	Phytochemicals: Astragalin, gallic acid, eufoliatin, eufoliatorin, eupatorin, euperfolin, euperfolitin, gallic acid, hyperoside, kaempferol, quercetin, rutin, tannic acid.
Borage (*Borago officinalis*)	Leaves, seeds.	Phytochemicals: Beta-carotene, rosmarinic acid, silicic acid, tannin. Nutrients: Calcium, choline, essential fatty acids, iron, magnesium, phosphorus, potassium, zinc, vitamins B_1, B_2, B_3, and C.
Boswellia (*Boswellia serrata*)	Gum resin.	Phytochemicals: Borneol, boswellic acids, carvone, caryophyllene, farnesol, geraniol, limonene.

ACTIONS AND USES	COMMENTS
Stimulates the appetite and stomach secretions. Heals the liver. Lessens inflammation, improves circulation, cleanses the blood, and strengthens the heart. May act as brain food. Good for female disorders and increases milk flow in nursing mothers.	Also called St. Benedict thistle, holy thistle. *Caution:* Should be handled with care to avoid toxic skin effects.
Eases muscle spasms and stimulates uterine contractions for childbirth. Useful for memory problems, menstrual disorders, and nervous disorders.	*Caution:* Should not be used during the first two trimesters of pregnancy.
Acts as a diuretic, laxative, antibiotic, liver tonic, and anti-inflammatory. Aids in the excretion of uric acid and stimulates digestion.	Used by indigenous peoples of Chile and Peru for liver ailments and gallstones.
Acts as a decongestant, laxative, anti-inflammatory, and diuretic. Loosens phlegm, reduces fever, increases perspiration, calms the body. Useful for colds, flu, bronchitis, and fever-induced aches and pains.	Also called white snakeroot. *Caution:* Do not use on a daily basis for more than one week, as long-term use can lead to toxicity.
Acts as an adrenal tonic and gland balancer. Contains valuable minerals and essential fatty acids needed for proper cardiovascular function and healthy skin and nails. May help reduce redness associated with acne.	The flowers of the borage plant are edible.
Acts as an anti-inflammatory, antiarthritic, antifungal, and antibacterial. Used topically for pain relief. Lowers cholesterol, protects the liver. Useful for arthritis, gout, low back pain, myositis, and fibromyalgia. Helps repair blood vessels damaged by inflammation. Traditionally used as a remedy for obesity, diarrhea, dysentery, pulmonary diseases, ringworm, and boils.	An Ayurvedic herb also known as Indian frankincense. An important herb in Ayurvedic medicine.

HERB (*SCIENTIFIC NAME*)	PART(S) USED	PHYTOCHEMICAL AND NUTRIENT CONTENT
Buchu (*Barosma betulina*)	Leaves.	Phytochemicals: Alpha-pinene, alpha-terpinene, barosma-camphor, diosphenol, hesperidin, limonene, menthone, pulegone, quercetin, quercetrin, rutin. Nutrients: Calcium, iron, magnesium, manganese, phosphorus, potassium, selenium, silicon, zinc, vitamins B_1, B_2, and B_3.
Burdock (*Arctium lappa*)	Plant, roots, seeds.	Phytochemicals: Acetic acid, arctigenin, arctiin, beta-carotene, butyric acid, caffeic acid, chlorogenic acid, costic acid, inulin, isovaleric acid, lauric acid, lignin, myristic acid, propionic acid, sitosterol, stigmasterol. Nutrients: Amino acids, calcium, chromium, copper, iron, magnesium, manganese, phosphorus, potassium, selenium, silicon, zinc, vitamins B_1, B_2, B_3, and C.
Butcher's broom (*Ruscus aculeatus*)	Plant, roots, seeds.	Phytochemicals: Beta-carotene, chrysophanic acid, glycolic acid, neoruscogenin, rutin, saponin. Nutrients: Calcium, chromium, iron, magnesium, manganese, phosphorus, potassium, selenium, silicon, zinc, vitamins B_1, B_2, B_3, and C.
Calendula (*Calendula officinalis*)	Flower petals.	Phytochemicals: Alpha-amyrin, beta-amyrin, beta-sitosterol, caffeic acid, campesterol, caryophyllene, chlorogenic acid, faradiol, galactose, gentisic acid, kaempferol, lutein, lycopene, malic acid, myristic acid, oleanolic acid, p-coumaric acid, phytofluene, quercetin, rutin, salicylic acid, saponin, stigmasterol, syringic acid, taraxasterol, vanillic acid, zeta-carotene. Nutrients: Calcium, coenzyme Q_{10}, vitamins C and E.

ACTIONS AND USES	COMMENTS
Lessens inflammation of the colon, gums, mucous membranes, prostate, sinuses, and vagina. Acts as a diuretic. Helps control bladder and kidney problems, diabetes, digestive disorders, fluid retention, and prostate disorders.	Do not boil buchu leaves.
Acts as an antioxidant. May help to protect against cancer by helping control cell mutation. Aids elimination of excess fluid, uric acid, and toxins. Has antibacterial and antifungal properties. Purifies the blood, restores liver and gallbladder function, and stimulates the digestive and immune systems. Helps skin disorders such as boils and carbuncles, and relieves gout and menopausal symptoms. Burdock root used as a hair rinse promotes scalp and hair health.	Also called bardana, beggar's buttons, clotbur, gobo, lappa, and thorny burr. *Caution:* Interferes with iron absorption when taken internally. Should not be used by pregnant or breast-feeding women, people with diabetes, or those with heart or cardiovascular conditions.
Reduces inflammation. Useful for carpal tunnel syndrome, circulatory disorders, edema, Ménière's disease, obesity, Raynaud's phenomenon, thrombophlebitis, varicose veins, and vertigo. Also good for the bladder and kidneys.	More effective if taken with vitamin C.
Reduces inflammation and is soothing to the skin. Helps regulate the menstrual cycle and lower fever. Useful for skin disorders, such as rashes and sunburn, as well as for neuritis and toothache. Good for diaper rash and other skin problems in small children.	Also called pot marigold. Usually nonirritating when used externally.

HERB (SCIENTIFIC NAME)	PART(S) USED	PHYTOCHEMICAL AND NUTRIENT CONTENT
Cascara sagrada (*Frangula purshiana*)	Bark.	Phytochemicals: Aloe-emodin, anthraquinones, barbaloin, beta-carotene, casanthranol, chrysophanic acid, chrysophanol, frangulin, malic acid, myristic acid. Nutrients: Calcium, iron, linoleic acid, magnesium, manganese, phosphorus, potassium, selenium, silicon, zinc, vitamins B_1, B_2, B_3, and C.
Catnip (*Nepeta cataria*)	Leaves.	Phytochemicals: Alpha-humulene, beta-elemene, camphor, carvacrol, caryophyllene, citral, citronellal, geraniol, myrcene, nepetalactone, piperitone, pulegone, rosmarinic acid, thymol. Nutrients: Calcium, chromium, iron, magnesium, manganese, phosphorus, potassium, selenium, silicon, zinc.
Cat's claw (*Uncaria tomentosa*)	Inner bark, roots.	Phytochemicals: Alloisopteropodine, allopteropodine, isomitraphylline, isopteropodine, mitraphylline, oleanolic acid, pteropodine, rhynchophylline, ursolic acid.
Cayenne (*Capsicum frutescens* or *C. annum*)	Berries.	Phytochemicals: Alpha-carotene, beta-carotene, beta-ionone, caffeic acid, campesterol, capsaicin, carvone, caryophyllene, chlorogenic acid, citric acid, cryptoxanthin, hesperidin, kaempferol, limonene, lutein, myristic acid, 1,8-cineole, p-coumaric acid, quercetin, scopoletin, stigmasterol, zeaxanthin. Nutrients: Amino acids, calcium, essential fatty acids, folate, iron, magnesium, phosphorus, potassium, zinc, vitamins B_1, B_2, B_3, B_5, B_6, C, and E.

ACTIONS AND USES	COMMENTS
Acts as a colon cleanser and laxative. Effective for colon disorders, constipation, and parasitic infestation.	Tastes very bitter taken as a tea.
Lowers fever (catnip tea enemas reduce fever quickly). Dispels gas and aids digestion and sleep; relieves stress; stimulates the appetite. Good for anxiety, colds and flu, inflammation, pain, and stress.	Can be given to children.
Acts as an antioxidant and anti-inflammatory. It may help with the management of arthritis. Stimulates the immune system. Cleanses the intestinal tract and enhances the action of white blood cells. Good for intestinal problems and viral infections. May help people with AIDS symptoms, arthritis, cancer, tumors, or ulcers.	Also called uña de gato. According to USDA research, cat's claw seeds contain an enzyme instrumental in converting saturated fats to unsaturated fats. *Caution:* Do not use during pregnancy.
Aids digestion, improves circulation, weight loss, and stops bleeding from ulcers. Acts as a catalyst for other herbs. Good for the heart, kidneys, lungs, pancreas, spleen, and stomach. Useful for arthritis and rheumatism. Helps to ward off colds, sinus infections, and sore throats. Good for pain when applied topically. Used with lobelia for nerves.	Also called capsicum, hot pepper, red pepper. *Caution:* Avoid contact with the eyes.

HERB (SCIENTIFIC NAME)	PART(S) USED	PHYTOCHEMICAL AND NUTRIENT CONTENT
Cedar (*Cedrus libani*)	Leaves, tops.	Phytochemicals: Borneol, quinic acid.
Celery (*Apium graveolens*)	Plant, roots, seeds.	Phytochemicals: Alpha-pinene, apigenin, bergapten, beta-carotene, caffeic acid, carvone, chlorogenic acid, coumarin, eugenol, ferulic acid, isoquercitrin, limonene, linalool, luteolin, mannitol, myristic acid, myristicin, p-coumaric acid, rutin, scopoletin, shikimic acid, thymol. Nutrients: Amino acids, boron, calcium, choline, essential fatty acids, folate, inositol, iron, magnesium, manganese, phosphorus, potassium, selenium, sulfur, zinc, vitamins A, B_1, B_2, B_3, B_5, B_6, C, E, and K.
Chamomile (*Matricaria recutita* or *M. chamomilla*)	Flowers, plant.	Phytochemicals: Alpha-bisabolol, apigenin, azulene, borneol, caffeic acid, chlorogenic acid, farnesol, gentisic acid, geraniol, hyperoside, kaempferol, luteolin, p-coumaric acid, perillyl alcohol, quercetin, rutin, salicylic acid, sinapic acid, tannin, umbelliferone. Nutrients: Choline, vitamins B_1, B_3, and C.
Chanca piedra (*Phyllanthus niruri*)	Entire plant.	Phytochemicals: Limonene, lupeol, methyl salicylate, quercetin, quercitrin, rutin, saponins.
Chaste tree (*Vitex agnus-castus*)	Fruit, leaf.	Phytochemicals: Alpha-pinene, alpha-terpineol, chrysosplenol, flavonoids, limonene, linalool, myrcene, 1,8-cineole, pinene, progesterone, testosterone.

ACTIONS AND USES	COMMENTS
Acts as an antiviral, antifungal, expectorant, lymphatic cleanser, and urinary antiseptic. Stimulates the immune system. Increases venous blood flow. Can be used externally for warts.	
Reduces blood pressure, relieves muscle spasms, and improves appetite. Good for arthritis, gout, and kidney problems. Acts as a diuretic, antioxidant, and sedative.	*Caution:* Do not use large amounts. Do not eat the seeds if you are pregnant.
Reduces inflammation, stimulates the appetite, and aids digestion and sleep. Acts as a diuretic and nerve tonic. Helpful for colitis, diverticulosis, fever, headaches, and pain. Good for menstrual cramps. A traditional remedy for stress and anxiety, indigestion, and insomnia. Useful as a mouthwash for minor mouth and gum infections. May help depressed people feel better.	Also called German chamomile, wild chamomile. Roman chamomile (*Chamaemelum nobile*) is also available but less common. *Caution:* Do not use it if allergic to ragweed. Do not use during pregnancy or nursing. It may interact with warfarin or cyclosporine, so patients taking these drugs should avoid it.
Fights inflammation and bacterial and viral infection. Acts as a diuretic. Useful for kidney stones, gallstones, colds, flu, digestion, asthma, bronchitis, diarrhea, pain relief, fever, sexually transmitted diseases, and muscle spasms.	A rainforest herb whose name means "stone crusher." Also known as seed-on-the-leaf.
Has a calming and soothing effect. Relieves muscle cramps. Regulates and normalizes hormone levels and menstrual cycles. Good for symptoms of PMS and menopause.	Also called chasteberry, vitex. *Caution:* Should not be used during pregnancy. Should not be given to children.

HERB (SCIENTIFIC NAME)	PART(S) USED	PHYTOCHEMICAL AND NUTRIENT CONTENT
Chickweed (*Stellaria media*)	Leaves, stems.	Phytochemicals: Beta-carotene, genistein, rutin. Nutrients: Calcium, essential fatty acids, iron, magnesium, manganese, phosphorus, potassium, selenium, silicon, sulfur, zinc, vitamins B_1, B_2, B_3, C, and E.
Chuchuhuasi (*Maytenus krukoviti*)	Bark, root, leaves.	Phytochemicals: Anthocyanidins, catechin, maytensine, nocotinyl, sesquiterpenes, triterpenes, tannins.
Cinnamon (*Cinnamomum verum*)	Bark, plant.	Phytochemicals: Alpha-pinene, benzaldehyde, beta-carotene, beta-pinene, borneol, camphor, caryophyllene, cinnamaldehyde, coumarin, cuminaldehyde, eugenol, farnesol, geraniol, limonene, linalool, mannitol, mucilage, 1,8-cineole, phellandrene, tannin, terpinolene, vanillin. Nutrients: Calcium, chromium, copper, iodine, iron, manganese, phosphorus, potassium, zinc, vitamins A, B_1, B_2, B_3, and C.
Clove (*Syzygium aromaticum*)	Flower buds, essential oil.	Phytochemicals: Beta-carotene, beta-pinene, beta-sitosterol, campesterol, carvone, caryophyllene, chavicol, cinnamaldehyde, ellagic acid, eugenol, gallic acid, kaempferol, linalool, methyleugenol, methylsalicylate, mucilage, oleanolic acid, stigmasterol, tannin, vanillin. Nutrients: Calcium, iron, magnesium, manganese, phosphorus, potassium, zinc, vitamins A, B_1, B_2, and C.

ACTIONS AND USES	COMMENTS
Relieves nasal congestion. May lower blood lipids. Useful for bronchitis, circulatory problems, colds, coughs, skin diseases, and warts (applied topically). A good source of vitamin C and other nutrients.	Also called starweed.
Fights inflammation and stimulates the immune system. Supports the adrenal system and balances and regulates menstrual cycles. Good for arthritis, rheumatism, back pain, muscle spasms, fever, skin tumors, bronchitis, diarrhea.	Also called chucchu huashu, chuchuasi, chuchasha, chuchuhuasha. Peruvian Amazon native name means "trembling back" for its value as an anti-arthritic drug. This rainforest herb also used traditionally to stimulate sexual desire and give energy.
Relieves diarrhea and nausea; counteracts congestion; aids peripheral circulation. Warms the body and enhances digestion, especially the metabolism of fats. Also fights fungal infection. Useful for diabetes, weight loss, yeast infection, and uterine hemorrhaging.	*Cinnamon cassia* is used for diabetes management but with varying degrees of success. *Caution:* Should not be used in large amounts during pregnancy.
Has antiseptic and antiparasitic properties, and acts as a digestive aid. Essential oil is applied topically for relief of toothache and mouth pain.	*Caution:* Clove oil is very strong and can cause irritation if used in its pure form. Diluting the oil in olive oil or distilled water is recommended. Essential oil should not be taken internally except under the careful supervision of a health care professional.

HERB (SCIENTIFIC NAME)	PART(S) USED	PHYTOCHEMICAL AND NUTRIENT CONTENT
Comfrey (*Symphytum officinale*)	Leaves, roots.	Phytochemicals: Allantoin, beta-carotene, caffeic acid, chlorogenic acid, rosmarinic acid, sitosterol, stigmasterol. Nutrients: Calcium, iron, magnesium, manganese, phosphorus, potassium, selenium, zinc, vitamins B_1, B_2, B_3, and C.
Corn silk (*Zea mays*)	Styles, stigmas ("tassels").	Phytochemicals: Benzaldehyde, beta-carotene, betaine, beta-sitosterol, caffeic acid, campesterol, carvacrol, caryophyllene, dioxycinnamic acid, geraniol, glycolic acid, limonene, 1,8-cineole, saponin, thymol, vitexin. Nutrients: Calcium, chromium, iron, magnesium, manganese, phosphorus, potassium, vitamins B_1, B_3, and C.
Cramp bark (*Viburnum opulus*)	Bark, root.	Phytochemicals: Esculetin, scopoletin, valerianic acid. Nutrients: Calcium, iron, magnesium, manganese, phosphorus, potassium, selenium, zinc.
Cranberry (*Vaccinium macrocarpon*)	Fruit.	Phytochemicals: Alpha-terpineol, anthocyanosides, benzaldehyde, benzoic acid, beta-carotene, chlorogenic acid, ellagic acid, eugenol, ferulic acid, lutein, malic acid, quercetin. Nutrients: Calcium, folate, iron, magnesium, manganese, phosphorus, potassium, selenium, sulfur, zinc, vitamins A, B_1, B_2, B_3, B_5, C, and E.
Damiana (*Turnera diffusa*)	Leaves.	Phytochemicals: Alpha-pinene, beta-carotene, beta-pinene, beta-sitosterol, 1,8-cineole, tannins, thymol. Nutrients: Calcium, iron, magnesium, manganese, phosphorus, potassium, selenium, zinc, vitamins B_1, B_2, B_3, and C.

ACTIONS AND USES	COMMENTS
Speeds healing of wounds and many skin conditions. Beneficial for bedsores, bites and stings, bruises, inflamed bunions, dermatitis, dry skin, bleeding hemorrhoids, leg ulcers, nosebleeds, psoriasis, scabies, skin rashes, and sunburn.	Also called knitbone. *Caution:* Recommended for external use only.
Acts as a diuretic. Aids the bladder, kidney, and small intestine. Lessens the incidence of bed-wetting when taken several hours before bedtime. Good for carpal tunnel syndrome, edema, obesity, premenstrual syndrome, and prostate disorders. Used in combination with other "kidney herbs," opens the urinary tract and removes mucus from the urine.	
Relieves muscle spasms and pain. Good for menstrual cramps. Useful for lower back and leg spasms.	Also called guelder rose. Closely related to black haw, which has the same medicinal properties. *Caution:* Should be avoided during pregnancy.
Acidifies the urine and prevents bacteria from adhering to bladder cells. Good for the kidneys, bladder, and skin. Has anticancer properties. Helpful for infections of the urinary tract. Shown to improve memory in older people (sixty years and older).	A good source of vitamin C. Cranberry juice cocktail products that contain sugar should be avoided.
Stimulates muscular contractions of the intestinal tract and delivery of oxygen to the genital area. Used as an energy tonic and aphrodisiac, and to remedy sexual and hormonal problems. A "sexuality tonic" for women.	*Caution:* Interferes with iron absorption when taken internally.

HERB (SCIENTIFIC NAME)	PART(S) USED	PHYTOCHEMICAL AND NUTRIENT CONTENT
Dandelion (*Taraxacum officinale*)	Flowers, leaves, roots, tops.	Phytochemicals: Beta-carotene, beta-sitosterol, caffeic acid, cryptoxanthin, lutein, mannitol, p-coumaric acid, saponin, stigmasterol. Nutrients: Calcium, iron, magnesium, manganese, phosphorus, potassium, selenium, zinc, vitamins B_1, B_2, B_3, and C.
Devil's claw (*Harpago-phytum procumbens*)	Rhizome.	Phytochemicals: Chlorogenic acid, cinnamic acid, harpagide, harpagoside, kaempferol, luteolin, oleanolic acid. Nutrients: Calcium, iron, magnesium, manganese, phosphorus, potassium, selenium, zinc.
Dong quai (*Angelica sinensis*)	Roots.	Phytochemicals: Alpha-pinene, bergapten, beta-carotene, beta-sitosterol, carvacrol, falcarinol, ferulic acid, ligustilide, myristic acid, p-cymene, scopoletin, umbelliferone, vanillic acid. Nutrients: Calcium, folate, iron, magnesium, manganese, phosphorus, potassium, selenium, zinc, vitamins B_1, B_2, B_5, and C.
Echinacea (*Echinacea species*)	Leaves, roots.	Phytochemicals: Alpha-pinene, apigenin, arabinogalactan, beta-carotene, beta-sitosterol, betaine, borneol, caffeic acid, caryophyllene, chlorogenic acid, cichoric acid, cynarin, echinacoside, ferulic acid, kaempferol, luteolin, quercetin, rutin, stigmasterol, vanillin, verbascoside. Nutrients: Calcium, iron, magnesium, manganese, phosphorus, potassium, selenium, zinc, vitamins B_1, B_2, B_3, and C.

ACTIONS AND USES	COMMENTS
Acts as a diuretic. Cleanses the blood and liver and increases bile production. Reduces serum cholesterol and uric acid levels. Improves functioning of the kidneys, pancreas, spleen, and stomach. Relieves menopausal symptoms. Useful for abscesses, anemia, boils, breast tumors, cirrhosis of the liver, constipation, fluid retention, hepatitis, jaundice, and rheumatism. Believed to help prevent age spots and breast cancer.	Leaves can be boiled and eaten like spinach (young leaves can be used in salads). *Caution:* Should not be combined with prescription diuretics. Not recommended for people with gallstones or biliary tract obstruction.
Relieves pain and reduces inflammation. Helps against pain in the hip and knee caused by osteoarthritis. Acts as a diuretic, sedative, and digestive stimulant. Good for back pain, arthritis, rheumatism, diabetes, allergies, liver, gallbladder and kidney disorders, arteriosclerosis, lumbago, gout, and menopausal symptoms. For backache, taking devil's claw allowed for a reduction in the use of rescue medications (i.e., pharmaceuticals for pain). When used by patients with arthritis there was less need for other medications. Migraine sufferers had a decreased number of headaches after one month.	Also called grapple plant, wood spider. *Caution:* Should not be used during pregnancy. Based on twenty studies, 3 percent of people reported side effects. Of that number, there were only a few cases—usually concerning gastrointestinal problems—that were severe enough to stop the use of the herb.
Acts as a mild sedative, laxative, diuretic, antispasmodic, and pain reliever. Improves the blood. Strengthens the reproductive system. Assists the body in using hormones. Used to treat female problems such as hot flashes and other menopausal symptoms, premenstrual syndrome, and vaginal dryness.	Also known as Chinese angelica. *Caution:* Should not be used during pregnancy. Should not be used by people who have diabetes or are light-sensitive. Dong quai enhances the action of the blood thinner warfarin, so the two should not be used together.
Fights inflammation and bacterial and viral infection. Stimulates certain white blood cells. Good for the immune system and the lymphatic system. Useful for allergies, colic, colds, flu, and other infectious illnesses. Results summarized from 234 studies showed that echinacea extracts were effective in preventing symptoms of the common cold compared to a placebo.	For internal use, a freeze-dried form or alcohol-free extract is recommended. *Caution:* Do not take for longer than three weeks. Should not be used by people who are allergic to ragweed.

HERB (SCIENTIFIC NAME)	PART(S) USED	PHYTOCHEMICAL AND NUTRIENT CONTENT
Elder (*Sambucus nigra*)	Flowers, fruit, inner bark, leaves, roots.	Phytochemicals: Alpha-amyrin, astragalin, beta-carotene, beta-sitosterol, betulin, caffeic acid, campesterol, chlorogenic acid, cycloartenol, ferulic acid, isoquercitrin, kaempferol, lupeol, malic acid, myristic acid, oleanolic acid, p-coumaric acid, pectin, quercetin, rutin, shikimic acid, stigmasterol, ursolic acid. Nutrients: Calcium, essential fatty acids, vitamins A, B_1, B_2, B_3, and C.
Ephedra (*Ephedra sinica*)	Stems.	Phytochemicals: Beta-carotene, d-norpseudoephedrine, ellagic acid, ephedrine, gallic acid. Nutrients: Calcium, iron, magnesium, manganese, phosphorus, potassium, selenium, zinc, vitamins B_1, B_2, B_3, and C.
Eucalyptus (*Eucalyptus globulus*)	Bark, essential oil, leaves.	Phytochemicals: Alpha-pinene, beta-pinene, caffeic acid, carvone, chlorogenic acid, ellagic acid, ferulic acid, gallic acid, gentisic acid, hyperoside, 1,8-cineole, p-cymene, protocatechuic acid, quercetin, quercitrin, rutin.
Eyebright (*Euphrasia officinalis*)	Entire plant, except the root.	Phytochemicals: Beta-carotene, caffeic acid, ferulic acid, tannins. Nutrients: Calcium, chromium, iron, magnesium, manganese, phosphorus, potassium, selenium, zinc, vitamins B_1, B_2, B_3, and C.

ACTIONS AND USES	COMMENTS
Combats free radicals and inflammation. Relieves coughs and congestion. Builds the blood, cleanses the system, eases constipation. Enhances immune system function. Increases perspiration, lowers fever, soothes the respiratory tract, and stimulates circulation. Effective against flu viruses. The flowers are used to soothe skin irritations.	Also called black elder, black elderberry, European elder. *Caution:* Should not be used during pregnancy. The stems of this plant should be *avoided*. They contain cyanide and can be very toxic.
	On February 6, 2004, the U.S. Food and Drug Administration (FDA) issued a final rule prohibiting the sale of dietary supplements containing ephedrine alkaloids (ephedra) because such supplements present an unreasonable risk of illness or injury. The ban was challenged in court in 2005, but it was ultimately upheld by a federal appellate court in 2006 and the U.S. Supreme Court refused to hear the case. As a result, the FDA ban is still in effect in the U.S.
Acts as a decongestant and mild antiseptic. Reduces swelling by helping to increase blood flow. Relaxes tired and sore muscles. Good for colds, coughs, and other respiratory disorders. Inhaling vapor from a few drops of the oil helps to break up mucus.	Recommended for external use only. Should not be used on broken skin or open cuts or wounds.
Prevents secretion of fluids and relieves discomfort from eyestrain or minor irritation. Used as an eyewash. Good for allergies, itchy and/or watery eyes, and runny nose. Combats hay fever.	

HERB (SCIENTIFIC NAME)	PART(S) USED	PHYTOCHEMICAL AND NUTRIENT CONTENT
False unicorn root (*Chamaelirium luteum*)	Roots.	Phytochemicals: Chamaelirin, helonin, saponins.
Fennel (*Foeniculum vulgare*)	Fruit, roots, leaves, stems.	Phytochemicals: Alpha-pinene, benzoic acid, bergapten, beta-carotene, beta-phellandrene, beta-sitosterol, caffeic acid, camphor, cinnamic acid, cynarin, ferulic acid, fumaric acid, isopimpinellin, isoquercitrin, kaempferol, limonene, linalool, myristicin, 1,8-cineole, p-coumaric acid, pectin, protocatechuic acid, psoralen, quercetin, rutin, scopoletin, sinapic acid, stigmasterol, umbelliferone, vanillic acid, vanillin, xanthotoxin. Nutrients: Amino acids, calcium, choline, essential fatty acids, iron, magnesium, manganese, phosphorus, potassium, selenium, vitamins B_1, B_2, B_3, C, and E.
Fenugreek (*Trigonella foenum-graecum*)	Seeds.	Phytochemicals: Beta-carotene, beta-sitosterol, coumarin, diosgenin, kaempferol, luteolin, p-coumaric acid, quercetin, rutin, saponin, trigonelline, vitexin. Nutrients: Amino acids, calcium, essential fatty acids, folate, iron, magnesium, manganese, phosphorus, potassium, selenium, zinc, vitamins B_1, B_2, B_3, and C.
Feverfew (*Chrysanthemum parthenium*)	Bark, dried flowers, leaves.	Phytochemicals: Beta-carotene, parthenolide, santamarin. Nutrients: Calcium, iron, magnesium, manganese, phosphorus, potassium, selenium, zinc, vitamins B_1, B_2, B_3, and C.

ACTIONS AND USES	COMMENTS
Balances sex hormones. Helps treat infertility, menstrual irregularities and pain, premenstrual syndrome, and prostate disorders. May help prevent miscarriage.	Also called helonias.
Used as an appetite suppressant and as an eyewash. Promotes the functioning of the kidneys, liver, and spleen, and also clears the lungs. Relieves abdominal pain, colon disorders, gas, and gastrointestinal tract spasms. Useful for acid stomach. Good after chemotherapy and/or radiation treatments for cancer.	The powdered plant can be used as a flea repellent.
Acts as a laxative, lubricates the intestines, and reduces fever. Helps lower cholesterol and blood sugar levels. Helps asthma and sinus problems by reducing mucus. Good for the eyes and for inflammation and lung disorders.	Oil of fenugreek has a maplelike flavor. *Caution:* Do not use if you are taking a blood thinner or have a hormone-sensitive cancer.
Combats inflammation and muscle spasms. Increases fluidity of lung and bronchial tube mucus, promotes menses, stimulates the appetite, and stimulates uterine contractions. Relieves nausea and vomiting. Good for arthritis, colitis, fever, headaches, mild and transient migraines, menstrual problems, muscle tension, and pain.	Chewing the leaves is a folk remedy, but this may cause mouth sores. Also called featherfew, featherfoil. *Caution:* Do not use when pregnant or nursing. People who take prescription blood-thinning medications or who regularly take over-the-counter painkillers should consult a health care provider before using feverfew, as the combination can result in internal bleeding.

HERB (SCIENTIFIC NAME)	PART(S) USED	PHYTOCHEMICAL AND NUTRIENT CONTENT
Flax (*Linum usitatissimum*)	Seeds, seed oil.	Phytochemicals: Apigenin, beta-carotene, beta-sitosterol, campesterol, chlorogenic acid, cycloartenol, lecithin, luteolin, myristic acid, squalene, stigmasterol, vitexin. Nutrients: Amino acids, calcium, essential fatty acids, iron, magnesium, manganese, phosphorus, potassium, sulfur, vanadium, zinc, vitamins B_1, B_2, B_3, B_5, and E.
Garlic (*Allium sativa*)	Bulb.	Phytochemicals: Allicin, beta-carotene, beta-sitosterol, caffeic acid, chlorogenic acid, diallyl-disulfide, ferulic acid, geraniol, kaempferol, linalool, oleanolic acid, p-coumaric acid, phloroglucinol, phytic acid, quercetin, rutin, s-allyl-cysteine, saponin, sinapic acid, stigmasterol. Nutrients: Calcium, folate, iron, magnesium, manganese, phosphorus, potassium, selenium, zinc, vitamins B_1, B_2, B_3, and C.
Gentian (*Gentiana lutea*)	Leaves, roots.	Phytochemicals: Caffeic acid, carvacrol, gentiopicrin, limonene, linalool, mangiferin, sinapic acid, swertiamarin. Nutrients: Calcium, iron, magnesium, manganese, phosphorus, potassium, selenium, zinc, vitamins B_1, B_2, B_3, and C.
Ginger (*Zingiber officinale*)	Rhizomes, roots.	Phytochemicals: Alpha-pinene, beta-carotene, beta-ionone, beta-sitosterol, caffeic acid, camphor, capsaicin, caryophyllene, chlorogenic acid, citral, curcumin, farnesol, ferulic acid, geraniol, gingerols, lecithin, 1,8-cineole, zingerone. Nutrients: Amino acids, calcium, essential fatty acids, iron, magnesium, manganese, phosphorus, potassium, selenium, zinc, vitamins B_1, B_2, B_3, B_6, and C. Ground ginger also contains vitamin A.

ACTIONS AND USES	COMMENTS
Promotes strong bones, nails, and teeth, as well as healthy skin. Useful for colon problems, female disorders, and inflammation. May help normalize hormones in postmenopausal women and thus could reduce the risk of breast cancer. Emerging evidence is showing a beneficial effect for people with high cholesterol levels and for those with diabetes.	The seeds are an excellent addition to a diet that is low in fiber. Flaxseed has the highest concentration of the phytoestrogen lignans of any other food. The lignans are removed during conversion to oil, so seeds are the only true source.
Detoxifies the body and protects against infection by enhancing immune function. Lowers blood pressure and improves circulation. Lowers blood lipid levels. Helps stabilize blood sugar levels. Aids in the treatment of arteriosclerosis, arthritis, asthma, cancer, circulatory problems, colds and flu, digestive problems, heart disorders, insomnia, liver disease, sinusitis, ulcers, and yeast infections. May prevent ulcers by inhibiting growth of *Helicobacter pylori*, the ulcer-causing bacterium. Good for virtually any disease or infection.	Garlic contains many sulfur compounds, which give it its healing properties. Odorless garlic supplements are available. Aged garlic extract (such as Kyolic) is good. *Caution:* Not recommended for people who take anticoagulants, as garlic has blood-thinning actions.
Aids digestion, stimulates appetite, and boosts circulation. Kills plasmodia (organisms that cause malaria) and worms. Good for circulatory problems and pancreatitis.	
Fights inflammation, cleanses the colon, reduces spasms and cramps, and stimulates circulation. A strong antioxidant and effective antimicrobial agent for sores and wounds. Protects the liver and stomach. Useful for bowel disorders, circulatory problems, arthritis, fever, headache, hot flashes, indigestion, morning sickness, motion sickness, muscle pain, nausea, and vomiting.	Can cause stomach distress if taken in large quantities. *Caution:* Not recommended for people who take anticoagulants or have gallstones. Not recommended for extended use during pregnancy.

HERB (SCIENTIFIC NAME)	PART(S) USED	PHYTOCHEMICAL AND NUTRIENT CONTENT
Ginkgo (*Ginkgo biloba*)	Leaves, seed.	Phytochemicals: Amentoflavone, apigenin, beta-carotene, bilobalide, ginkgetin, isorhamnetin, kaempferol, luteolin, myristic acid, p-coumaric acid, procyanidin, quercetin, shikimic acid, stigmasterol, tannin, thymol. Nutrients: Amino acids, calcium, iron, magnesium, manganese, phosphorus, potassium, zinc, vitamins A, B_1, B_2, B_3, B_5, and C.
Ginseng (*Panax quinquefolius*) [American ginseng], (*P. ginseng*) [Chinese or Korean ginseng]	Roots.	Phytochemicals: Beta-sitosterol, campesterols, caryophyllene, cinnamic acid, escin (*P. quinquefolius*), ferulic acid, fumaric acid, ginsenosides, kaempferol, oleanolic acid, panaxic acid, panaxin, saponin, stigmasterol, vanillic acid. Nutrients: Calcium, choline, fiber, folate, iron, magnesium, manganese, phosphorus, potassium, silicon, zinc, vitamins B_1, B_2, B_3, B_5, and C.
Goldenseal (*Hydrastis canadensis*)	Rhizomes, roots.	Phytochemicals: Berberine, beta-carotene, canadine, chlorogenic acid. Nutrients: Calcium, iron, magnesium, manganese, phosphorus, potassium, selenium, zinc, vitamins B_1, B_2, B_3, and C.

ACTIONS AND USES	COMMENTS
Improves brain functioning by increasing cerebral and peripheral circulation and tissue oxygenation. Has antioxidant properties. May slow the progression of Alzheimer's disease, and may relieve leg cramps by improving circulation. Beneficial for asthma, dementia, depression, eczema, headaches, heart and kidney disorders, memory loss, and tinnitus (ringing in the ears). Shows promise as a treatment for vascular-related impotence.	Can take at least two weeks to see results. *Caution:* Should not be used by people who have bleeding disorders, or who are scheduled for surgery or a dental procedure.
Strengthens the adrenal and reproductive glands. Enhances immune function, promotes lung functioning, and stimulates the appetite. Useful for bronchitis, circulatory problems, diabetes, infertility, lack of energy, and stress; to ease withdrawal from cocaine; and to protect against the effects of radiation exposure. In a laboratory study, enhanced breast-cancer-cell suppression in combination with standard treatment. Used by athletes for overall body strengthening. May help improve drug- or alcohol-induced liver dysfunction in older adults.	Siberian ginseng (*Eleutherococcus senticosus*) belongs to a different botanical family than American and Korean ginseng, but its properties are similar, and all are commonly referred to simply as ginseng. *Caution:* Should not be used by people who have high blood pressure, are pregnant, or are nursing. Also avoid if taking insulin or MAOIs (monoamine oxidase inhibitors) for depression.
Fights infection and inflammation. Cleanses the body. Increases the effectiveness of insulin and strengthens the immune system, colon, liver, pancreas, spleen, and lymphatic and respiratory systems. Improves digestion, regulates menses, decreases uterine bleeding, and stimulates the central nervous system. Good for allergies, ulcers, and disorders affecting the bladder, prostate, stomach, and vagina. Used at the first sign of possible symptoms, can stop a cold, flu, or sore throat from developing.	Alternating with echinacea or other herbs is recommended. Alcohol-free extract is the best form. *Caution:* Do not take goldenseal internally on a daily basis for more than one week at a time. Do not use it during pregnancy or if you are breast-feeding, and use with caution if you are allergic to ragweed. If you have a history of cardiovascular disease, diabetes, or glaucoma, use it only under a doctor's supervision.

HERB (SCIENTIFIC NAME)	PART(S) USED	PHYTOCHEMICAL AND NUTRIENT CONTENT
Gotu kola (*Centella asiatica*)	Nuts, roots, seeds.	Phytochemicals: Beta-carotene, beta-sitosterol, campesterol, camphor, kaempferol, saponin, stigmasterol. Nutrients: Calcium, iron, magnesium, manganese, phosphorus, potassium, selenium, zinc, vitamins B_1, B_2, B_3, and C.
Gravel root (*Eupatorium purpureum*)	Flowers, root.	Phytochemicals: Euparin, eupatorin, resin.
Green tea (*Camellia sinensis*)	Leaves.	Phytochemicals: Apigenin, astragalin, benzaldehyde, beta-carotene, beta-ionone, beta-sitosterol, caffeic acid, caffeine, carvacrol, catechins, chlorogenic acid, cinnamic acid, cryptoxanthin, epicatechin, epigallocatechin, eugenol, farnesol, gallic acid, geraniol, hyperoside, indole, isoquercitrin, kaempferol, lutein, lycopene, myrcene, myricetin, myristic acid, naringenin, polyphenols, procyanidins, quercetin, quercitrin, rutin, salicylic acid, tannic acid, thymol, vitexin, zeaxanthin. Nutrients: Amino acids, calcium, iron, magnesium, manganese, phosphorus, potassium, zinc, vitamins B_1, B_2, B_3, B_5, and C.
Guarana (*Paullinia cupana*)	Seeds.	Phytochemicals: Adenine, caffeine, D-catechin, saponin, tannins, theobromine, theophylline.

ACTIONS AND USES	COMMENTS
Helps eliminate excess fluids, decreases fatigue and depression, increases sex drive, shrinks tissues, and stimulates the central nervous system. May neutralize blood acids and lower body temperature. Promotes wound healing, and is good for varicose veins and for heart and liver function. Useful for cardiovascular and circulatory disorders, fatigue, connective tissue disorders, kidney stones, poor appetite, and sleep disorders.	May cause dermatitis if applied topically.
Acts as a diuretic and urinary tract tonic. Combats prostate disorders, kidney stones, and problems related to fluid retention.	Also called joe-pye weed, queen-of-the meadow.
Acts as an antioxidant and helps to protect against cancer. Lowers cholesterol levels, reduces the clotting tendency of the blood, stimulates the immune system, fights tooth decay, helps regulate blood sugar and insulin levels, combats mental fatigue, and may delay the onset of atherosclerosis. Good for asthma. Studies show promise as a weight-loss aid, but the green tea must not be decaffeinated. May help prevent enlarged prostate.	To get green tea's antioxidant benefits, drink it without milk (milk may bind with the beneficial compounds, making them unavailable to the body). *Caution:* Contains a small amount of caffeine. Should not be used in large quantities by pregnant women or nursing mothers. Persons with anxiety disorder or irregular heartbeat should limit their intake to no more than 2 cups daily.
Acts as a general tonic, stimulant, and intestinal cleanser. Increases mental alertness as well as speed and accuracy when reading. Improves stamina and endurance. Reduces fatigue. Useful for headaches, urinary tract irritation, diarrhea. Also shown to improve mood.	Also called Brazilian cocoa, uabano. *Caution:* Due to guarana's caffeine content, taking more than 400 mg a day is not recommended. Not recommended for people with high blood pressure or heart conditions.

HERB (SCIENTIFIC NAME)	PART(S) USED	PHYTOCHEMICAL AND NUTRIENT CONTENT
Hawthorn (*Crataegus laevigata*)	Flowers, fruit, leaves.	Phytochemicals: Acetylcholine, adenine, adenosine, anthocyanidins, beta-carotene, beta-sitosterol, caffeic acid, catechin, chlorogenic acid, epicatechin, esculin, hyperoside, pectin, quercitrin, rutin, ursolic acid, vitexin. Nutrients: Amino acids, calcium, choline, chromium, essential fatty acids, iron, magnesium, manganese, phosphorus, potassium, selenium, silicon, zinc, vitamins B_1, B_2, B_3, and C.
Hops (*Humulus lupulus*)	Flowers, fruit, leaves.	Phytochemicals: Alpha-pinene, alpha-terpineol, beta-carotene, beta-eudesmol, beta-sitosterol, caffeic acid, campesterol, catechin, chlorogenic acid, citral, eugenol, ferulic acid, limonene, p-cymene, piperidine, procyanidins, quercetin, tannins. Nutrients: Amino acids, calcium, chromium, magnesium, potassium, selenium, silicon, zinc, vitamins B_1, B_3, and C.
Horehound (*Marrubium vulgare*)	Flowers, leaves.	Phytochemicals: Alpha-pinene, apigenin, beta-sitosterol, caffeic acid, gallic acid, limonene, luteolin, pectin, tannic acid, tannins, ursolic acid. Nutrients: B-complex vitamins, iron, potassium, vitamins A, C, and E.
Horse chestnut (*Aesculus hippocastanum*)	Bark, leaves, oil, seeds.	Phytochemicals: Allantoin, citric acid, epicatechin, escin, esculetin, esculin, fraxetin, fraxin, isoquercitrin, kaempferol, leucocyanidin, myricetin, quercetin, quercitrin, rutin, saponin, scopoletin, tannin.

ACTIONS AND USES	COMMENTS
Dilates the coronary blood vessels, lowers blood pressure and cholesterol levels, and restores heart muscle. Decreases fat deposit levels. Increases intracellular vitamin C levels. Useful for anemia, cardiovascular and circulatory disorders, high cholesterol, and lowered immunity. Patients with diabetes who were already using blood pressure medicine experienced a greater drop in blood pressure with hawthorn.	*Caution:* Do not use if you take medication for heart disease.
Relieves anxiety. Stimulates the appetite. Useful for cardiovascular disorders, hyperactivity, insomnia, nervousness, pain, restlessness, shock, stress, toothaches, and ulcers. May help people with diabetes lower blood sugar and help reduce hot flashes in menopausal women.	Placed inside a pillowcase, aids sleep. *Caution:* Should not be used by people who take antidepressants.
Decreases thickness and increases fluidity of mucus in the bronchial tubes and lungs. Boosts the immune system. Useful for indigestion, loss of appetite, bloating, and hay fever, sinusitis, and other respiratory disorders.	*Caution:* Large doses may cause irregular heart rhythms.
Protects against vascular damage, makes capillary walls less porous, shields against UV radiation damage. Good for varicose veins, reducing excess tissue fluids, and easing nighttime muscle spasms in the legs. For chronic venous insufficiency, horse chestnut was effective at reducing leg pain and allowed for less blood to pool in the lower limbs. Used topically, reduces pain and swelling, and prevents bruising.	*Caution:* If you are taking warfarin, aspirin, or other blood thinners, horse chestnut products that contain esculin may increase the risk of bleeding. Check to make sure that your horse chestnut product is esculin-free.

HERB (SCIENTIFIC NAME)	PART(S) USED	PHYTOCHEMICAL AND NUTRIENT CONTENT
Hydrangea (*Hydrangea arborescens*)	Rhizomes, roots.	Phytochemicals: Kaempferol, quercetin, rutin, saponin. Nutrients: Calcium, iron, magnesium, manganese, phosphorus, potassium, selenium, zinc.
Hyssop (*Hyssopus officinalis*)	Flowers, leaves, shoots.	Phytochemicals: Alpha-pinene, benzaldehyde, beta-ionone, beta-sitosterol, borneol, caffeic acid, camphor, carvacrol, eugenol, ferulic acid, geraniol, hesperidin, limonene, linalool, marrubiin, oleanolic acid, 1,8-cineole, rosmarinic acid, thymol, ursolic acid. Nutrients: Choline.
Irish moss (*Chondrus crispus*)	Entire plant.	Phytochemicals: Beta-carotene. Nutrients: Calcium, iron, magnesium, manganese, phosphorus, potassium, selenium, zinc, vitamins B_1, B_2, B_3, and C.
Jaborandi (*Pilocarpus jaborandi*)	Leaves.	Phytochemicals: Alpha-pinene, limonene, myrcene, pilocarpine.
Jatoba (*Hymenaea courbaril*)	Bark, leaves, fruit.	Phytochemicals: Beta-sitosterol, caryophyllene, delta-cadinene, epicatechin.
Juniper (*Juniperus communis*)	Fruit.	Phytochemicals: Alpha-pinene, beta-carotene, beta-pinene, betulin, borneol, camphor, caryophyllene, catechin, farnesol, epicatechin, glycolic acid, limonene, linalool, menthol, rutin, tannins, umbelliferone. Nutrients: Calcium, chromium, iron, magnesium, manganese, phosphorus, potassium, selenium, zinc, vitamins B_1, B_2, B_3, and C.

ACTIONS AND USES	COMMENTS
Stimulates the kidneys and acts as a diuretic. Good for bladder infection, kidney disease, obesity, and prostate disorders. Combined with gravel root, good for kidney stones.	*Caution:* The leaves of this plant should *not* be consumed. They contain cyanide and can be toxic.
Promotes expulsion of mucus from the respiratory tract, relieves congestion, regulates blood pressure, and dispels gas. Used externally, helpful for wound healing. Good for circulatory problems, epilepsy, fever, gout, and weight problems. Poultices made from fresh green hyssop help heal cuts.	*Caution:* Should not be used during pregnancy.
Acts as an expectorant and aids in the formation of stools. Good for bronchitis and many intestinal disorders. Also used in skin lotions and in hair rinses for dry hair.	
Fights inflammation and acts as a diuretic. Helps stimulate milk production and flow in nursing mothers. Beneficial for fever, colds and flu, bronchitis, colon disorders, and edema. Topically, useful for baldness and for promoting circulation in the capillaries.	A rainforest herb whose active compound, pilocarpine, has been used for over 120 years to relieve intraocular pressure in glaucoma.
Fights inflammation, free radicals, and bacterial and fungal infection. Increases energy. Beneficial for asthma, bronchitis, bursitis, bladder infection, candida and other fungal infections, arthritis, and prostatitis.	A rainforest herb with a wide range of traditional uses.
Acts as a diuretic, anti-inflammatory, and decongestant. Helps regulate blood sugar levels. Helpful in treatment of asthma, bladder infection, fluid retention, gout, obesity, and prostate disorders.	*Caution:* May interfere with absorption of iron and other minerals when taken internally. Should not be used during pregnancy. Should not be used by persons with kidney disease.

HERB (SCIENTIFIC NAME)	PART(S) USED	PHYTOCHEMICAL AND NUTRIENT CONTENT
Kava kava (*Piper methysticum*)	Roots.	Phytochemicals: Cinnamic acid, kavalactones (including kawain, dihydrokawain, methysticin, dihydromethysticin, and yangonin).
Kudzu (*Pueraria lobata*)	Leaves, roots, shoots.	Phytochemicals: Daidzein, daidzin, genistein, p-coumaric acid, puerarin, quercetin. Nutrients: Calcium, iron, magnesium, phosphorus, potassium, vitamin B_2.
Lady's-mantle (*Achillea millefolium*)	Entire plant, except the root.	Phytochemicals: Achilleine, alpha-pinene, apigenin, azulene, beta-carotene, betaine, beta-pinene, beta-sitosterol, betonicine, borneol, caffeic acid, camphor, caryophyllene, chamazulene, coumarins, eugenol, guaiazulene, isorhamnetin, limonene, luteolin, mannitol, menthol, myrcene, myristic acid, 1,8-cineole, p-cymene, quercetin, quercitrin, rutin, salicylic acid, stigmasterol, tannin, thujone. Nutrients: Amino acids, calcium, essential fatty acids, folate, iron, magnesium, manganese, phosphorus, potassium, selenium, zinc, vitamins B_1, B_2, B_3, and C.
Lavender (*Lavandula angustifolia*)	Flowers.	Phytochemicals: Alpha-pinene, beta-pinene, beta-santalene, borneol, camphor, caryophyllene, coumarin, geraniol, limonene, linalool, luteolin, 1,8-cineole, rosmarinic acid, tannin, umbelliferone, ursolic acid.

ACTIONS AND USES	COMMENTS
Induces physical and mental relaxation. Acts as a diuretic, genitourinary antiseptic, and gastrointestinal tonic. Relieves muscle spasms and eases pain. Helpful for anxiety and anxiety disorders, insomnia, stress-related disorders, menopausal symptoms, and urinary tract infections. It has been shown to be an analgesic and an anticonvulsive and protects the nervous system. Usually begins working within two hours, but multiple (about three times a day) dosing is needed to maintain blood levels.	Also called kava. *Caution:* Can cause drowsiness. If this occurs, discontinue use or reduce the dosage. Should not be combined with alcohol. Not recommended for persons under the age of eighteen, pregnant women, nursing mothers, individuals who suffer from depression or take certain prescription drugs, especially antianxiety drugs, or those with liver or skin diseases. Kava taken in large amounts for extended periods of time may worsen liver function tests.
Suppresses alcohol cravings. Lowers blood pressure and relieves headache, stiff neck, vertigo, and tinnitus. Useful for treating alcoholism, colds, flu, and gastrointestinal problems.	In China and Japan, kudzu has been used as a food starch and medicine for centuries. The Chinese use kudzu extract to treat angina pectoris.
Wound dressing. Has anti-inflammatory, diuretic, and antiviral effects. Helps to heal mucous membranes, improve blood clotting, and increase perspiration. Helps to regulate menstruation, reduce excessive bleeding, and ease cramps. Useful for muscle spasms, fever, gastrointestinal disorders, inflammatory disorders, and viral infections. Applied topically, stops bleeding and promotes healing. Good as a douche for vaginal irritation.	Also called milfoil, old man's pepper, soldier's woundwort, knight's milfoil, herba militaris, thousand-leaf, nosebleed, carpenter's weed, bloodwort, staunchweed, devil's nettle, devil's plaything, bad man's plaything, yarroway. *Caution:* Interferes with iron absorption and other minerals. Topical use may cause irritation. Individuals who are sun sensitive should avoid it. Not to be used by pregnant women.
Relieves stress and depression. Beneficial for the skin. Good for headaches, psoriasis, and other skin problems.	Essential oil of lavender is very popular in aromatherapy. *Caution:* Should not be used during pregnancy. Lavender oil should not be taken internally.

HERB (SCIENTIFIC NAME)	PART(S) USED	PHYTOCHEMICAL AND NUTRIENT CONTENT
Lemongrass (*Cymbopogon citratus*)	Leaves, stems.	Phytochemicals: Alpha-pinene, beta-pinene, beta-santalene, borneol, camphor, caryophyllene, coumarin, geraniol, limonene, linalool, luteolin, 1,8-cineole, rosmarinic acid, tannin, umbelliferone, ursolic acid. Phytochemicals: Alpha-pinene, beta-sitosterol, caryophyllene, citral, farnesol, geraniol, limonene, luteolin, myrcene, 1,8-cineole, quercetin, rutin, saponin, triacontanol. Nutrients: Calcium, iron, magnesium, manganese, phosphorus, potassium, selenium, zinc.
Licorice (*Glycyrrhiza glabra*)	Roots.	Phytochemicals: Apigenin, benzaldehyde, beta-carotene, beta-sitosterol, betaine, camphor, carvacrol, estriol, eugenol, ferulic acid, formononetin, geraniol, glabrene, glabridin, glabrol, glycyrrhetinic acid, glycyrrhizin, isoliquiritigenin, isoliquiritin, isoquercitrin, lignin, mannitol, phenol, quercetin, salicylic acid, sinapic acid, stigmasterol, thymol, umbelliferone, vitexin. Nutrients: Calcium, choline, iron, magnesium, manganese, phosphorus, potassium, selenium, silicon, zinc, vitamins B_1, B_2, B_3, and C.

ACTIONS AND USES

COMMENTS

Acts as an astringent, tonic, and digestive aid. Good for the skin and nails. Useful for fever, flu, headaches, and intestinal irritations.

Used in perfumes and other products as a fragrance.

Side effects:
Oral: Dizziness, drowsiness, dry mouth, excess urination, and increased appetite. In high doses, essential oil of lemongrass can damage liver and stomach mucous membranes. Excessive intake of lemongrass tea may also affect kidney function.
Topical: Skin rash with the use of lemongrass essential oils.

Fights inflammation and viral, bacterial, and parasitic infection. Stimulates the production of interferon and may help inhibit replication of HIV. Cleanses the colon. Reduces muscle spasms, increases fluidity of mucus in the lungs and bronchial tubes, and promotes adrenal gland function. Has estrogen- and progesterone-like effects; may change the pitch of the voice. Helps to inhibit the formation of plaque and prevent bacteria from sticking to tooth enamel. Beneficial for allergies, asthma, chronic fatigue syndrome, depression, emphysema, enlarged prostate, fever, herpesvirus infection, hypoglycemia, glandular functions, inflammatory bowel disorders, premenstrual syndrome, menopausal symptoms, and upper respiratory infections. May prevent hepatitis C from causing liver cancer and cirrhosis and protect against atherosclerosis. Deglycyrrhizinated licorice may stimulate natural defense mechanisms that prevent the occurrence of ulcers by increasing the number of mucus-secreting cells in the digestive tract. This improves the quality of mucus, lengthens intestinal cell life, and enhances microcirculation in the gastrointestinal lining. Cancer patients who took licorice and a soup containing tonic vegetables had less pain. The plant has been shown to have anticancer properties.

Licorice derivatives have been recommended as a standard support for ulcer sufferers in Europe. Licorice-flavored candy does not work for medicinal purposes because it is mostly made with anise, not licorice.

Caution: Should not be used during pregnancy, nor by persons with diabetes, glaucoma, heart disease, high blood pressure, severe menstrual problems, or a history of stroke.

HERB (SCIENTIFIC NAME)	PART(S) USED	PHYTOCHEMICAL AND NUTRIENT CONTENT
Maca (*Lepidium meyenii*)	Roots.	Phytochemicals: Beta-sitosterol, saponin, stigmasterol, tannins. Nutrients: Amino acids, calcium, iron, magnesium, phosphorus, zinc, vitamins B_1, B_2, B_{12}, C, and E.
Macela (*Achyrocline satureoides*)	Aerial parts.	Phytochemicals: Alpha-pinene, caffeic acid, caryophyllene, chlorogenic acid, coumarin, delta-cadinene, galangin, luteolin, 1,8-cineole, quercetagetin, quercetin, scoparone.
Marshmallow (*Althaea officinalis*)	Flowers, leaves, roots.	Phytochemicals: Beta-carotene, betaine, caffeic acid, chlorogenic acid, ferulic acid, kaempferol, mucilage, paraffin, p-coumaric acid, pectin, phytosterols, quercetin, salicylic acid, scopoletin, sorbitol, tannins, vanillic acid. Nutrients: Amino acids, calcium, iron, magnesium, manganese, phosphorus, potassium, selenium, zinc, vitamins B_1, B_2, B_3, and C.
Meadowsweet (*Filipendula ulmaria*)	Leaves, flower tops.	Phytochemicals: Anthocyanidin, avicularin, coumarin, hyperoside, methyl salicylate, quercetin, rutin, salicin, salicylic acid, vanillin.

ACTIONS AND USES	COMMENTS
Increases energy and supports the immune system. Good for anemia, chronic fatigue syndrome, impotence, fertility, menopausal symptoms, and menstrual problems.	A rainforest herb that is a member of the potato family. An important food in the diet of native Peruvians for over 2,000 years, it is rich in amino acids and high in protein.
	Caution: People with liver or heart disease should avoid high doses, as it has been shown to worsen liver blood tests and raise blood pressure.
Acts as an anti-inflammatory, antiseptic, antiviral, and antiparasitic. Stimulates and supports the immune system. Good for gastrointestinal and respiratory disorders. Useful in treating cancer, Crohn's disease, colds and flu, diabetes, menstrual problems and menopausal symptoms, and muscle aches and spasms.	A rainforest herb that has been found to have potential anti-HIV properties.
Aids the body in expelling excess fluid and mucus. Soothes and heals skin, mucous membranes, and other tissues, externally and internally. Good for bladder infection, digestive upsets, fluid retention, headache, intestinal disorders, kidney problems, sinusitis, and sore throat.	Often used as a filler in the compounding of pills.
Tightens tissues and promotes elimination of excess fluid. Reduces inflammation and strengthens and tones the system. Good for colds, flu, nausea, digestive disorders, muscle cramps and aches, and diarrhea.	The word *aspirin* is derived from an old name for this plant, *spirea.*
	Caution: Because this plant contains compounds related to aspirin, it should not be used by pregnant women, and it should not be given to children with fever due to cold, flu, measles, chickenpox, or any other viral infection, as this increases the risk of Reye's syndrome, a dangerous complication that can alter or damage the liver, brain, and heart.

HERB (SCIENTIFIC NAME)	PART(S) USED	PHYTOCHEMICAL AND NUTRIENT CONTENT
Milk thistle (*Silybum marianum*)	Fruit, leaves, seeds.	Phytochemicals: Apigenin, beta-carotene, fumaric acid, kaempferol, naringenin, quercetin, silandrin, silybin, silychristin, silydianin, silymarin, silymonin, taxifolin. Nutrients: Calcium, essential fatty acids, iron, magnesium, manganese, phosphorus, potassium, selenium, zinc.
Motherwort (*Leonurus cardiaca*)	Leaves, flowers, stems.	Phytochemicals: Alpha-pinene, benzaldehyde, caryophyllene, catechin, hyperoside, isoquercitrin, limonene, linalool, marrubiin, oleanolic acid, quercetin, quercitrin, rutin, saponin, stachydrine, tannin, ursolic acid. Nutrients: Vitamin C.
Muira puama (*Ptychopetalum olacoides*)	Bark, roots.	Phytochemicals: Beta-sitosterol, campesterol, coumarin, lupeol.
Mullein (*Verbascum thapsus*)	Leaves.	Phytochemicals: Beta-carotene, beta-sitosterol, coumarin, hesperidin, saponins. Nutrients: Calcium, iron, magnesium, manganese, phosphorus, potassium, selenium, zinc, vitamins B_1, B_2, B_3, and C.
Mustard (*Brassica nigra*)	Seeds.	Phytochemicals: Allyl isothiocyanate, caffeic acid, chlorogenic acid, ferulic acid, p-coumaric acid, protocatechuic acid, sinapic acid, vanillic acid.

ACTIONS AND USES	COMMENTS
Protects the liver from toxins and pollutants by preventing free radical damage and stimulates the production of new liver cells. People with liver disease who used silymarin had fewer liver-related symptoms and better quality-of-life scores. Also protects the kidneys. Good for gallbladder and adrenal disorders, inflammatory bowel disorders, psoriasis, weakened immune system, and all liver disorders. Has shown anticancer effects against prostate cancer and breast cancer. Silymarin inhibits COX-2 formation.	Also called Mary thistle or wild artichoke. Because milk thistle has poor water solubility, it is not effective as a tea. A concentrated capsule or extract form is best.
Traditionally used to relieve childbirth pain and as a tranquilizer. Helpful for menstrual disorders, menopausal symptoms, vaginitis, thyroid and rheumatic problems. Has a tonic effect on the heart. Useful for headache, insomnia, and vertigo.	*Caution:* Should not be used during pregnancy (until the onset of labor), as it can stimulate uterine contractions. Check with your health care provider before using it during the birthing process. Not recommended for persons with clotting disorders, high blood pressure, or heart disease.
Helps relieve pain, acts as a mild laxative and detoxifier, and supports the heart. Has a general tonic effect and balances sex hormones. Beneficial in treating nervous system disorders, impotence, depression, stress, rheumatism, hair loss, asthma, and menopausal and menstrual problems.	An alcohol-based extract is believed to be the best form of this rainforest herb, as the active constituents are neither water soluble nor broken down in the digestive process.
Acts as a laxative, painkiller, and sleep aid. Taken internally, aids in getting rid of warts. Clears congestion. Useful for asthma, bronchitis, difficulty breathing, earache, hay fever, and swollen glands. Used in kidney formulas to soothe inflammation.	
Improves digestion and aids in the metabolism of fat. Applied externally, helpful for chest congestion, inflammation, injuries, and joint pain.	*Caution:* Can be irritating when applied directly to the skin. Not recommended for use on children under the age of six.

HERB (SCIENTIFIC NAME)	PART(S) USED	PHYTOCHEMICAL AND NUTRIENT CONTENT
Myrrh (*Commiphora myrrha*)	Resin from stems.	Phytochemicals: Acetic acid, beta-sitosterol, campesterol, cinnamaldehyde, cuminaldehyde, dipentene, eugenol, limonene, m-cresol.
Nettle (*Urtica dioica*)	Flowers, leaves, roots.	Phytochemicals: Acetic acid, beta-carotene, betaine, caffeic acid, ferulic acid, lecithin, lycopene, p-coumaric acid, scopoletin. Nutrients: Calcium, copper, essential fatty acids, folate, iron, magnesium, manganese, phosphorus, potassium, selenium, sulfur, zinc, vitamins B_1, B_2, B_3, B_5, C, and E.
Oat straw (*Avena sativa*)	Whole plant.	Phytochemicals: Benzaldehyde, beta-carotene, beta-ionone, beta-sitosterol, betaine, caffeic acid, campesterol, caryophyllene, chlorophyll, ferulic acid, lignin, limonene, p-coumaric acid, quercetin, scopoletin, sinapic acid, stigmasterol, vanillic acid, vanillin. Nutrients: Calcium, folate, iron, magnesium, manganese, phosphorus, potassium, selenium, zinc, vitamins A, B_1, B_2, B_3, B_5, B_6, and E.
Olive leaf (*Olea europaea*)	Extract from leaves.	Phytochemicals: Apigenin, beta-sitosterol glucoside, cinchonidine, esculetin, kaempferol, luteolin, mannitol, maslinic acid, oleanic acid, oleuropein, quercetin, rutin, tannins. Nutrient: Calcium.
Oregon grape (*Mahonia aquifolia*)	Roots.	Phytochemicals: Berberine, tannins.

ACTIONS AND USES

COMMENTS

Acts as an antiseptic, disinfectant, expectorant, and deodorizer. Stimulates the immune system and gastric secretions. Tones and stimulates mucous tissue. Helps to fight harmful bacteria in the mouth. Good for bad breath, periodontal disease, skin disorders, asthma, bronchitis, colds, flu, sinusitis, sore throat, herpes simplex, and ulcers. Topically, useful for abscesses, boils, sores, and wounds.

Used in many perfumes and in incense for its aromatic properties.

Acts as a diuretic, expectorant, pain reliever, and tonic. Good for benign prostatic hyperplasia, anemia, arthritis, rheumatism, hay fever, and other allergic disorders, kidney problems, and malabsorption syndrome. Improves goiter, inflammatory conditions, and mucous conditions of the lungs. Used in hair care products, helps stimulate hair follicles and regulate scalp oil buildup.

Also called stinging nettle.

Caution: Do not take if you are taking diuretics or hypotensive drugs (can have additive effects) or cytochrome P450 substrate drugs (can increase the risk of side effects).

Acts as an antidepressant and restorative nerve tonic. Increases perspiration. Helps to ease insomnia. Good for bed-wetting, depression, stress, and skin disorders.

Fights all types of bacteria, viruses, fungi, and parasites. Helps stave off colds and flu. May have antioxidant properties. Has shown potential for lowering high blood pressure. Good for virtually any infectious disease, as well as for chronic fatigue syndrome, diarrheal diseases, inflammatory arthritis, and psoriasis.

Caution: Do not take if you are using blood pressure medicines or insulin and other medications that lower blood pressure.

Purifies the blood and cleanses the liver. Acts as a laxative. Good for many skin conditions, from acne to psoriasis.

Has actions similar to those of goldenseal and barberry.

HERB (SCIENTIFIC NAME)	PART(S) USED	PHYTOCHEMICAL AND NUTRIENT CONTENT
Papaya (*Carica papaya*)	Fruit, leaves.	Phytochemicals: Benzaldehyde, beta-carotene, caryophyllene, linalool, lycopene, malic acid, methyl salicylate, myristic acid, papain, phytofluene, zeaxanthin. Nutrients: Calcium, iron, magnesium, manganese, phosphorus, potassium, zinc, vitamins B_1, B_2, B_3, B_5, and C.
Parsley (*Petroselinum crispum*)	Fruit, leaves, roots, stems.	Phytochemicals: Alpha-pinene, apigenin, apiole, benzaldehyde, bergapten, beta-carotene, caffeic acid, chlorogenic acid, geraniol, glycolic acid, kaempferol, limonene, linalool, lutein, myristic acid, myristicin, naringenin, p-coumaric acid, psoralen, quercetin, rosmarinic acid, rutin, xanthotoxin. Nutrients: Calcium, folate, iron, magnesium, manganese, phosphorus, potassium, selenium, zinc, vitamins A, B_1, B_2, B_3, B_5, C, and E.
Passionflower (*Passiflora incarnata*)	Flowers, leaves, shoots, stems.	Phytochemicals: Apigenin, flavonoids, harmaline, kaempferol, luteolin, maltol, quercetin, rutin, scopoletin, stigmasterol, umbelliferone, vitexin. Nutrients: Amino acids, calcium.
Pau d'arco (*Tabebuia heptaphylla*)	Inner bark.	Phytochemicals: Beta-carotene, beta-sitosterol, lapachol.

ACTIONS AND USES	COMMENTS
Stimulates the appetite and aids digestion. Good for heartburn, indigestion, and inflammatory bowel disorders.	The leaves can be used to tenderize meat.
Contains a substance that prevents the multiplication of tumor cells. Expels worms, relieves gas, stimulates normal activity of the digestive system, and freshens breath. Helps bladder, kidney, liver, lung, stomach, and thyroid function. Good for bed-wetting, fluid retention, gas, halitosis, high blood pressure, indigestion, kidney disease, obesity, and prostate disorders.	Contains more vitamin C than oranges by weight.
Has a gentle sedative effect and helps lower blood pressure. Helpful for anxiety, hyperactivity, insomnia, neuritis, and stress-related disorders.	Also called maypop. *Caution:* Should not be used during pregnancy, as it may stimulate the uterus.
Fights bacterial and viral infection. Cleanses the blood. Good for candidiasis, smoker's cough, warts, and all types of infection. Helpful for AIDS symptoms, allergies, cancer, cardiovascular problems, inflammatory bowel disease, rheumatism, tumors, and ulcers. Another species, *Tabebuia avellanedae*, may help restore skin after exposure to fungi and yeasts.	Also called lapacho and taheebo and was first used by the ancient Paraguayans.

HERB (*SCIENTIFIC NAME*)	PART(S) USED	PHYTOCHEMICAL AND NUTRIENT CONTENT
Peppermint (*Mentha piperita*)	Flowering tops, oil, leaves.	Phytochemicals: Acetic acid, alpha-carotene, alpha-pinene, azulene, beta-carotene, beta-ionone, betaine, caffeic acid, carvacrol, carvone, chlorogenic acid, coumarin, eugenol, hesperetin, limonene, linalool, luteolin, menthol, 1,8-cineole, p-coumaric acid, pectin, rosmarinic acid, rutin, tannin, thymol, vanillin. Nutrients: Calcium, choline, iron, magnesium, manganese, phosphorus, potassium, selenium, zinc, vitamins B_1, B_2, B_3, and E.
Plantain (*Plantago major*)	Leaves.	Phytochemicals: Adenine, allantoin, aucubin, apigenin, benzoic acid, caffeic acid, chlorogenic acid, cinnamic acid, ferulic acid, fiber, luteolin, oleanolic acid, p-coumaric acid, salicylic acid, tannin, ursolic acid, vanillic acid. Nutrients: Potassium, vitamin A.
Pleurisy root (*Asclepias tuberosa*)	Rhizome.	Phytochemicals: Alpha-amyrin, asclepiadin, beta-amyrin, isorhamnetin, kaempferol, lupeol, quercetin, rutin, viburnitol.
Primrose (*Oenothera biennis*)	Seed oil.	Phytochemicals: Beta-sitosterol, caffeic acid, campesterol, ellagic acid, gallic acid, kaempferol, lignin, p-coumaric acid, phytosterols, quercetin, tannin. Nutrients: Amino acids, calcium, essential fatty acids, iron, magnesium, manganese, phosphorus, potassium, zinc, vitamin E.

ACTIONS AND USES	COMMENTS
Increases stomach acidity, aiding digestion. Slightly anesthetizes mucous membranes and the gastrointestinal tract. Useful for chills, colic, diarrhea, headache, heart trouble, indigestion, irritable bowel syndrome, nausea, poor appetite, rheumatism, and spasms. Patients with irritable bowel syndrome who took peppermint had less abdominal pain, flatulence, and diarrhea.	*Caution:* May interfere with iron absorption. Should not be used by pregnant or nursing women. Do not ingest pure menthol or pure peppermint leaves.
Acts as a diuretic and is soothing to the lungs and urinary tract. May slow the growth of tuberculosis bacteria. Has a healing, antibiotic, and styptic effect when used topically for sores and wounds. Useful for indigestion and heartburn. Applied in a poultice, good for bee stings and any kind of bite.	This is not the bananalike fruit. Young leaves are tasty and can be eaten in salads. *Caution:* Do not mistake plantain for foxglove (*Digitalis lanata*), which has a similar appearance.
Reduces inflammation of the pleural membranes of the lungs, enhances secretion of healthy lung fluids, and stimulates the lymphatic system. Has antispasmodic properties. Induces sweating and aids expectoration. Beneficial for pleurisy, pneumonia, bronchitis, flu, and coughs.	Also called butterfly weed.
Promotes cardiovascular health. Aids in weight loss and reduces high blood pressure. Acts as a natural estrogen promoter. Helpful in treating alcoholism, arthritis, hot flashes, menstrual problems such as cramps and heavy bleeding, multiple sclerosis, and skin disorders.	Also called evening primrose. *Caution:* Primrose *root* should not be used during pregnancy.

HERB (*SCIENTIFIC NAME*)	PART(S) USED	PHYTOCHEMICAL AND NUTRIENT CONTENT
Pumpkin (*Cucurbita pepo*)	Flesh, seed.	Phytochemicals: Astragalin, beta-carotene, beta-sitosterol, caffeic acid, chlorogenin, cryptoxanthin, diosgenin, ferulic acid, gitogenin, kaempferol, lutein, mannitol, myristic acid, phytosterols, quercetin, ruscogenin, salicylic acid, zeaxanthin. Nutrients: Amino acids, calcium, essential fatty acids, iron, magnesium, manganese, phosphorus, potassium, selenium, zinc, vitamins A, C, and E.
Puncture vine (*Tribulus terrestris*)	Flowers, fruit, leaves, stems.	Phytochemicals: Astragalin, beta-sitosterol, campesterol, chlorogenin, diosgenin, gitogenin, kaempferol, quercetin, ruscogenin, rutin, stigmasterol. Nutrients: Amino acids, calcium, essential fatty acids, iron, phosphorus, potassium, vitamin C.
Pygeum (*Pygeum africanum*)	Bark.	Phytochemicals: Beta-sitosterol, oleanic acid, ursolic acid.
Red clover (*Trifolium pratense*)	Flowers.	Phytochemicals: Beta-carotene, beta-sitosterol, biochanin, caffeic acid, campesterol, chlorogenic acid, coumarin, coumestrol, daidzein, eugenol, formononetin, genistein, isorhamnetin, methyl salicylate, myricetin, p-coumaric acid, salicylic acid. Nutrients: Calcium, iron, magnesium, manganese, phosphorus, potassium, selenium, zinc, vitamins B_3, C, and E.

ACTIONS AND USES	COMMENTS
Useful for prostate disorders and irritable bladder.	
Improves sex drive. Eases menopausal symptoms. Stimulates production of and balances male and female hormones. Enhances the immune system. Helps build muscles and increase stamina and endurance. Has antifungal, antibacterial, and anti-inflammatory actions. Useful as a general tonic and revitalizer for the liver, kidneys, and urinary tract.	Also called caltrop.
Reduces inflammation and congestion. Lowers levels of inflammatory compounds in the prostate. Effective in reducing prostate enlargement and symptoms associated with benign prostatic hyperplasia such as urinary hesitancy, weak urine flow, nighttime urination, and recurrent urinary infections.	Used clinically in Europe to treat benign prostatic hyperplasia (BPH); the beneficial effect may take several weeks.
Fights infection, suppresses appetite, and purifies the blood. Has expectorant, antispasmodic, and relaxing effects. Relieves menopausal symptoms such as hot flashes. Good for bacterial infections, coughs, bronchitis, inflamed lungs, inflammatory bowel disorders, kidney problems, liver disease, skin disorders, and weakened immune system.	Do not take if you have a hormone-sensitive disease, are taking methotrexate, or are using blood thinners.

HERB (SCIENTIFIC NAME)	PART(S) USED	PHYTOCHEMICAL AND NUTRIENT CONTENT
Red raspberry (*Rubus idaeus*)	Bark, leaves, roots.	Phytochemicals: Alpha-carotene, benzaldehyde, beta-carotene, beta-ionone, caffeic acid, ellagic acid, farnesol, ferulic acid, gallic acid, geraniol, lutein, tannin. Nutrients: Calcium, iron, magnesium, manganese, phosphorus, potassium, selenium, silicon, zinc, vitamins B_1, B_2, B_3, C, and E.
Rhubarb (*Rheum rhabarbarum*)	Roots, stalks.	Phytochemicals: Acetic acid, beta-carotene, caffeic acid, chrysophanol, emodin, epicatechin, ferulic acid, fumaric acid, gallic acid, isoquercitrin, lutein, p-coumaric acid, protocatechuic acid, rutin, sinapic acid, vanillic acid. Nutrients: Calcium, iron, magnesium, manganese, phosphorus, potassium, selenium, sulfur, zinc, vitamins B_1, B_2, B_3, B_5, C, and E.
Rose (*Rosa canina*)	Fruit (hips).	Phytochemicals: Beta-carotene, betulin, catechin, epicatechin, flavonoids, isoquercitrin, lycopene, malic acid, pectin, tannin, vanillin, zeaxanthin. Nutrients: Calcium, iron, magnesium, manganese, phosphorus, potassium, selenium, zinc, vitamins B_1, B_2, B_3, C, and E.
Rosemary (*Rosmarinus officinalis*)	Leaves.	Phytochemicals: Alpha-pinene, apigenin, beta-carotene, beta-sitosterol, betulinic acid, borneol, caffeic acid, camphor, carnosol, carvacrol, carvone, caryophyllene, chlorogenic acid, diosmin, genkwanin, geraniol, hesperidin, limonene, linalool, luteolin, oleanolic acid, 1,8-cineole, phytosterols, rosmanol, rosmarinic acid, salicylates, squalene, tannin, thymol, ursolic acid. Nutrients: Calcium, iron, magnesium, manganese, phosphorus, potassium, zinc, vitamins B_1, B_3, and C.

ACTIONS AND USES

COMMENTS

Reduces menstrual bleeding, relaxes uterine and intestinal spasms, and strengthens uterine walls. Promotes healthy nails, bones, teeth, and skin. Good for diarrhea and for female disorders such as morning sickness, hot flashes, and menstrual cramps. Also heals canker sores. Combined with peppermint, good for morning sickness.

Fights infection and eliminates worms. Enhances gallbladder function and promotes healing of duodenal ulcers. Good for constipation, malabsorption, and disorders of the colon, spleen, and liver.

Caution: Should not be used during pregnancy.

Good for bladder problems and all infections. A good source of vitamin C when used fresh. Rose hip tea is good for diarrhea.

Many vitamins and other supplements are derived from rose hips.

Fights free radicals, inflammation (COX-2 enzyme), bacteria, and fungi. Relaxes the stomach, stimulates circulation and digestion, and acts as an astringent and decongestant. Improves circulation to the brain. Also helps detoxify the liver and has anticancer and antitumor properties. Good for headaches, high and low blood pressure, circulatory problems, and menstrual cramps. Can be used as an antiseptic gargle. Rosemary oil impedes the growth of food-borne bacteria and fungi, and someday may be used to prolong the shelf life of foods.

Makes a good food preservative.

Caution: Should not be used during pregnancy.

HERB (SCIENTIFIC NAME)	PART(S) USED	PHYTOCHEMICAL AND NUTRIENT CONTENT
Sage (*Salvia officinalis*)	Leaves.	Phytochemicals: Alpha-amyrin, alpha-pinene, alpha-terpineol, apigenin, beta-carotene, beta-sitosterol, betulin, borneol, caffeic acid, campesterol, camphene, camphor, carnosolic acid, caryophyllene, catechin, chlorogenic acid, citral, farnesol, ferulic acid, gallic acid, genkwanin, geraniol, hispidulin, limonene, linalool, luteolin, maslinic acid, oleanolic acid, 1,8-cineole, p-coumaric acid, pinene, rosmarinic acid, saponin, stigmasterol, tannins, terpineol, thymol, ursolic acid, vanillic acid. Nutrients: Boron, calcium, iron, magnesium, manganese, phosphorus, potassium, selenium, zinc, vitamins B_1, B_2, B_3, B_5, and C.
St. John's wort (*Hypericum perforatum*)	Flowers, leaves, stems, oil.	Phytochemicals: Carotenoids, caryophyllene, chlorophyll, flavonoids, hyperoside, isoquercitrin, limonene, lutein, mannitol, myristic acid, phenol, phloroglucinol, phytosterols, quercetin, quercitrin, rutin, saponin, tannins. Nutrients: Vitamin C.

ACTIONS AND USES

COMMENTS

Stimulates the central nervous system and digestive tract and has estrogenic effects on the body. Reduces sweating and salivation. Good for hot flashes and other symptoms of estrogen deficiency, whether in menopause or following hysterectomy. Beneficial for disorders affecting the mouth and throat, such as tonsillitis. In tea form, can be used as a hair rinse to promote shine (especially for dark hair) and hair growth. Also used to dry up milk when women wish to stop nursing.

Caution: Interferes with the absorption of iron and other minerals when taken internally. Decreases milk supply in nursing mothers. Should not be taken by individuals with seizure disorders or high blood pressure. Should not be taken during pregnancy or while nursing.

Good for depression and nerve pain. It has been shown to help patients with mild depression get over an acute episode and recover. Helps control stress. In laboratory studies, protects bone marrow and intestinal mucosa from X-ray damage. Applied topically, the oil aids wound healing. It has not been shown to be effective for children with ADHD (attention deficit hyperactivity disorder).

Caution: May increase sensitivity to sunlight. It may also produce anxiety, gastrointestinal symptoms, and headaches. It can interact with some drugs, including antidepressants, birth control pills, and anticoagulants.

Avoid use of St. John's wort in addition to other prescription antidepressants, as it may create a serious condition of excess serotonin in the body.

Use of this supplement should also be avoided if taking other supplements such as 5-HTP or SAMe because these products may also affect serotonin levels.

HERB (SCIENTIFIC NAME)	PART(S) USED	PHYTOCHEMICAL AND NUTRIENT CONTENT
Sangre de grado (*Croton lechleri*)	Bark, resin.	Phytochemicals: Alpha-pinene, betaine, beta-pinene, borneol, camphene, dipentene, eugenol, gamma-terpinene, lignin, linalool, myrcene, p-cymene, tannins, taspine, vanillin.
Sarsaparilla (*Smilax species*)	Roots, rhizomes.	Phytochemicals: Beta-sitosterol, saponin, stigmasterol. Nutrients: Iron, magnesium, manganese, phosphorus, potassium, selenium, zinc.
Saw palmetto (*Serenoa repens*)	Berries, seeds.	Phytochemicals: Beta-carotene, beta-sitosterol, ferulic acid, mannitol, myristic acid, tannins, vanillic acid, vanillin.
Skullcap (*Scutellaria laterfolia*)	Leaves, shoots.	Phytochemicals: Beta-carotene, lignin, tannins. Nutrients: Calcium, iron, magnesium, manganese, phosphorus, potassium, selenium, zinc, vitamins B_1, B_2, B_3, and C.
Slippery elm (*Ulmus rubra*)	Inner bark.	Phytochemicals: Beta-carotene, campesterol, mucilage, starch, tannin. Nutrients: Calcium, iron, magnesium, manganese, phosphorus, potassium, selenium, zinc, vitamins B_1, B_2, B_3, and C.
Squawvine (*Mitchella repens*)	Leaves, stems.	Phytochemicals: Alkaloids, glycosides, mucilage, saponins, tannins.

ACTIONS AND USES	COMMENTS
Fights free radicals, inflammation, and bacterial, viral, and fungal infection. Helps heal wounds and stop bleeding. Good for respiratory and skin disorders, mouth and skin ulcers, sore throat, colds and flu, candida, psoriasis, herpes, and vaginitis.	A rainforest herb whose name means dragon's blood.
Promotes excretion of fluids, increases energy, protects against harm from radiation exposure, and regulates hormones. Useful for female sexual dysfunction, hives, impotence, infertility, nervous system disorders, premenstrual syndrome, psoriasis, rheumatoid arthritis, and disorders caused by blood impurities.	Also called Chinese root, small spikenard.
Acts as a diuretic, urinary antiseptic, and appetite stimulant. Inhibits production of dihydrotestosterone, a form of testosterone that contributes to enlargement of the prostate. Shown to improve lower urinary tract symptoms in men with benign prostatic hyperplasia. May also enhance sexual functioning and sexual desire.	Used clinically in Europe to treat benign prostatic hyperplasia (BPH). Can be combined with nettle root. Common side effects include gastrointestinal upset, diarrhea, fatigue, headache, decreased libido, and rhinitis. Most effects are reported as mild and similar to effects with placebo.
Aids sleep, improves circulation, and strengthens the heart muscle. Relieves muscle cramps, pain, spasms, and stress. Good for anxiety, fatigue, cardiovascular disease, headache, hyperactivity, nervous disorders, and rheumatism. Useful in treating barbiturate addiction and drug withdrawal.	*Caution:* Should not be given to children under six.
Soothes inflamed mucous membranes of the bowels, stomach, and urinary tract. Good for diarrhea and ulcers and for treatment of colds, flu, and sore throat. Beneficial for Crohn's disease, ulcerative colitis, diverticulosis, diverticulitis, and gastritis.	Also called moose elm, red elm.
Relieves pelvic congestion and soothes the nervous system. Good for menstrual cramps.	Also called partridgeberry.

HERB (SCIENTIFIC NAME)	PART(S) USED	PHYTOCHEMICAL AND NUTRIENT CONTENT
Stone root (*Collinsonia canadensis*)	Whole plant, fresh root.	Phytochemicals: Alpha-pinene, caffeic acid, caryophyllene, limonene. Nutrients: Magnesium.
Suma (*Pfaffia paniculata*)	Bark, berries, leaves, roots.	Phytochemicals: Beta-sitosterol, saponin, stigmasterol. Nutrients: Iron, magnesium, zinc, vitamins A, B_1, B_2, B_5, E, and K.
Tea tree (*Melaleuca alternifolia*)	Essential oil.	Phytochemicals: Alpha-pinene, alpha-terpineol, aromadendrene, beta-pinene, camphor, caryophyllene, limonene, linalool, 1,8-cineole, p-cymene, terpinenes, terpinolene.
Thyme (*Thymus vulgaris*)	Berries, flowers, leaves.	Phytochemicals: Alpha-pinene, apigenin, beta-carotene, borneol, caffeic acid, camphor, caprylic acid, carvacrol, carvone, chlorogenic acid, cinnamic acid, citral, eugenol, ferulic acid, gallic acid, geraniol, kaempferol, lauric acid, limonene, linalool, luteolin, myristic acid, naringenin, oleanolic acid, p-coumaric acid, p-cymene, phytosterols, rosmarinic acid, salicylates, tannin, thymol, ursolic acid, vanillic acid. Nutrients: Amino acids, calcium, essential fatty acids, iron, magnesium, manganese, phosphorus, potassium, selenium, zinc, vitamins B_1, B_2, B_3, and C.

ACTIONS AND USES	COMMENTS
Acts as a diuretic, sedative, antispasmodic, astringent, and tonic. Good for the urinary tract. Breaks up mucus. Helpful for bronchitis, headache, cramps, indigestion, and hemorrhoids.	Also known as heal-all, horse balm, knob root, and rich weed.
Fights inflammation, boosts the immune system, and combats anemia, fatigue, and stress. Good for arthritis, cancer, liver disease, menopausal symptoms, high blood pressure, Epstein-Barr virus, and weakened immune system.	Also known as Brazilian ginseng.
Used topically, disinfects wounds and heals virtually all skin conditions, including acne, athlete's foot, boils, cuts and scrapes, earache, fungal infections, hair and scalp problems, herpes outbreaks, insect and spider bites, scabies, and warts. Added to water, can be used as a douche for vaginitis and a gargle for colds, sore throats, and mouth sores (do not swallow it, however).	*Caution:* Should not be taken internally; can be toxic. If irritation occurs, discontinue use or dilute with distilled water, vegetable oil, primrose oil, or vitamin E oil. If irritation persists after dilution, discontinue use.
Eliminates gas and reduces fever, headache, and mucus. Has strong antiseptic properties. Lowers cholesterol levels. Good for asthma, bronchitis, croup, and other respiratory problems, and for fever, headache, and liver disease. Eliminates scalp itching and flaking.	

HERB (SCIENTIFIC NAME)	PART(S) USED	PHYTOCHEMICAL AND NUTRIENT CONTENT
Turmeric (*Curcuma longa*)	Rhizomes.	Phytochemicals: Alpha-pinene, alpha-terpineol, azulene, beta-carotene, borneol, caffeic acid, caryophyllene, cinnamic acid, curcumin, eugenol, guaiacol, limonene, linalool, 1,8-cineole, p-coumaric acid, p-cymene, turmerone, vanillic acid. Nutrients: Calcium, iron, manganese, phosphorus, potassium, zinc, vitamins B_1, B_2, B_3, and C.
Uva ursi (*Arctostaphylos uva-ursi*)	Leaves.	Phytochemicals: Arbutin, beta-carotene, beta-sitosterol, ellagic acid, gallic acid, hyperin, isoquercitrin, myricetin, oleanolic acid, quercetin, quercitrin, ursolic acid. Nutrients: Calcium, iron, magnesium, manganese, phosphorus, potassium, selenium, zinc, vitamins B_1, B_2, B_3, and C.
Valerian (*Valeriana officinalis*)	Rhizomes, roots.	Phytochemicals: Azulene, beta-carotene, beta-ionone, beta-sitosterol, borneol, bornyl acetate, caffeic acid, caryophyllene, chlorogenic acid, isovaleric acid, kaempferol, limonene, p-coumaric acid, quercetin, valepotriates, valerenic acid, valerenone, valeric acid. Nutrients: Calcium, choline, essential fatty acids, iron, magnesium, manganese, phosphorus, potassium, selenium, zinc, vitamins B_1, B_2, B_3, and C.
Vervain (*Verbena officinalis*)	Flowers, leaves, shoots, stems.	Phytochemicals: Adenosine, aucubin, beta-carotene, caffeic acid, citral, tannin, ursolic acid, verbenalin, verbenin.

ACTIONS AND USES	COMMENTS
Curcumin, the yellow pigment in turmeric, is the active ingredient. Fights free radicals, protects the liver against toxins, inhibits platelet aggregation, aids circulation, lowers cholesterol levels, and improves blood vessel health. Has antibiotic, anticancer, and anti-inflammatory (COX-2 enzyme) properties. Good for all arthritic conditions. Curcumin has been shown to stop the proliferation of rapidly dividing cancer cells. Under investigation for treating pancreatic and other cancers, and psoriasis.	Used as a seasoning and the main ingredient in curry powder. Has inhibited the spread of HIV in laboratory tests. *Caution:* Extended use can result in stomach distress. Not recommended for persons with biliary tract obstruction, as curcumin stimulates bile secretion. Some medications may have a lesser effect if turmeric is regularly used (e.g., aspirin, ibuprofen, and blood thinners).
Promotes excretion of fluids, fights bacteria, and strengthens heart muscle. Good for disorders of the spleen, liver, pancreas, and small intestine. Useful for bladder and kidney infections, diabetes, and prostate disorders.	Also called bearberry. *Caution:* Not recommended for women who are pregnant or nursing, or for children under twelve.
Acts as a sedative, improves circulation, and reduces mucus from colds. Good for anxiety, fatigue, high blood pressure, insomnia, irritable bowel syndrome, menstrual and muscle cramps, nervousness, pain, spasms, stress, and ulcers. Shown to promote better sleep quality and longer sleeping periods, and to reduce the number of times people get up at night. Combining valerian with hops can also promote a better quality of sleep and induce deeper sleep.	A water-soluble extract form is best. *Caution:* Should not be combined with alcohol. Other cautions about use are for those taking anti-anxiety medication or for those who have gallbladder, pancreatic, or liver disease, are pregnant or nursing, or are operating heavy machinery.
Strengthens the nervous system. Promotes liver and gallbladder health. Reduces tension and stress. Induces sweating. Promotes menstruation and increases mother's milk. Useful for mild depression, insomnia, headache, toothache, wounds, colds, and fever.	*Caution:* Should not be used during pregnancy, as it stimulates uterine contractions.

HERB (SCIENTIFIC NAME)	PART(S) USED	PHYTOCHEMICAL AND NUTRIENT CONTENT
White oak (*Quercus alba*)	Bark.	Phytochemicals: Beta-carotene, beta-sitosterol, catechin, gallic acid, pectin, quercetin, quercitrin, tannin. Nutrients: Calcium, iron, magnesium, manganese, phosphorus, potassium, selenium, zinc, vitamins B$_1$, B$_2$, B$_3$, and C.
White willow (*Salix alba*)	Bark.	Phytochemicals: Apigenin, beta-carotene, catechin, isoquercitrin, lignin, p-coumaric acid, quercetin, rutin, salicin, salicylic acid, tannin. Nutrients: Calcium, iron, magnesium, manganese, phosphorus, potassium, selenium, zinc, vitamins B$_1$, B$_2$, B$_3$, and C.
Wild cherry (*Prunus serotina*)	Inner bark, root bark.	Phytochemicals: Benzaldehyde, caffeic acid, kaempferol, p-coumaric acid, quercetin, scopoletin, tannin, ursolic acid. Nutrients: Calcium, iron, magnesium, phosphorus, potassium, zinc.
Wild oregano (*Origanum vulgare*)	Leaves, shoots, stems.	Phytochemicals: Alpha-pinene, apigenin, beta-carotene, borneol, caffeic acid, camphor, capric acid, carvacrol, caryophyllene, catechol, chlorogenic acid, cinnamic acid, eriodictyol, eugenol, geraniol, kaempferol, limonene, linalool, luteolin, myristic acid, naringenin, naringin, oleanolic acid, 1,8-cineole, p-coumaric acid, phytosterols, quercetin, rosmarinic acid, rutin, tannins, thymol, ursolic acid, vanillic acid, vitexin. Nutrients: Calcium, essential fatty acids, iron, magnesium, manganese, phosphorus, potassium, zinc, vitamins A, B$_1$, B$_3$, and C.

ACTIONS AND USES	COMMENTS
Acts as an antiseptic. Good for skin wounds, bee stings, burns, diarrhea, fevers and cold, bronchitis, nosebleed, poison ivy, and varicose veins. Also good for the teeth. Can be used in enemas and douches.	
Relieves pain. Good for allergies, headache, backache, nerve pain, joint pain, inflammation, menstrual cramps, toothache, and injuries. For backache, use of white willow allowed for a reduction in the use of pain medications.	Contains compounds from which aspirin was derived. *Caution:* Not recommended for use during pregnancy. May interfere with absorption of iron and other minerals when taken internally. Should not be used by people who are allergic to aspirin.
Acts as an expectorant and mild sedative. Good for coughs, colds, bronchitis, asthma, digestive disorders, and diarrhea.	Also called chokecherry, wild black cherry, Virginia prune. *Caution:* Wild cherry bark should not be used during pregnancy. Also, the leaves, bark, and fruit pits contain hydrocyanic acid, which can be poisonous. A commercially prepared syrup or tincture is best.
Fights free radicals, inflammation, and bacterial, viral, and fungal infection. Boosts the immune system. Useful for acne, allergies, animal bites, arthritis, asthma, athlete's foot, bee stings, bronchitis, chronic infections, cold, cough, diarrhea, digestive problems, earache, eczema, fatigue, gum disease, headache, menstrual irregularities, muscle pain, parasitic infections, psoriasis, sinusitis, skin infections, urinary tract disorders, and wounds.	Oregano sold in supermarkets is usually a combination of several oregano species. It does not have the medicinal benefits of *Origanum vulgare*.

HERB (SCIENTIFIC NAME)	PART(S) USED	PHYTOCHEMICAL AND NUTRIENT CONTENT
Wild yam (*Dioscorea villosa*)	Rhizomes, roots.	Phytochemicals: Beta-carotene, diosgenin. Nutrients: Calcium, chromium, iron, magnesium, manganese, phosphorus, potassium, selenium, zinc, vitamins B_1, B_2, B_3, and C.
Wintergreen (*Gaultheria procumbens*)	Leaves, roots, stems.	Phytochemicals: Caffeic acid, ferulic acid, gallic acid, p-coumaric acid, methyl salicylate, tannin, vanillic acid.
Witch hazel (*Hamamelis virginiana*)	Bark, leaves, twigs.	Phytochemials: Beta-ionone, gallic acid, isoquercitrin, kaempferol, leucodelphinidin, myrcetin, phenol, quercetin, quercetrin, saponins, tannins.
Wood betony (*Stachys officinalis*)	Leaves.	Phytochemicals: Betaine, caffeic acid, chlorogenic acid, rosmarinic acid, stachydrine, tannin. Nutrients: Choline, magnesium, manganese, phosphorus.
Wormwood (*Artemisia absinthium*)	Leaves, tops.	Phytochemicals: Beta-carotene, chamazulene, chlorogenic acid, isoquercitrin, p-coumaric acid, rutin, salicylic acid, tannins, vanillic acid. Nutrients: Vitamin C.

ACTIONS AND USES	COMMENTS
Relaxes muscle spasms, reduces inflammation, and promotes perspiration. Contains compounds similar to the hormone progesterone. Good for colic, gallbladder disorders, hypoglycemia, irritable bowel syndrome, kidney stones, neuralgia, rheumatism, and female disorders, including premenstrual syndrome and menopause-related symptoms. In one study, postmenopausal women who consumed yam experienced an improvement in the levels of sex hormones, blood lipids, and antioxidants.	Many yam-based products are extracted from plants treated with fertilizers and pesticides, which may end up in the final products. The selection, cleansing, and processing of the raw materials is very important. *Caution:* Should not be used during pregnancy and lactation. For use in children, check with your pediatrician.
Relieves pain and reduces inflammation. Stimulates circulation. Good for arthritis, headache, toothache, muscle pain, and rheumatic complaints.	Oil distilled from the leaves is used in perfumes and as a flavoring. Contains a compound composed of 90 percent methyl salicylate, a substance similar to aspirin.
Applied topically, has astringent and healing properties, and relieves itching. Good for hemorrhoids, mouth and skin inflammation, and phlebitis. Very useful in skin care.	
Stimulates the heart and relaxes muscles. Improves digestion and appreciation of food. Good for cardiovascular disorders, hyperactivity, nerve pain, headaches, and anxiety attacks.	Also called betony. *Caution:* Should not be used during pregnancy.
Acts as a mild sedative, eliminates worms, increases stomach acidity, and lowers fever. Useful for loss of appetite and for liver, gallbladder, gastric, and vascular disorders, including migraines. Applied topically, good for healing wounds, skin ulcers and blemishes, and insect bites.	Ingredient of absinthe liquor, banned in many countries. Often used with black walnut for removal of parasites. *Caution:* Do not use in high doses or for extended periods because it contains the chemical component thujune, which can be poisonous. Should not be used by those who suffer from any type of seizure disorder, or who are pregnant or nursing.

HERB (SCIENTIFIC NAME)	PART(S) USED	PHYTOCHEMICAL AND NUTRIENT CONTENT
Yellow dock (*Rumex crispus*)	Roots.	Phytochemicals: Beta-carotene, hyperoside, quercetin, quercitrin, rutin, tannin. Nutrients: Calcium, iron, magnesium, manganese, phosphorus, potassium, selenium, zinc, vitamins B_1, B_2, B_3, and C.
Yerba maté (*Ilex paraguariensis*)	Leaves.	Phytochemicals: Caffeine, chlorogenic acid, chlorophyll, rutin, tannin, theobromine, theophylline, ursolic acid, vanillin. Nutrients: Choline, inositol, nicotinic acid, pyridoxine, trace minerals, vitamins B_3, B_5, B_6, C, and E.
Yohimbe (*Pausinystalia yohimbe*)	Bark.	Phytochemicals: Ajmaline, corynantheine, corynanthine, tannin, yohimbine.
Yucca (*Yucca baccata*)	Roots.	Phytochemicals: Beta-carotene, sarsapogenin, tannin. Nutrients: Calcium, iron, magnesium, manganese, phosphorus, potassium, selenium, zinc, vitamins B_1, B_2, B_3, and C.

ACTIONS AND USES	COMMENTS
Acts as a blood purifier and cleanser, and as a general tonic. Improves colon and liver function. Good for inflammation of the nasal passages and respiratory tract, anemia, liver disease, and skin disorders such as eczema, hives, psoriasis, and rashes. Combined with sarsaparilla, makes a tea for chronic skin disorders.	Also called curled dock. *Caution:* Yellow dock leaves should not be consumed in soups or salads. They are high in oxalates and may cause oxalic acid poisoning.
Fights free radicals, cleanses the blood, and suppresses appetite. Fights aging, stimulates the mind, stimulates the production of cortisone, and tones the nervous system. Enhances the healing powers of other herbs. When combined with guarana, it was useful at slowing the rate that food left the stomach, thereby promoting a longer sense of fullness. This led to a significant weight loss compared to a control group. Useful for allergies, constipation, and inflammatory bowel disorders.	Also called maté, Paraguay tea, South American holly. *Caution:* Should not be used by people who suffer from insomnia.
Increases libido and blood flow to erectile tissue. May increase testosterone levels.	Yohimbine, a key component of this herb, is sold as a prescription medication. Available in a wide variety of bodybuilding and sexual aid supplements. *Caution:* Yohimbe should not be used by women who are pregnant or nursing. Do not use yohimbe if you have high blood pressure, heart disease, stomach ulcers, depression, or other psychiatric conditions. There have been cases of people dying from taking too much yohimbe.
Purifies the blood. Beneficial in treating arthritis, osteoporosis, and inflammatory disorders.	Routinely prescribed for arthritis in some clinics. Can be cut up, added to water (1 cup of yucca in 2 cups of water), and used as a soap or shampoo substitute. Can also be added to shampoo.

Medicinal Herbs by Actions and Targets in the Body

Different medicinal herbs have different types of effects and tend to exert their activities on different body systems and organs. The following table classifies some of the best-known herbs according to their actions and areas of prime activity.

ACTION(S)	HERBS
Antibacterial/antiviral	Aloe, anise, annatto, astragalus, black walnut, boneset, boswellia, burdock, catnip, cat's claw, cayenne, cedar, chanca piedra, chickweed, echinacea, elder, eucalyptus, garlic, goldenseal, jaborandi, jatoba, kudzu, lady's-mantle, lemongrass, licorice, macela, meadowsweet, myrrh, olive leaf, pau d'arco, pleurisy root, puncture vine, red clover, rose, rosemary, sangre de grado, slippery elm, suma, tea tree, turmeric, uva ursi, valerian, white oak, wild oregano.
Anticancer/antitumor	Astragalus, birch, burdock, cat's claw, chuchuhuasi, cranberry, dandelion, fennel, garlic, green tea, licorice, macela, milk thistle, parsley, pau d'arco, rosemary, suma, turmeric.
Antifungal	Acerola, alfalfa, aloe, black walnut, boswellia, burdock, cedar, cinnamon, jatoba, puncture vine, rosemary, sangre de grado, tea tree, wild oregano.
Anti-inflammatory	Alfalfa, aloe, annatto, ashwagandha, bilberry, birch, blessed thistle, boldo, boneset, boswellia, buchu, butcher's broom, calendula, catnip, cat's claw, chamomile, chanca piedra, chuchuhuasi, devil's claw, echinacea, elder, fenugreek, feverfew, flax, ginger, goldenseal, jaborandi, jatoba, juniper, lady's-mantle, licorice, macela, meadowsweet, mullein, mustard, pleurisy root, puncture vine, pygeum, rosemary, sangre de grado, suma, turmeric, white willow, wild oregano, wild yam, wintergreen, witch hazel, yellow dock.

ACTION(S)	HERBS
Antioxidant	Acerola, annatto, bilberry, burdock, cat's claw, celery, elder, ginger, ginkgo, green tea, jatoba, milk thistle, olive leaf, rosemary, sangre de grado, turmeric, wild oregano, yerba maté.
Cleanser/detoxifier	Alfalfa, black walnut, blessed thistle, cascara sagrada, cat's claw, cedar, dandelion, elder, garlic, ginger, goldenseal, guarana, licorice, muira puama, Oregon grape, pau d'arco, rosemary, yellow dock, yerba maté.
Bones/joints	Alfalfa, black cohosh, boswellia, cat's claw, cayenne, celery, chuchuhuasi, dandelion, devil's claw, feverfew, flax, garlic, ginger, jatoba, muira puama, nettle, olive leaf, pau d'arco, peppermint, primrose, red raspberry, St. John's wort, sarsaparilla, skullcap, suma, wild oregano, wild yam, wintergreen, yucca.
Brain/nervous system	Ashwagandha, astragalus, bayberry, bilberry, blessed thistle, blue cohosh, catnip, celery, chamomile, chaste tree, devil's claw, dong quai, eyebright, fennel, fenugreek, feverfew, ginger, ginseng, goldenseal, gotu kola, guarana, hops, jaborandi, kava kava, kudzu, lavender, lemongrass, licorice, marshmallow, motherwort, muira puama, oat straw, passionflower, peppermint, plantain, rosemary, sage, St. John's wort, sarsaparilla, skullcap, squawvine, stone root, suma, thyme, valerian, vervain, white willow, wild cherry, wild oregano, wintergreen, wood betony, wormwood, yerba maté.
Circulatory/cardiovascular systems	Aloe, barberry, bayberry, bilberry, black cohosh, black walnut, blessed thistle, borage, boswellia, butcher's broom, cayenne, celery, chickweed, cinnamon, devil's claw, elder, garlic, gentian, ginger, ginkgo, ginseng, gotu kola, green tea, hawthorn, hops, horse chestnut, hyssop, jaborandi, kudzu, licorice, motherwort, muira puama, olive leaf, parsley, passionflower, pau d'arco, peppermint, primrose, rosemary, skullcap, suma, uva ursi, valerian, white oak, wintergreen, wood betony.

ACTION(S)	HERBS
Gastrointestinal/digestive systems	Acerola, alfalfa, aloe, anise, annatto, bilberry, black walnut, blessed thistle, boldo, boswellia, buchu, burdock, cascara sagrada, catnip, cayenne, chamomile, chanca piedra, chuchuhuasi, cinnamon, clove, dandelion, devil's claw, fennel, fenugreek, flax, garlic, gentian, ginger, ginseng, goldenseal, gotu kola, green tea, guarana, horehound, jaborandi, juniper, kava kava, kudzu, lady's-mantle, lemongrass, licorice, macela, marshmallow, meadowsweet, muira puama, mustard, olive leaf, Oregon grape, papaya, parsley, pau d'arco, peppermint, plantain, puncture vine, red clover, red raspberry, rosemary, sage, slippery elm, stone root, suma, thyme, turmeric, uva ursi, valerian, vervain, white oak, wild cherry, wild oregano, wood betony, wormwood, yellow dock, yerba maté.
Hair/nails/teeth	Borage, burdock, clove, hops, Irish moss, lemongrass, muira puama, nettle, red raspberry, sage, tea tree, vervain, white willow, wintergreen.
Immune system	Ashwagandha, astragalus, bayberry, burdock, cat's claw, cedar, chuchuhuasi, devil's claw, echinacea, eyebright, elder, garlic, ginseng, goldenseal, green tea, horehound, licorice, maca, macela, milk thistle, myrrh, pau d'arco, puncture vine, red clover, suma, white willow, wild oregano, yerba maté.
Muscles	Blue cohosh, celery, chanca piedra, chuchuhuasi, eucalyptus, feverfew, ginger, hawthorn, horse chestnut, kava kava, lady's-mantle, licorice, macela, meadowsweet, puncture vine, skullcap, uva ursi, valerian, wild oregano, wild yam, wintergreen, wood betony.

ACTION(S)	HERBS
Reproductive system	*Menopause:* Chaste tree, dandelion, devil's claw, kava kava, licorice, motherwort, puncture vine, sage, suma, wild yam. *Menstruation:* Black cohosh, blue cohosh, calendula, chamomile, chaste tree, chuchuhuasi, corn silk, crampbark, dong quai, false unicorn root, feverfew, licorice, maca, macela, motherwort, muira puama, primrose, red raspberry, rosemary, sarsaparilla, squawvine, valerian, white willow, wild oregano, wild yam. *Prostate:* Buchu, goldenseal, gravel root, hydrangea, juniper, licorice, milk thistle, parsley, pumpkin, pygeum, saw palmetto, uva ursi. *Sexual function/hormones:* Alfalfa, ashwagandha, chaste tree, chuchuhuasi, damiana, dong quai, false unicorn root, gotu kola, muira puama, puncture vine, sarsaparilla, saw palmetto, yohimbe (not recommended).
Respiratory tract	Anise, astragalus, boneset, boswellia, catnip, cayenne, chanca piedra, chuchuhuasi, chickweed, elder, eucalyptus, fennel, fenugreek, feverfew, garlic, ginkgo, ginseng, goldenseal, green tea, horehound, Irish moss, jaborandi, jatoba, juniper, licorice, macela, muira puama, mullein, mustard, myrrh, nettle, parsley, plantain, pleurisy root, red clover, stone root, thyme, white oak, wild cherry, wild oregano, yellow dock.
Skin	Acerola, alfalfa, aloe, annatto, barberry, borage, boswellia, calendula, chickweed, chuchuhuasi, comfrey, cranberry, elder, flax, green tea, Irish moss, lavender, lemongrass, marshmallow, milk thistle, myrrh, oat straw, olive leaf, Oregon grape, primrose, red clover, red raspberry, sangre de grado, sarsaparilla, tea tree, white oak, wild oregano, witch hazel, wormwood, yellow dock.
Urinary tract	Annatto, bilberry, birch, buchu, butcher's broom, cayenne, cedar, celery, chanca piedra, corn silk, cranberry, dandelion, devil's claw, fennel, ginkgo, goldenseal, gotu kola, gravel root, guarana, hydrangea, jatoba, juniper, kava kava, marshmallow, milk thistle, mullein, nettle, parsley, plantain, puncture vine, pumpkin, rose, red clover, saw palmetto, slippery elm, stone root, uva ursi, wild oregano, wild yam.

Drug
Interactions

INTRODUCTION

Mixing two or more drugs together in the body can sometimes create havoc, and instead of a health benefit the patient suffers a setback. Worse, you may be confronted with a health crisis. Most people think these unintended effects apply only to prescription drugs. However, dietary supplements and even the food we eat can interact with each other, or with over-the-counter (OTC) or prescription drugs, to cause problems. Herbs and vitamins, while not drugs in the strictest sense, are still complex organic chemicals that react with one another and with other chemicals in the body. This is, of course, how they work.

Types of drug interactions that you need to be concerned with can basically be summarized as follows:

- *Drugs interacting with drugs.* Both prescription and over-the-counter medications are included in this category. For instance, taking OTC antacids during a course of the antibiotic ciprofloxacin (Cipro) lowers the effectiveness of the antibiotic. If you take birth control pills, you should know that the antibiotic rifampin could lower their effectiveness. Miconazole (the active ingredient in Monistat and other products), an OTC drug for yeast infections, should not be used with warfarin (Coumadin) or bleeding and bruising could occur. Sildenafil (Viagra) should not be mixed with nitrates (such as nitroglycerin) used to treat heart disease, and certain antidepressants can interfere with blood pressure medicine.

- *Drugs interacting with dietary supplements.* There are many documented cases of herbs and vitamins interacting with prescription and OTC drugs. For example, St. John's wort can interfere with the action of irinotecan, a standard chemotherapy drug. St. John's wort also acts with the blood thinner warfarin and the heart medicine digitalis (Digoxin, Lanoxin), making them less effective. St. John's wort also lowers levels of theophylline, an asthma drug. Taking large doses of vitamin K can nullify the action of any blood-thinning medication a person might be taking. The list goes on and on. The five most common natural products with potential interaction are garlic, valerian, kava, ginkgo, and St. John's wort, according to a study at the Mayo Clinic. Children and adults can experience problems with dietary supplements. In one study, which tracked the adverse drug reaction (ADR) calls to the California Poison Control System, 28 percent were for children. The most common products involved with ADRs were zinc, echinacea, chromium picolinate, and witch hazel. As of 2009, all dietary supplement labels include a company name to report any adverse events. This information is logged by the company and shared with the FDA if the problem is serious.

- *Drugs interacting with food and beverages.* Taking ciprofloxacin with coffee, chocolate, or even a cola drink that contains caffeine may cause excess nervousness or manic behavior. If foods containing tyramine, such as cheese or soy sauce, are mixed with some MAO inhibitors (a class of medication most often prescribed for mood disorders), there can be a fatal increase in blood pressure. Do not drink grapefruit juice along with blood pressure medications or cyclosporine (a transplant drug); doing this may increase the effect of these drugs. It was discovered in 1991 that grapefruit juice has the ability to inhibit an enzyme that metabolizes many drugs, thus allowing levels of the drugs to build up in the body. Older adults may have a special susceptibility to this reaction.

The U.S. Food and Drug Administration (FDA) has been trying to understand more about drug interactions, particularly in the past few decades, and has been developing laboratory testing programs to reveal possible problems early in the game. Because clinical trials with humans are generally based on small numbers of people, the safety profile of a proposed drug is not close to complete until the drug actually gets to market and a larger number of people get to try it under real-life conditions. A problem that is relatively rare in nature might not become apparent until several hundred thousand people have taken the drug. While there is a lot of emotion attached to this issue, it is simply impossible to predict beforehand every possible drug reaction and interaction. If people demand that kind of perfection, they have unrealistic expectations. Development costs, already unreasonably high, would certainly skyrocket, and development of new drugs that would benefit millions might be delayed indefinitely or even curtailed.

WHY ARE THERE DRUG INTERACTIONS?

Over the past few years researchers have learned that there is a class of enzymes, called the CYP family of enzymes, that plays an essential role in the metabolism and detoxification of drugs. These enzymes act primarily in the liver, but also in the intestinal tract and other areas. For instance, there is a single enzyme (of the five known CYP enzymes) that plays a key role in metabolizing over half the drugs prescribed today. It is called CYP3A4 (or cytochrome P450). So, any substance—no matter whether it is another prescription drug, a common food, an OTC product, or an herbal or vitamin supplement—that either inhibits the action of this enzyme (or, conversely, increases its activity) will have a significant effect on how drugs are metabolized in the body. If more enzymes are produced, the drug is removed from the body too quickly and its effectiveness is lessened. If fewer enzymes are produced, the drug may build up in the body to toxic levels.

Furthermore, many drugs operate within a fairly narrow "window" of concentration. That is, there must be enough of the drug to be effective, but only a little bit more can be toxic to the body.

Now that we know about these five enzymes, drugs can be tested by simply seeing if the drug interacts with each of the enzymes in a test tube. Knowing which enzyme actually metabolizes the new drug, researchers can then compare the drug with other drugs metabolized by the same enzyme and eventually build up a list of possible interactions. If two drugs use the same enzyme, it is possible that together there might be a conflict.

Test-tube studies certainly cannot tell the whole story, but they do point the way for targeted trials that might shed more light on possible problems before a new drug gets to market. There are race, gender, age, and other issues involved, too. Members of some ethnic groups may tend to produce very little of one enzyme but lots of the others. That means certain people might not be able to metabolize a new drug, and they can be tentatively identified beforehand.

Herbs and Drug Interactions

We have already noted that St. John's wort has the capacity to affect the activity of certain drugs. It does so notably through its potential to affect the enzyme CYP3A4. What about other herbs? We know that herbs are not routinely tested like prescription drugs. There are no FDA Phase 1, Phase 2, or Phase 3 trials for herbal remedies.

Additional investigations have found that kava kava extract made from *Piper methysticum* showed the ability to affect CYP3A4, and certain kavalactone compounds additionally affected CYP3A23. Kava also worsens the side effects of certain anesthetics, as does valerian. The plant sterol echinacea (*Echi-*

nacea purpurea) appears to have some effect on one or more of the metabolizing enzymes. Echinacea may reverse the effects of certain steroids. Caffeine, a phytochemical found in a number of plants, certainly has a proven effect. Obviously, much more research is needed to see how herbs might interact with other substances and with prescription drugs.

Mineral and Drug Interactions

Minerals can form complexes, or chelates, with some drugs. This creates insoluble structures that the body cannot absorb. Antibiotics and calcium are a known interactive pair. Calcium-fortified orange juice has caused chelation with ciprofloxacin (Cipro), gatifloxacin (Tequin), and levofloxacin (Levaquin). These antibiotics were made less effective by the calcium, as was the antibiotic tetracycline. Tetracyclines also bind with aluminum and magnesium, among others.

Calcium carbonate, as used in common antacids, binds with the thyroid hormone levothyroxine. Calcium carbonate should be taken at least four hours before taking the medication.

Iron forms complexes with ciprofloxacin, as well as with the quinolone antibiotics nalidixic acid and norfloxacin. Iron also binds with the Parkinson's disease medication levodopa (L-dopa). This binding reduces the effectiveness of all these drugs. Copper, manganese, magnesium, and zinc have similar effects on the quinolone antibiotics. Magnesium hydroxide appears to enhance the activity of ibuprofen (found in Advil, Motrin, and other over-the-counter and prescription products), possibly by increasing the gastric pH and creating an environment conducive to absorption. Caution should be used when combining ibuprofen and magnesium hydroxide, as prolonged use has been shown to increase the risk of gastrointestinal irritation.

Vitamin and Drug Interactions

Interaction between vitamins and prescription and OTC drugs is a wide-open field that needs to be explored. We have already noted that vitamin K counteracts the effects of the blood thinner warfarin. It is also known that vitamin B_6 (pyridoxine) reduces blood levels of the Parkinson's disease drug levodopa. Vitamin A supplements, although not at levels typically found in multivitamins, may react badly with isotretinoin (Accutane), an acne medication.

Dietary Supplements and Drug Interactions

Several interactions have been reported between dietary supplements and prescription medications. Work in rats showed that policosanol increased the antiulcer effects of cimetidine (Tagamet). Use of conjugated linoleic acid (CLA) may interfere with hepatic enzyme function and tamoxifen (a breast cancer drug). Some drugs—propranolol and tricyclic antidepressants, for example—lower coenzyme Q_{10} levels.

Several drugs have been shown to lower carnitine levels, including sodium valproate, pivampicillin, and isotretinoin. Some patients using these drugs benefit from supplements of carnitine. Melatonin has been reported to interact with a number of prescription drugs. For example, serum melatonin levels increase faster taking fluvoxamine, reducing CYP3A4 enzyme activity. Melatonin interacts with nifedipine, increasing blood pressure and heart rate. Chondroitin may provoke autoimmune dysfunction and interact with the drug warfarin, increasing the time it takes your blood to clot.

Foods and Drug Activity

As has been noted throughout this book, supplemental fiber products can significantly delay the absorption of drugs and nutrients (vitamins and minerals). Psyllium-based products used in bulk laxatives, for example, should be taken at least two hours before or after taking medication or nutrients. Some products, such as bran fiber, bulk laxatives, and pectin-containing foods such as apples and pears, should not be consumed along with the heart drug digoxin. These lower the effect of the drug by binding with it and lowering its concentration.

Many articles have been written about the effects of grapefruit juice. Because people often drink grapefruit juice in the United States, we have cut right to the chase. In short, it has been found that grapefruit juice increases the bioavailability of many drugs (makes their concentration higher in the body) by inhibiting the CYP3A4 enzyme in the small intestine.

Here are examples of some types of drugs that grapefruit juice can cause problems with (interact):

- Some statin drugs to lower cholesterol, such as simvastatin (Zocor) and atorvastatin (Lipitor).

- Some drugs that treat high blood pressure, such as nifedipine (Procardia and Adalat CC).

- Some organ-transplant rejection drugs, such as cyclosporine (Sandimmune and Neoral).

- Some anti-anxiety drugs, such as buspirone.

- Some corticosteroids that treat Crohn's disease or ulcerative colitis, such as budesonide (Entocort EC and Uceris).

- Some drugs that treat abnormal heart rhythms, such as amiodarone (Pacerone and Nexterone).

- Some antihistamines, such as fexofenadine (Allegra).

Grapefruit juice does not affect all the drugs in the categories above. The severity of the interaction can be different depending on the person, the drug, and the amount of grapefruit juice you drink. Discuss this with your doctor, pharmacist, or other health care provider and read any information provided with your prescription or OTC drug.

Reducing Your Risk of Interactions

There are many things you, as a consumer, can do to reduce your risk. First of all, be aware that drug interactions do exist, and that nutrients and vitamins, along with food and beverages, must be included in the equation. Second, always read labels carefully on both your prescription drugs and any over-the-counter products you buy. Learn about any warnings that apply to drugs you are taking. These warnings are available in the drug packaging, on the labels in abbreviated form, and on the internet.

There are programs on the internet that will allow you to check for drug interactions by typing in the names of the drugs you are going to take and letting the computer find any adverse interactions. One example of such a program can be found at www.drugdigest.org.

Do not trust any verbal advice unless it comes from a pharmacist or other health care practitioner. What worked for your friend or neighbor might not be best for *you*. Your doctor is a good source of information, but your pharmacist frankly knows more about the actions of drugs and might be a better source.

Before even filling a prescription, make sure your medical record is updated with everything you normally take, and ensure that your doctor is aware of any over-the-counter medications you normally use *plus* any herbal, vitamin, or mineral supplements.

Keep good records of all your medications and their dosages, such as how many milligrams or capsules and how often you take them. Be sure to include the name of the manufacturer. Make a list and keep it in your wallet. You may also want to keep a copy in your home. It's a good idea to let another family member know where you keep these "drug lists."

Ask your doctor if there are any foods, beverages, or supplements you should avoid when getting new medication prescribed. When your doctor writes a new prescription for you, be sure to mention the other drugs you are now taking (or show your list to the doctor). Don't forget to mention any OTC drugs you are taking.

If possible, it's best to use only one pharmacy to get all of your prescriptions. Pharmacies have computer-assisted drug interaction programs that will raise a red flag if the pharmacist punches in a new prescription and it will interact badly with your other drugs already in the computer. But all of your drugs have to be on the same computer network for this to work properly.

Notes

NUTRITION, DIET, AND WELLNESS

4: **food labels on packaged foods.** https://www.fda.gov/food/food-labeling-nutrition/changes-nutrition-facts-label.

8: **diet rich in high GI foods.** Barclay AW, Petocz P, McMillan-Price J, et al. Glycemic index, glycemic load, and chronic disease risk—a meta-analysis of observational studies, *American Journal of Clinical Nutrition* 87, no. 3 (2008): 627–37. https://doi.org/10.1093/ajcn/87.3.627.

12: **eating red meat shortens life.** Yeng Y, Li Y, Satija A, Pan A, et al. Association of changes in red meat consumption with total and cause specific mortality among US women and men: two prospective cohort studies. *BMJ* 365 (2019): l2110. http://dx.doi.org/10.1136/bmj.l2110.

13: **Americans consume too few essential amino acids.** Rodriguez NR. Introduction to Protein Summit 2.0: continued exploration of the impact of high-quality protein on optimal health. *American Journal of Clinical Nutrition* 101 (Suppl) (2015): 1317S–19S. https://academic.oup.com/ajcn/article/101/6/1317S/4564491; https://doi.org/10.3945/ajcn.114.083980.

15: **saturated fats be kept below 7 percent.** National Cholesterol Education Program: Executive summary. https://www.nhlbi.nih.gov/files/docs/guidelines/atp3xsum.pdf.

16: **fat intake should contribute 25 to 35 percent.** National Cholesterol Education Program: Executive summary.

17: **monounsaturated fats can be up to 20 percent.** National Cholesterol Education Program: Executive summary.

18: **serve as the basis of the DVs.** Food and Nutrition Board, National Academy of Sciences. https://www.nap.edu/author/FNB/health-and-medicine-division/food-and-nutrition-board.

20: **people just aren't eating nutrient-rich foods.** Dietary Guidelines for Americans 2015–2020. 8th edition. https://health.gov/our-work/food-nutrition/2015-2020-dietary-guidelines/guidelines/.

21: **put an NSF-certified sticker on.** https://www.nsf.org/about-nsf.

22: **convert IU to the newer system.** Dietary Supplement Ingredient Database. National Institutes of Health, Office of Dietary Supplements. https://dsid.od.nih.gov/Conversions.php.

25: **WHO Technical Report Series 935, 2002.** Joint FAO/WHO/UNU Expert Consultation on Protein and Amino Acid Requirements in Human Nutrition (2002: Geneva, Switzerland). Protein and amino acid requirements in human nutrition. WHO Technical Report Series No. 935. https://apps.who.int/iris/handle/10665/43411.

27: **40 percent of men and 29 percent of women.** Ames BN. Low micronutrient intake may accelerate the degenerative diseases of aging through allocation of scarce micronutrients by triage. *Proceedings of the National Academy of Sciences of the USA* 103, no. 47 (2006): 17589–594. Published online 2006 Nov 13. doi: 10.1073/pnas.0608757103.

27: **90 percent of people don't get enough folate.** Ames BN. Low micronutrient intake may accelerate the degenerative diseases of aging through allocation of scarce micronutrients by triage.

27: **In children, more than 80 percent are deficient.** Bailey RL, Fulgoni VL III, Keast DR, et al. Do dietary supplements improve micronutrient sufficiency in children and adolescents? *Journal of Pediatrics* 161, no. 5 (2012): 837–42. doi: 10.1016/j.jpeds.2012.05.009.

27: **nutrients that are most underconsumed.** Blumberg JB, Frei BB, Fulgoni VL, et al. Impact of frequency of multi-vitamin/multi-mineral supplement intake on nutritional adequacy and nutrient deficiencies in U.S. adults. *Nutrients* 9, no. 8 (2017): 849. doi: 10.3390/nu9080849.

29: **coffee has been shown to prolong life.** Ming D, Satija A, Bhupathiraju SN, et al. Association of coffee consumption with total and cause-specific mortality in three large prospective cohorts. *Circulation* 132, no. 24 (2015): 2305–15, doi: 10.1161/CIRCULATIONAHA.115.017341.

30: **EAT-Lancet diet offers a sound way.** Willett W, Rockstrom J, Loken B, et al. Food in the Anthropocene: The EAT–*Lancet* Commission on healthy diets from sustainable food systems. *The Lancet* 393, no. 10170 (2019): P447–P492. http://dx.doi.org/10.1016/S0140-6736(18)31788-4.

33: **consuming a flavonoid-rich diet over a lifetime.** Shishtar E, Rogers GT, Blumberg JB, et al. Long-term dietary flavonoid intake and risk of Alzheimer disease and related dementias in the Framingham Offspring Cohort. *American Journal of Clinical Nutrition* 112, no. 2 (2020): 343–53. https://doi.org/10.1093/ajcn/nqaa079.

34: **Carotenoids like those found in tomatoes.** Zwilling CE, Tanveer T, Zamroziewicz, Barbe AK. Nutrient biomarker patterns, cognitive function, and fMRI measures of network efficiency in the aging brain. *Neuroimage* 188 (2019): 239–51. https://www.sciencedirect.com/science/article/abs/pii/S1053811918321517?via%3Dihub.

34: **flavonoid content of foods.** Bhagwat S, Haytowitz DB. (2016). USDA Database for the Flavonoid Content of Selected Foods. Release 3.2 (November 2015). Nutrient Data Laboratory, Beltsville Human Nutrition Research Center, ARS, USDA. https://doi.org/10.15482/USDA.ADC/1324465.

36: **sugar consumption is six cups.** NH DHHS-DPHS-Health Promotion in Motion. How much sugar do you eat? https://www.dhhs.nh.gov/dphs/nhp/documents/sugar.pdf.

36: **no impact on blood sugar levels.** U.S. FDA. Additional Information about High-Intensity Sweeteners Permitted for Use in Food in the United States. Reviewed February 8, 2018. https://www.fda.gov/food/ingredientspackaginglabeling/foodadditivesingredients/ucm397725.htm.

36: **crude stevia extracts are not permitted for sale.** Muth ND. The truth about stevia—the so-called "healthy" alternative sweetener. https://www.acefitness.org/certifiednewsarticle/1644/the-truth-about-stevia-the-so-called-quot-healthy/.

36: **Reb A does not cause cancer.** Muth ND. The truth about stevia.

37: **It has no known side effects.** Why everyone's going mad for monk fruit. http://www.healthline.com/health/food-nutrition/monk-fruit-health-benefits#overview1.

37: **monk fruit has only a few calories.** Levy J. Monk fruit: nature's best sweetener? https://draxe.com/nutrition/monk-fruit/.

40: **1,500 milligrams of sodium a day.** How much sodium should I eat per day? https://www.heart.org/en/healthy-living/healthy-eating/eat-smart/nutrition-basics/aha-diet-and-lifestyle-recommendations.

VITAMINS

42: **tomato paste was absorbed the same.** Cohn W, Thürmann P, Tenter U, et al. Comparative multiple dose plasma kinetics of lycopene administered in tomato juice, tomato soup or lycopene tablets. *European Journal of Nutrition* 43 (2004): 304–12. https://doi.org/10.1007/s00394-004-0476-0.

43: **50 percent of Americans are now taking supplements.** Blumberg JB, Frei BB, Fulgoni VL, et al. Impact of frequency of multi-vitamin/multi-mineral supplement intake on nutritional adequacy and nutrient deficiencies in U.S. adults. *Nutrients* 9, no. 8 (2017): 849. doi: 10.3390/nu9080849.

45: **Girls with frequent urinary tract infections benefited from vitamin A.** Kahbazi M, Sharafkhah M, Yousefichaijan P, et al. Vitamin A supplementation is effective for improving the clinical symptoms of urinary tract infections and reducing renal scarring in girls with acute pyelonephritis: A randomized, double-blind placebo-controlled, clinical trial study. *Complementary Therapies in Medicine* 42 (2019): 429–37. doi: 10.1016/j.ctim.2018.12.007. Epub 2018 Dec 12.

47: **Betatene is the trade name.** Betatene: natural beta-carotene. https://nutrition.basf.com/global/en/human-nutrition/products/betatene-naturalbeta-carotene.html.

50: **Thiamine has been helpful in treating young patients.** Ghaleiha A, Davari H, Jahangard L, et al. Adjuvant thiamine improved standard treatment in patients with major depressive disorder: Results from a randomized, double-blind, and placebo-controlled clinical trial. *European Archives of Psychiatry and Clinical Neuroscience* 8 (2016): 695–702. doi: 10.1007/s00406-016-0685-6. Epub 2016 Mar 16.

50: **Thiamine may also support heart function.** Schoenenberger AW, Schoenenberger-Berzins R, der Maur CA, et al. Thiamine supplementation in symptomatic chronic heart failure: a randomized, double-blind, placebo-controlled, cross-over pilot study. *Clinical Research in Cardiology* 101, no. 3 (2012): 159–64. doi: 10.1007/s00392-011-0376-2. Epub 2011 Nov 5.

51: **People over the age of sixty years are more likely.** Jungert A, McNulty H, Hoey L, et al. Riboflavin is an important determinant of vitamin B-6 status in healthy adults. *Journal of Nutrition* 150, no. 10 (2020): 2699–706. https://doi.org/10.1093/jn/nxaa225.

51: **magnesium had fewer migraine days per month.** Gaul C, Diener HC, Danesch U. Migravent® Study Group. Improvement of migraine symptoms with a proprietary supplement containing riboflavin, magnesium and Q10: a randomized, placebo-controlled, double-blind, multicenter trial. *Journal of Headache and Pain* 16 (2015): 516. doi: 10.1186/s10194-015-0516-6. Epub 2015 Apr 3.

52: **low intake may impair mental and physical performance.** Wang X, Hui Z, Dai X, et al. Micronutrient-fortified milk and academic performance among Chinese middle school students: A cluster-randomized controlled trial. *Nutrients* 9, no. 3 (2017): 226. doi: 10.3390/nu9030226.

54: **People who are anxious should avoid large amounts of niacin.** Allan NP, Saulnier KG, Cooper D, et al. Niacin biological challenge: A paradigm to evaluate social concerns. *Journal of Behavior Therapy and Experimental Psychiatry* 65 (2019): 101489. doi: 10.1016/j.jbtep.2019.101489. Epub 2019 May 30.

58: **benefits of B$_{12}$ in older patients with peripheral and central nerve problems.** Miles LM, Allen E, Clarke R, et al. Impact of baseline vitamin B12 status on the effect of vitamin B12 supplementation on neurologic function in older people: secondary analysis of data from the OPEN randomised controlled trial. *European Journal of Clinical Nutrition* 71, no. 10 (2017): 1166–72. doi: 10.1038/ejcn.2017.7. Epub 2017 Feb 22.

59: **patients with COPD had B$_{12}$ deficiencies.** Paulin FV, Zagatto AM, Chiappa GR, et al. Addition of vitamin B$_{12}$ to exercise training improves cycle ergometer endurance in advanced COPD patients: A randomized and controlled study. *Respiratory Medicine* 122 (2017): 23–29. doi: 10.1016/j.rmed.2016.11.015. Epub 2016 Nov 22.

60: **brittle nails who received a topical lacquer treatment and biotin.** Chiavetta A, Mazzurco S, Secolo MP, et al. Treatment of brittle nail with a hydroxypropyl chitosan-based lacquer, alone or in combination with oral biotin: A randomized, assessor-blinded trial. *Dermatologic Therapy* 32, no. 5 (2019): e13028. doi: 10.1111/dth.13028. Epub 2019 Jul 31.

60: **promise for patients with progressive multiple sclerosis.** Tourbah A, Lebrun-Frenay C, Edan G, et al.; MS-SPI study group. MD1003 (high-dose biotin) for the treatment of progressive multiple sclerosis: A randomised, double-blind, placebo-controlled study. *Multiple Schlerosis Journal* 22, no. 13 (2016): 1719–31. doi: 10.1177/1352458516667568. Epub 2016 Sep 1.

61: **dietary choline requires estrogen.** Fischer LM, da Costa KA, Kwock L, et al. Dietary choline requirements of women: effects of estrogen and genetic variation. *American Journal of Clinical Nutrition* 92, no. (2010): 1113–119. doi: 10.3945/ajcn.2010.30064. Epub 2010 Sep 22.

62: **People with Alzheimer's disease who received supplemental folic acid.** Chen H, Liu S, Ji L, et al. Folic acid supplementation mitigates Alzheimer's disease by reducing inflammation: A randomized controlled trial. *Mediators of Inflammation* 2016: 5912146. doi: 10.1155/2016/5912146. Epub 2016 Jun 2.

63: **Folic acid may help reduce the risk of stroke.** Huo Y, Li J, Qin X, et al.; CSPPT Investigators. Efficacy of folic acid therapy in primary prevention of stroke among adults with hypertension in China: The CSPPT randomized clinical trial. *JAMA* 313, no. 13 (2015): 1325–35. doi: 10.1001/jama.2015.2274.

65: **Inositol coupled with alpha-lipoic acid.** Capasso I, Esposito E, Maurea N, et al. Combination of inositol and alpha lipoic acid in metabolic syndrome-affected women: A randomized placebo-controlled trial. *Trials* 14 (2013): 273. doi: 10.1186/1745-6215-14-273.

67: **vitamin C reduced the number of colds by 36 percent.** Johnston CS, Barkyoumb GM, Schumacher SS. Vitamin C supplementation slightly improves physical activity levels and reduces cold incidence in men with marginal vitamin C status: A randomized controlled trial. *Nutrients* 6, no. 7 (2014): 2572–83. doi: 10.3390/nu6072572.

67: **both benefited from 500 mg of vitamin C.** Ellulu MS, Rahmat A, Patimah I, et al. Effect of vitamin C on inflammation and metabolic markers in hypertensive and/or diabetic obese adults: A randomized controlled trial. *Drug Design, Development and Therapy* 9 (2015): 3405–12. doi: 10.2147/DDDT.S83144.

67: **patients with the coronavirus who are in the intensive care unit.** Liu F, Zhu Y, Zhang J, et al. Intravenous high-dose vitamin C for the treatment of severe COVID-19: Study protocol for a multicentre randomised controlled trial. *BMJ Open* 10, no. 7 (2020): e039519. doi: 10.1136/bmjopen-2020-039519.

70: **With aging, vitamin C intake may decline.** Lewis LN, Hayhoe RPG, Mulligan AA, et al. Lower dietary and circulating vitamin c in middle- and older-aged men and women are associated with lower estimated skeletal muscle mass. *Journal of Nutrition* 150, no. 10 (2020): 2789–98. doi: 10.1093/jn/nxaa221.

72: low vitamin D levels were more likely to contract the coronavirus. Ilie PC, Stefanescu S, Smith L. The role of vitamin D in the prevention of coronavirus disease 2019 infection and mortality. *Aging Clinical and Experimental Research* 32, no. 7 (2020): 1195–98. doi: 10.1007/s40520-020-01570-8. Epub 2020 May 6.

72: mitigated with adequate blood vitamin D. Weir EK, Thenappan T, Bhargava M, et al. Does vitamin D deficiency increase the severity of COVID-19? *Clinical Medicine* (London) 20, no. 4 (2020): e107–e108. doi: 10.7861/clinmed.2020-0301. Epub 2020 Jun 5.

73: no benefit from taking large amounts of vitamin D. Manson JE, Cook NR, Lee IM, et al.; VITAL Research Group. Vitamin D supplements and prevention of cancer and cardiovascular disease. *New England Journal of Medicine* 380, no. 1 (2019): 33–44. doi: 10.1056/NEJMoa1809944. Epub 2018 Nov 10.

76: echoed over the past several years. Peh HY, Tan WS, Liao W, et al. Vitamin E therapy beyond cancer: Tocopherol versus tocotrienol. *Pharmacology Therapy* 162 (2016): 152–69. doi: 10.1016/j.pharmthera.2015.12.003. Epub 2015 Dec 17.

78: current DRIs may be insufficient. Theuwissen E, Magdeleyns EJ, Braam LA, et al. Vitamin K status in healthy volunteers. *Food & Function* 2 (2014): 229–34. doi: 10.1039/c3fo60464k.

81: oxidative stress, and coenzyme Q_{10} may be beneficial. Mousavinejad E, Ghaffari MA, Riahi F, et al. Coenzyme Q_{10} supplementation reduces oxidative stress and decreases antioxidant enzyme activity in children with autism spectrum disorders. *Psychiatry Research* 265 (2018): 62–69. doi: 10.1016/j.psychres.2018.03.061. Epub 2018 Apr 4.

82: coenzyme Q_{10} reduced a marker of oxidative stress. Rivara MB, Yeung CK, Robinson-Cohen C, et al. Effect of Coenzyme Q_{10} on biomarkers of oxidative stress and cardiac function in hemodialysis patients: The CoQ_{10} Biomarker Trial. *American Journal of Kidney Diseases* 69, no. 3 (2017): 389–99. doi: 10.1053/j.ajkd.2016.08.041. Epub 2016 Dec 4.

MINERALS

87: Boron may exert anti-inflammatory properties. Nikkhah S, Dolatian M, Naghii MR, et al. Effects of boron supplementation on the severity and duration of pain in primary dysmenorrhea. *Complementary Therapies in Clinical Practice* 21, no. 2 (2015): 79–83. doi: 10.1016/j.ctcp.2015.03.005. Epub 2015 Apr 4.

88: improve bone mass in postmenopausal women. Nakamura K, Saito T, Kobayashi R, et al. Physical activity modifies the effect of calcium supplements on bone loss in perimenopausal and postmenopausal women: Subgroup analysis of a randomized controlled trial. *Archives of Osteoporosis* 14, no. 1 (2019): 17. doi: 10.1007/s11657-019-0575-4.

88: **calcium and vitamin D was shown to promote weight loss.** Subih HS, Zueter Z, Obeidat BM, et al. A high weekly dose of cholecalciferol and calcium supplement enhances weight loss and improves health biomarkers in obese women. *Nutrition Research* 59 (2018): 53–64. doi: 10.1016/j.nutres.2018.07.011. Epub 2018 Jul 25.

94: **Chromium was of benefit to people with a binge-eating.** Brownley KA, Von Holle A, Hamer RM, et al. A double-blind, randomized pilot trial of chromium picolinate for binge eating disorder: Results of the Binge Eating and Chromium (BEACh) study. *Journal of Psychosomatic Research* 75, no. 1 (2013): 36–42. doi: 10.1016/j.jpsychores.2013.03.092. Epub 2013 Apr 22.

95: **hemoglobin A1c went down after four months.** Paiva AN, Lima JG, Medeiros AC, et al. Beneficial effects of oral chromium picolinate supplementation on glycemic control in patients with type 2 diabetes: A randomized clinical study. *Journal of Trace Elements in Medicine and Biology* 32 (2015): 66–72. doi: 10.1016/j.jtemb.2015.05.006. Epub 2015 May 28.

98: **Paleo diet may develop iodine deficiency.** Manousou S, Stål M, Larsson C, et al. A Paleolithic-type diet results in iodine deficiency: A 2-year randomized trial in postmenopausal obese women. *European Journal of Clinical Nutrition* 72, no. 1 (2018): 124–29. doi: 10.1038/ejcn.2017.134. Epub 2017 Sep 13.

99: **Elite athletes may benefit from supplemental iron.** Ishibashi A, Maeda N, Kamei A, et al. Iron supplementation during three consecutive days of endurance training augmented hepcidin levels. *Nutrients* 9, no. 8 (2017): 820. doi: 10.3390/nu9080820.

100: **present in 30 to 83 percent of people with heart disease.** Mistry R, Hosoya H, Kohut A, et al. Iron deficiency in heart failure, an underdiagnosed and undertreated condition during hospitalization. *Annals of Hematology* 98, no. 10 (2019): 2293–97. doi: 10.1007/s00277-019-03777-w. Epub 2019 Aug 12.

101: **shown to be beneficial to the microbiome.** Tang M, Frank DN, Sherlock L, et al. Effect of vitamin E with therapeutic iron supplementation on iron repletion and gut microbiome in US iron deficient infants and toddlers. *Journal of Pediatric Gastroenterology and Nutrition* 63, no. 3 (2016): 379–85. doi: 10.1097/MPG.0000000000001154.

103: **magnesium is related to depression.** Tarleton EK, Littenberg B, MacLean CD, et al. Role of magnesium supplementation in the treatment of depression: A randomized clinical trial. *PLoS One* 12, no. 6 (2017): e0180067. doi: 10.1371/journal.pone.0180067.

105: **high manganese intake was shown to increase.** Kresovich JK, Bulka CM, Joyce BT, et al. The inflammatory potential of dietary manganese in a cohort of elderly men. *Biological Trace Element Research* 183, no. 1 (2018): 49–57. doi: 10.1007/s12011-017-1127-7. Epub 2017 Aug 18.

106: **increased energy expenditure was noted in both.** Assaad M, El
      Mallah C, Obeid O. Phosphorus ingestion with a high-carbohydrate
      meal increased the postprandial energy expenditure of obese and
      lean individuals. *Nutrition* 57 (2019): 59–62. doi: 10.1016/j.
      nut.2018.05.019. Epub 2018 Jun 19.

108: **a diet high in potassium lowered it.** Gijsbers L, Dower JI, Mensink
      M, et al. Effects of sodium and potassium supplementation on blood
      pressure and arterial stiffness: A fully controlled dietary intervention
      study. *Journal of Human Hypertension* 29, no. 10 (2015): 592–98. doi:
      10.1038/jhh.2015.3. Epub 2015 Feb 12.

108: **nutrient-rich foods resulted in the lowering of blood pressure.**
      Wijendran V, Bauer K, Baker R, et al. Dietary intervention with nutrient-
      dense, portion-controlled functional foods improves blood pressure in
      adults. *Novel Techniques in Nutrition and Food Science* 4, no. 4 (2019).
      https://crimsonpublishers.com/ntnf/pdf/NTNF.000594.pdf. doi:
      10.31031/NTNF.2019.04.000594.

108: **potassium-to-sodium ratio of more than 1.** Wijendran V, Bell SJ.
      Relationship of dietary sodium, potassium and the sodium-to-potassium
      ratio to blood pressure. *Journal of Medical-Clinical Research and Reviews*
      3, no. 5 (2019): 1–5. https://www.scivisionpub.com/pdfs/relationship-
      of-dietary-sodium-potassium-and-the-sodiumtopotassium-ratio-to-blood-
      pressure-952.pdf.

110: **Selenium also lowered cholesterol and blood sugar.** Tamtaji OR,
      Heidari-Soureshjani R, Mirhosseini N, et al. Probiotic and selenium
      co-supplementation, and the effects on clinical, metabolic and genetic
      status in Alzheimer's disease: A randomized, double-blind, controlled
      trial. *Clinical Nutrition* 38, no. 6 (2019): 2569–75. doi: 10.1016/j.
      clnu.2018.11.034. Epub 2018 Dec 10.

113: **high blood pressure is called the DASH.** Juraschek SP, Miller ER
      3rd, Weaver CM, et al. Effects of sodium reduction and the DASH Diet
      in relation to baseline blood pressure. *Journal of the American College of
      Cardiology* 70, no. 23 (2017): 2841–48. doi: 10.1016/j.jacc.2017.10.011.
      Epub 2017 Nov 12.

AIR

120: **The coronavirus spreads more easily indoors.** Centers for Disease
      Control and Prevention. Participate in outdoor and indoor activities.
      https://www.cdc.gov/coronavirus/2019-ncov/daily-life-coping/outdoor-
      activities.html.

WATER

131: **Fear of contracting the coronavirus from tap water.** Environmental
      Protection Agency. Coronavirus and drinking water and wastewater.
      https://www.epa.gov/coronavirus/coronavirus-and-drinking-water-
      and-wastewater.

140: **quality regulations for bottled waters.** Posnick, LM, Kim H. Bottled water regulation and the FDA. *Food Safety Magazine,* August 1, 2002. https://www.food-safety.com/articles/4373-bottled-water-regulation-and-the-fda.

AMINO ACIDS

155: **Arginine has also been shown to improve sports performance.** Pahlavani N, Entezari MH, Nasiri M, et al. The effect of l-arginine supplementation on body composition and performance in male athletes: A double-blinded randomized clinical trial. *European Journal of Clinical Nutrition* 71, no. 4 (2017): 544–48. doi: 10.1038/ejcn.2016.266. Epub 2017 Jan 25.

156: **Aspartic acid was thought to increase testosterone.** Melville GW, Siegler JC, Marshall PWM. The effects of d-aspartic acid supplementation in resistance-trained men over a three month training period: A randomised controlled trial. *PLoS One* 12, no. 8 (2017): e0182630. doi: 10.1371/journal.pone.0182630.

158: **different pattern of microbes in the intestine.** Koeth RA, Lam-Galvez BR, Kirsop J, et al. L-carnitine in omnivorous diets induces an atherogenic gut microbial pathway in humans. *Journal of Clinical Investigation* 129, no. 1 (2019): 373–87. doi: 10.1172/JCI94601. Epub 2018 Dec 10.

161: **NAC was thought to help children with autism.** Dean OM, Gray KM, Villagonzalo KA, et al. A randomised, double blind, placebo-controlled trial of a fixed dose of N-acetyl cysteine in children with autistic disorder. *Australian and New Zealand Journal of Psychiatry* 51, no. 3 (2017): 241–49. doi: 10.1177/0004867416652735. Epub 2016 Jul 11.

165: **Glutathione likely works as an antioxidant.** Richie JP Jr, Nichenametla S, Neidig W, et al. Randomized controlled trial of oral glutathione supplementation on body stores of glutathione. *European Journal of Nutrition* 54, no. 2 (2015): 251–63. doi: 10.1007/s00394-014-0706-z. Epub 2014 May 5.

167: **Histidine looks promising for treating obesity.** Feng RN, Niu YC, Sun XW, et al. Histidine supplementation improves insulin resistance through suppressed inflammation in obese women with the metabolic syndrome: A randomised controlled trial. *Diabetologia* 56, no. 5 (2013): 985–94. doi: 10.1007/s00125-013-2839-7. Epub 2013 Jan 30.

168: **homocysteine were associated with cognitive decline.** Christine CW, Auinger P, Joslin A, et al.; Parkinson Study Group–DATATOP Investigators. Vitamin B_{12} and homocysteine levels predict different outcomes in early Parkinson's disease. *Movement Disorders* 33, no. 5 (2018): 762–70. doi: 10.1002/mds.27301. Epub 2018 Mar 6.

169: **a small amount of protein containing 3 grams of leucine.** Devries MC, McGlory C, Bolster DR, et al. Leucine, not total protein, content of a supplement is the primary determinant of muscle protein anabolic responses in healthy older women. *Journal of Nutrition* 148, no. 7 (2019): 208–95. doi: 10.1093/jn/nxy091. Epub 2019 Mar 1.

171: **methionine is a pro-aging amino acid.** Stekovic S, Hofer SJ, Tripolt N, et al. Alternate day fasting improves physiological and molecular markers of aging in healthy, non-obese humans. *Cell Metabolism* 30, no. 3 (2019): 462–76.e6. doi: 10.1016/j.cmet.2019.07.016. Epub 2019 Aug 27.

172: **ornithine has been shown to mitigate stress.** Miyake M, Kirisako T, Kokubo T, et al. Randomised controlled trial of the effects of L-ornithine on stress markers and sleep quality in healthy workers. *Nutrition Journal* 13 (2014): 53. doi: 10.1186/1475-2891-13-53.

173: **D-serine improved memory.** Avellar M, Scoriels L, Madeira C, et al. The effect of D-serine administration on cognition and mood in older adults. *Oncotarget* 7, no. 11 (2016): 11881–88. doi: 10.18632/oncotarget.7691.

175: **People with cirrhosis caused by alcohol often experience severe leg cramping.** Vidot H, Cvejic E, Carey S, et al. Randomised clinical trial: Oral taurine supplementation versus placebo reduces muscle cramps in patients with chronic liver disease. *Alimentary Pharmacology & Therapeutics* 48, no. 7 (2018): 704–12. doi: 10.1111/apt.14950. Epub 2018 Aug 23.

176: **depressed young adults took tryptophan.** Tsujita N, Akamatsu Y, Nishida MM, et al. Effect of tryptophan, vitamin B_6, and nicotinamide-containing supplement loading between meals on mood and autonomic nervous system activity in young adults with subclinical depression: A randomized, double-blind, and placebo-controlled study. *Journal of Nutritional Science and Vitaminology* (Tokyo) 65, no. 6 (2019): 507–14. doi: 10.3177/jnsv.65.507.

178: **valine was taken along with arginine and serine.** Tsuda Y, Yamaguchi M, Noma T, et al. Combined effect of arginine, valine, and serine on exercise-induced fatigue in healthy volunteers: A randomized, double-blinded, placebo-controlled crossover study. *Nutrients* 11, no. 4 (2019): 862. doi: 10.3390/nu11040862.

ANTIOXIDANTS

181: **people with diabetes also develop a painful neuropathy.** Agathos E, Tentolouris A, Eleftheriadou I, et al. Effect of α-lipoic acid on symptoms and quality of life in patients with painful diabetic neuropathy. *Journal of International Medical Research* 46, no. 5 (2018): 1779–90. doi: 10.1177/0300060518756540. Epub 2018 Mar 8.

181: **less oxidative stress as measured by the lower oxidation of LDL cholesterol.** Arevström L, Bergh C, Landberg R, et al. Freeze-dried bilberry (Vaccinium myrtillus) dietary supplement improves walking distance and lipids after myocardial infarction: An open-label randomized clinical trial. *Nutrition Research* 62 (2019): 13–22. doi: 10.1016/j.nutres.2018.11.008. Epub 2018 Nov 17.

183: **coenzyme Q$_{10}$ has been shown to improve the lives of people with chronic heart disease.** Mortensen SA, Rosenfeldt F, Kumar A, et al.; Q-SYMBIO Study Investigators. The effect of coenzyme Q$_{10}$ on morbidity and mortality in chronic heart failure: Results from Q-SYMBIO: A randomized double-blind trial. *JACC: Heart Failure* 2, no. 6 (2014): 641–49. doi: 10.1016/j.jchf.2014.06.008. Epub 2014 Oct 1.

183: **Impressive findings were noted for people with prediabetes.** Chuengsamarn S, Rattanamongkolgul S, Luechapudiporn R, et al. Curcumin extract for prevention of type 2 diabetes. *Diabetes Care* 35, no. 11 (2012): 2121–27. doi: 10.2337/dc12-0116. Epub 2012 Jul 6.

184: **a high flavonoid intake is associated with a blood-pressure-lowering effect.** Ottaviani JI, Britten A, Lucarelli D, et al. Biomarker-estimated flavan-3-ol intake is associated with lower blood pressure in cross-sectional analysis in EPIC Norfolk. *Scientific Reports* 10, no. 1 (2020): 17964. doi: 10.1038/s41598-020-74863-7.

185: **aged garlic extract was shown to boost immune function.** Percival SS. Aged garlic extract modifies human immunity. *Journal of Nutrition* 146, no. 2 (2016): 433S–436S. doi: 10.3945/jn.115.210427. Epub 2016 Jan 13.

188: **adolescents with ADHD who took 80 to 120 milligrams per day of ginkgo biloba.** Shakibaei F, Radmanesh M, Salari E, et al. Ginkgo biloba in the treatment of attention-deficit/hyperactivity disorder in children and adolescents. A randomized, placebo-controlled, trial. *Complementary Therapies in Clinical Practice* 21, no. 2 (2015): 61–67. doi: 10.1016/j.ctcp.2015.04.001. Epub 2015 Apr 18.

189: **green tea extract containing 858.6 milligrams of EGCG.** Chen IJ, Liu CY, Chiu JP, et al. Therapeutic effect of high-dose green tea extract on weight reduction: A randomized, double-blind, placebo-controlled clinical trial. *Clinical Nutrition* 35, no. 3 (2016): 592–99. doi: 10.1016/j.clnu.2015.05.003. Epub 2015 May 29.

191: **Infertile men benefited from taking 600 milligrams of NAC.** Jannatifar R, Parivar K, Roodbari NH, et al. Effects of N-acetyl-cysteine supplementation on sperm quality, chromatin integrity and level of oxidative stress in infertile men. *Reproductive Biology and Endocrinology* 17, no. 1 (2019): 24. doi: 10.1186/s12958-019-0468-9.

192: **OPC supplementation demonstrated fewer areas of gum bleeding.** Díaz Sánchez RM, Castillo-Dalí G, Fernández-Olavarría A, et al. A prospective, double-blind, randomized, controlled clinical trial in the gingivitis prevention with an oligomeric proanthocyanidin nutritional supplement. *Mediators of Inflammation* 2017 (2017): 7460780. doi: 10.1155/2017/7460780. Epub 2017 Dec 10.

193: **300 micrograms or more of selenium for ten years had a 60 percent.** Rayman MP, Winther KH, Pastor-Barriuso R, et al. Effect of long-term selenium supplementation on mortality: Results from a multiple-dose, randomised controlled trial. *Free*

Radical Biology & Medicine 127 (2018): 46–54. doi: 10.1016/j. freeradbiomed.2018.02.015. Epub 2018 Feb 14.

194: **A newer study confirmed these findings in people with type 2 diabetes.** Ebrahimpour-Koujan S, Gargari BP, Mobasseri M, et al. Lower glycemic indices and lipid profile among type 2 diabetes mellitus patients who received novel dose of *Silybum marianum* (L.) Gaertn. (silymarin) extract supplement: A triple-blinded randomized controlled clinical trial. *Phytomedicine* 44 (2018): 39–44. doi: 10.1016/j. phymed.2018.03.050. Epub 2018 Mar 19.

195: **lutein (10 milligrams) and zeaxanthin (4 milligrams) daily.** Piermarocchi S, Saviano S, Parisi V, et al.; Carmis Study Group. Carotenoids in Age-Related Maculopathy Italian Study (CARMIS): Two-year results of a randomized study. *European Journal of Ophthalmology* 22, no. 2 (2012): 216–25. doi: 10.5301/ejo.5000069.

NATURAL FOOD SUPPLEMENTS

211: **People with gastroesophageal reflux disease (GERD) benefited from taking aloe vera.** Panahi Y, Khedmat H, Valizadegan G, et al. Efficacy and safety of Aloe vera syrup for the treatment of gastroesophageal reflux disease: A pilot randomized positive-controlled trial. *Journal of Traditional Chinese Medicine* 35, no. 6 (2015): 632–36. doi: 10.1016/ s0254-6272(15)30151-5.

212: **bee propolis may help people with type 2 diabetes.** Samadi N, Mozaffari-Khosravi H, Rahmanian M, et al. Effects of bee propolis supplementation on glycemic control, lipid profile and insulin resistance indices in patients with type 2 diabetes: A randomized, double-blind clinical trial. *Journal of Integrative Medicine* 15, no. 2 (2017): 124–34. doi: 10.1016/S2095-4964(17)60315-7.

213: **Yeast beta-glucan (900 milligrams a day) taken during cold and flu season.** Dharsono T, Rudnicka K, Wilhelm M, et al. Effects of yeast (1,3)-(1,6)-beta-glucan on severity of upper respiratory tract infections: A double-blind, randomized, placebo-controlled study in healthy subjects. *Journal of the American College of Nutrition* 38, no. 1 (2019): 40–50. doi: 10.1080/07315724.2018.1478339. Epub 2018 Sep 10.

214: **one strain of bifidobacteria (MIMBb75).** Guglielmetti S, Mora D, Gschwender M, et al. Randomised clinical trial: *Bifidobacterium bifidum* MIMBb75 significantly alleviates irritable bowel syndrome and improves quality of life—a double-blind, placebo-controlled study. *Alimentary Pharmacology & Therapeutics* 33, no. 10 (2011): 1123–32. doi: 10.1111/j.1365-2036.2011.04633.x. Epub 2011 Mar 21.

216: **women with painful menstrual periods, chlorella.** Haidari F, Homayouni F, Helli B, et al. Effect of chlorella supplementation on systematic symptoms and serum levels of prostaglandins, inflammatory and oxidative markers in women with primary dysmenorrhea. *European Journal of Obstetrics & Gynecology and Reproductive Biology* 299 (2018): 185–89. doi: 10.1016/j.ejogrb.2018.08.578. Epub 2018 Aug 27.

219: **bovine colostrum (60 grams) was better at increasing leg muscle strength.** Duff WR, Chilibeck PD, Rooke JJ, et al. The effect of bovine colostrum supplementation in older adults during resistance training. *International Journal of Sport Nutrition and Exercise Metabolism* 24, no. 3 (2014): 276–85. doi: 10.1123/ijsnem.2013-0182. Epub 2013 Nov 25.

220: **Vegetarians who received 20 grams daily of creatine.** Benton D, Donohoe R. The influence of creatine supplementation on the cognitive functioning of vegetarians and omnivores. *British Journal of Nutrition* 105, no. 7 (2011): 1100–105. doi: 10.1017/S0007114510004733. Epub 2010 Dec 1.

221: **DHEA is on the banned substance list.** Collomp K, Buisson C, Gravisse N, et al. Effects of short-term DHEA intake on hormonal responses in young recreationally trained athletes: Modulation by gender. *Endocrine* 59, no. 3 (2018): 538–46. doi: 10.1007/s12020-017-1514-z. Epub 2018 Jan 10.

227: **grape seed extract was helpful at reducing blood pressure.** Odai T, Terauchi M, Kato K, et al. Effects of grape seed proanthocyanidin extract on vascular endothelial function in participants with prehypertension: A randomized, double-blind, placebo-controlled study. *Nutrients* 11, no. 12 (2019): 2844. doi: 10.3390/nu11122844.

227: **Women in menopause reaped benefit from taking 500 milligrams of evening primrose oil.** Farzaneh F, Fatehi S, Sohrabi MR, et al. The effect of oral evening primrose oil on menopausal hot flashes: A randomized clinical trial. *Archives of Gynecology and Obstetrics* 288, no. 5 (2013): 1075–79. doi: 10.1007/s00404-013-2852-6. Epub 2013 Apr 27.

232: **depression benefited within two weeks from taking 5-HTP.** Jangid P, Malik P, Singh P, et al. Comparative study of efficacy of l-5-hydroxytryptophan and fluoxetine in patients presenting with first depressive episode. *Asian Journal of Psychiatry* 6, no. 1 (2013): 29–34. doi: 10.1016/j.ajp.2012.05.011. Epub 2012 Jul 12.

233: **garlic had special benefit during cold and flu season.** Nantz MP, Rowe CA, Muller CE, et al. Supplementation with aged garlic extract improves both NK and γδ-T cell function and reduces the severity of cold and flu symptoms: A randomized, double-blind, placebo-controlled nutrition intervention. *Clinical Nutrition* 31, no. 3 (2012): 337–44. doi: 10.1016/j.clnu.2011.11.019. Epub 2012 Jan 24.

234: **ginkgo biloba did not reduce the likelihood of developing Alzheimer's disease.** Vellas B, Coley N, Ousset PJ, et al.; GuidAge Study Group. Long-term use of standardised Ginkgo biloba extract for the prevention of Alzheimer's disease (GuidAge): A randomised placebo-controlled trial. *Lancet Neurology* 11, no. 10 (2012): 851–59. doi: 10.1016/S1474-4422(12)70206-5. Epub 2012 Sep 6.

235: **500 milligrams of ginseng daily experienced improved quality of life.** Ghorbani Z, Mirghafourvand M, Charandabi SM, et al. The effect of ginseng on sexual dysfunction in menopausal women: A double-blind, randomized, controlled trial. *Complementary Therapies in Medicine* 45 (2019): 57–64. doi: 10.1016/j.ctim.2019.05.015. Epub 2019 May 22.

245: Women aged forty to sixty benefited from a high dose of lecithin.
Hirose A, Terauchi M, Osaka Y, et al. Effect of soy lecithin on fatigue
and menopausal symptoms in middle-aged women: A randomized,
double-blind, placebo-controlled study. *Nutrition Journal* 17, no. 1
(2018): 4. doi: 10.1186/s12937-018-0314-5.

246: percentage of women who ovulated was not statistically different.
Chen JT, Tominaga K, Sato Y, et al. Maitake mushroom (*Grifola
frondosa*) extract induces ovulation in patients with polycystic ovary
syndrome: A possible monotherapy and a combination therapy after
failure with first-line clomiphene citrate. *Journal of Alternative and
Complementary Medicine* 16, no. 12 (2010): 1295–99. doi: 10.1089/
acm.2009.0696. Epub 2010 Oct 29.

248: migraines (two to eight per month) tried melatonin. Gonçalves AL,
Martini Ferreira A, Ribeiro RT, et al. Randomised clinical trial comparing
melatonin 3 mg, amitriptyline 25 mg and placebo for migraine
prevention. *Journal of Neurology, Neurosurgery, and Psychiatry* 87, no. 10
(2016): 1127–32. doi: 10.1136/jnnp-2016-313458. Epub 2016 May 10.

253: tested perilla oil in people with mild to moderate dementia.
Kamalashiran C, Sriyakul K, Pattaraarchachai J, et al. Outcomes of
perilla seed oil as an additional neuroprotective therapy in patients
with mild to moderate dementia: A randomized control trial. *Current
Alzheimer Research* 16, no. 2 (2019): 146–55. doi: 10.2174/156720501
6666181212153720.

257: menopause benefited from taking 1,000 milligrams. Sharif
SN, Darsareh F. Effect of royal jelly on menopausal symptoms: A
randomized placebo-controlled clinical trial. *Complementary Therapies
in Clinical Practice* 37 (2019): 47–50. doi: 10.1016/j.ctcp.2019.08.006.
Epub 2019 Aug 22.

258: SAMe alone without other medications was not effective. Sarris J,
Murphy J, Stough C, et al. S-adenosylmethionine (SAMe) monotherapy
for depression: An 8-week double-blind, randomised, controlled trial.
Psychopharmacology (Berlin) 237, no. 1 (2020): 209–18. doi: 10.1007/
s00213-019-05358-1. Epub 2019 Nov 11.

262: spirulina helped promote weight loss. Szulinska M, Gibas-Dorna M,
Miller-Kasprzak E, et al. Spirulina maxima improves insulin sensitivity,
lipid profile, and total antioxidant status in obese patients with well-
treated hypertension: A randomized double-blind placebo-controlled
study. *European Review for Medical and Pharmacological Sciences* 21, no.
10 (2017): 2473–81. PMID: 28617537.

HERBS

281: Helps healing of burn wounds. Shahzad MN, Ahmed N. Effectiveness
of Aloe Vera gel compared with 1% silver sulphadiazine cream as burn
wound dressing in second degree burns. *Journal of Pakistan Medical
Association* 63, no. 2 (2013): 225–30. https://pubmed.ncbi.nlm.nih.
gov/23894900/.

283: **normalize thyroid hormones.** Sharma AK, Basu I, Singh S. Efficacy and safety of ashwagandha root extract in subclinical hypothyroid patients: A double-blind, randomized placebo-controlled trial. *Journal of Alternative and Complementary Medicine* 24, no. 3 (2018): 243–48. doi: 10.1089/acm.2017.0183. Epub 2017 Aug 22.

283: **May reduce heart disease risk in people with type 2 diabetes.** Lazavi F, Mirmiran P, Sohrab G, et al. The barberry juice effects on metabolic factors and oxidative stress in patients with type 2 diabetes: A randomized clinical trial. *Complementary Therapies in Clinical Practice* 31 (2018): 170–74. doi: 10.1016/j.ctcp.2018.01.009. Epub 2018 Feb 17.

285: **beneficial for people who recently had a heart attack.** Arevstrom L, Bergh C, Landberg R, et al. Freeze-dried bilberry (*Vaccinium myrtillus*) dietary supplement improves walking distance and lipids after myocardial infarction: An open-label randomized clinical trial. *Nutrition Research* 62 (2019): 13–22. doi: 10.1016/j.nutres.2018.11.008. Epub 2018 Nov 17.

287: **reduce redness associated with acne.** Jung JY, Kwon HH, Hong JS, et al. Effect of dietary supplementation with omega-3 fatty acid and gamma-linolenic acid on acne vulgaris: A randomised, double-blind, controlled trial. *Acta Dermato-Venereologica* 94, no. 5 (2014): 521–25. doi: 10.2340/00015555-1802.

293: **May help depressed people feel better.** Amsterdam JD, Shults J, Soeller I, et al. Chamomile (Matricaria recutita) may provide antidepressant activity in anxious, depressed humans: An exploratory study. *Alternative Therapies in Health and Medicine* 18, no. 5 (2012): 44–49. https://pubmed.ncbi.nlm.nih.gov/22894890/.

299: **Helps against pain in the hip and knee.** Devil's claw. Purported Uses. https://www.mskcc.org/cancer-care/integrative-medicine/herbs/devil-claw.

303: **Do not use if you are taking a blood thinner.** Fenugreek. Do not take if. https://www.mskcc.org/cancer-care/integrative-medicine/herbs/fenugreek.

305: **help normalize hormones in postmenopausal women.** Flax. Purported uses. https://www.mskcc.org/cancer-care/integrative-medicine/herbs/flaxseed.

307: **avoid if taking insulin or MAOIs.** Asian ginseng. Do not take if. https://www.mskcc.org/cancer-care/integrative-medicine/herbs/ginseng-asian.

309: **taking more than 400 mg a day is not recommended.** Mayo Clinic Staff. Caffeine: How much is too much? https://www.mayoclinic.org/healthy-lifestyle/nutrition-and-healthy-eating/in-depth/caffeine/art-20045678#:~:text=Up%20to%20400%20milligrams%20(mg,widely%2C%20especially%20among%20energy%20drinks.

311: **help reduce hot flashes in menopausal women.** Hops and purported uses. https://www.mskcc.org/cancer-care/integrative-medicine/herbs/hops.

311: **horse chestnut product is esculin-free.** Horse chestnut. Do not take if. https://www.mskcc.org/cancer-care/integrative-medicine/herbs/horse-chestnut.

317: **Skin rash with the use of lemongrass essential oils.** Lemongrass. Side effects. https://www.mskcc.org/cancer-care/integrative-medicine/ herbs/lemongrass.

323: **Do not take if you are taking diuretics or hypotensive drugs.** Nettle. Do not use if. https://www.mskcc.org/cancer-care/integrative- medicine/herbs/nettle.

323: **Do not take if you are using blood pressure medicines or insulin.** Olive leaf. Do not use if. https://www.mskcc.org/cancer-care/ integrative-medicine/herbs/olive-leaf.

329: **Used clinically in Europe to treat benign prostatic hyperplasia.** Pygeum. Special point. https://www.mskcc.org/cancer-care/integrative- medicine/herbs/pygeum.

329: **methotrexate, or are using blood thinners.** Red clover. Do not use if. https://www.mskcc.org/cancer-care/integrative-medicine/herbs/red- clover.

333: **5-HTP or SAMe because these products may also affect serotonin levels.** St. John's wort. Patient cautions. https://www.mskcc.org/ cancer-care/integrative-medicine/herbs/st-john-wort.

335: **effects are reported as mild and similar to effects with placebo.** Saw palmetto. Side effects. https://www.mskcc.org/cancer-care/integrative- medicine/herbs/saw-palmetto.

339: **medications may have a lesser effect if turmeric is regularly used.** Turmeric: What else do I need to know? https://www.mskcc.org/ cancer-care/integrative-medicine/herbs/turmeric.

339: **anti-anxiety medications or for those who have gallbladder, pancreatic, or liver disease.** Valerian. Do not take if. https://www. mskcc.org/cancer-care/integrative-medicine/herbs/valerian.

DRUG INTERACTIONS

356: **drugs that grapefruit juice can cause problems.** Food and Drug Administration. Grapefruit juice and some drugs don't mix. https:// www.fda.gov/consumers/consumer-updates/grapefruit-juice-and-some- drugs-dont-mix.

Index

Note: Italicized page numbers indicate material in tables.